Digital Image Processing for Medical Applications

The influence and impact of digital images on modern society is tremendous, and image processing is now a critical component in science and technology. The rapid progress in computerized medical image reconstruction, and the associated developments in analysis methods and computer-aided diagnosis, has propelled medical imaging into one of the most important sub-fields in scientific imaging.

This text is intended for use in a first course in image processing and analysis for final-year undergraduate or first-year graduate students. It takes its motivation from medical applications and uses real medical images and situations to clarify concepts and to build intuition and understanding. Designed for readers who will become end users of digital image processing, the effective use of image processing tools is emphasized. An overview of the fundamentals of the most important clinical imaging modalities in use is included to provide a context, and to illustrate how the images are produced and acquired. Through using this text, students will understand why they are undertaking particular operations, and practical computer-based activities will enable them to see in real time how operations affect real images.

Geoff Dougherty is Professor of Applied Physics and Medical Imaging at California State University, Channel Islands, where he teaches both undergraduate and graduate courses in image processing, medical imaging and pattern recognition. He has been conducting research in the applications of image processing and analysis to medical images for over 15 years, and is the author of more than 60 publications. He is a Senior Member of the IEEE, a Fellow of the IET and a Member of the American Association of Physicists in Medicine (AAPM).

Digital Image Processing for Medical Applications

GEOFF DOUGHERTY

California State University, Channel Islands

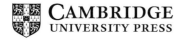
CAMBRIDGE
UNIVERSITY PRESS

CAMBRIDGE UNIVERSITY PRESS
Cambridge, New York, Melbourne, Madrid, Cape Town, Singapore,
São Paulo, Delhi, Dubai, Tokyo, Mexico City

Cambridge University Press
The Edinburgh Building, Cambridge CB2 8RU, UK

Published in the United States of America by Cambridge University Press, New York

www.cambridge.org
Information on this title: www.cambridge.org/9780521860857

First published 2009
Reprinted with corrections 2011

Printed in the United Kingdom at the University Press, Cambridge

A catalog record for this publication is available from the British Library

Library of Congress Cataloguing in Publication data
Dougherty, Geoff, 1950–
Digital image processing for medical applications / Geoff Dougherty.
 p. ; cm.
Includes bibliographical references and index.
ISBN 978-0-521-86085-7 (hardback)
1. Diagnostic imaging – Digital techniques.   2. Image processing – Digital techniques   I. Title.
[DNLM: 1. Diagnostic Imaging.   2. Image Processing, Computer-Assisted.   3. Medical Informatics
Applications.   WN 180 D732d   2009]
RC78.7.D53D72   2009
16.07′54′–dc22
                                                                      2008031555

ISBN 978-0-521-86085-7 Hardback
Additional resources for this publication at www.cambridge.org/dougherty

Contents

The color plates are situated between pages 178 and 179.

Preface

The influence and impact of digital images on modern society, science, technology and art are tremendous. Image processing has become such a critical component in contemporary science and technology that many tasks would not be attempted without it. It is a truly interdisciplinary subject that draws from synergistic developments involving many disciplines and is used in medical imaging, microscopy, astronomy, computer vision, geology and many other fields.

The rapid and continuing progress in computerized medical image reconstruction, and the associated developments in analysis methods and computer-aided diagnosis, have propelled medical imaging into one of the most important sub-fields in scientific imaging. This book takes its motivation from medical applications and uses real medical images and situations to clarify and consolidate concepts and to build intuition, insight and understanding. An overview of the fundamentals of the most important clinical imaging modalities in use is included to provide a context, and to illustrate how the images are produced and acquired.

This is a text for use in a first practical course in image processing and analysis, for final-year undergraduate or first-year graduate students with a background in biomedical engineering, computer science, radiologic sciences or physics. Designed for readers who will become "end users" of digital image processing in the biomedical sciences, it emphasizes the conceptual framework and the effective use of image processing tools and uses mathematics as a tool, minimizing the advanced mathematical development of other textbooks.

Discussions of the major medical imaging modalities enable students to understand the diagnostic tasks for which images are needed and the typical distortions and artifacts associated with each modality. This knowledge then motivates the presentation of the techniques needed to reverse distortions, minimize artifacts and enhance important features. Students understand *why* they are undertaking particular operations, and the practical activities enable them to see in real time *how* operations affect real images. Image processing is a hands-on discipline, and the best way to learn is by doing. Theory and practice are linked, each reinforcing the other.

The key distinguishing features of the book are as follows.

- Its pedagogical approach combines intuition with problem-solving, and emphasizes conceptual learning, i.e. understanding the "big picture," rather than getting overwhelmed with the details.
- Overviews summarize the essential purpose of the material covered in each chapter.
- Learning objectives list the specific knowledge and skills to be acquired.

- Practical computer-based activities, referred to in each chapter, build intuition, skills and confidence. They can be used by the instructor for class demonstrations and/or by the students as hands-on activities.
- Accessible end-of-chapter problems reinforce and consolidate understanding.
- Only a modest background in mathematics and science, at the level of College/University entry, is assumed.

Courses supported and organization of the text

The text is based on courses in image analysis, pattern recognition and medical imaging that I teach at California State University, Channel Islands, and have taught previously at the Health Sciences Center, Kuwait University. The material is more than can comfortably be covered in a single-semester course, and can be fine-tuned to specific courses and audiences. The book can be used to support several different courses, by emphasizing different chapters and skimming or avoiding others altogether. For example, a course for biomedical engineers or radiologic science students would include all the material from Chapters 3 and 4, and might skim through Chapters 10 and 11. It would benefit from an early visit to a local hospital or imaging center to view image acquisition and analysis in a clinical setting. A few invited talks from medical professionals, such as radiologists, pathologists or oncologists, could be included to add to the clinical perspective. A course in image analysis for computer scientists or physicists would probably downplay Chapters 3–4, omit Chapters 13 and 14, skim through Chapter 11, and ensure that all the activities and end-of-chapter problems were attempted. And a course in pattern recognition, or a graduate course, would concentrate on Chapters 9–12 and the material in the appendices.

Each chapter starts with an overview of its contents and a list of its objectives. Concepts, techniques and algorithms are introduced and then applied to typical medical imaging problems. The material is integrated with a number of practical computer-based activities, arranged at the end of each chapter, and supplemented by exercises, mostly numerical, for the reader to verify his/her understanding. Worked examples are included in separate boxed sections.

The book comprises four parts. Part I is an introduction to image processing. It provides an overview of the field and its many applications (Chapter 1), explains how digital images are acquired and discusses their characteristics (Chapter 2). It explains how medical images are produced, using both ionizing (Chapter 3) and non-ionizing radiation (Chapter 4), and discusses the most important clinical imaging modalities.

Part II explains the fundamental concepts of image processing. Gray-level histograms are introduced, and display look-up tables (LUTs) discussed in terms of changing image appearance (Chapter 5). Image enhancement in both the spatial and frequency domains is addressed in Chapters 6 and 7, respectively. Chapter 8 discusses techniques which aim to restore a degraded image to its original condition.

Part III deals with image analysis and visualization. Morphology is introduced as an image analysis tool in Chapter 9, illustrating its applicability to medical imaging problems.

Segmentation techniques are discussed in Chapter 10, which leads into feature extraction and classification in Chapter 11. Chapter 12 discusses how the three-dimensional structure of internal organs can be visualized and displayed convincingly on a two-dimensional computer monitor.

Part IV discusses a number of specific applications in medicine, indicating the image analysis techniques that are being used (Chapter 13), and considers the trends and ongoing developments in medical imaging (Chapter 14).

Three appendices provide further details (on the Fourier transform, set theory and probability, and shape and texture) relevant to the techniques explored.

Computer-based activities

ImageJ is a very popular public domain (http://rsb.info.nih.gov/ij/) Java image processing and analysis program that was developed at the National Institutes of Health. It has a convenient and intuitive graphical user interface (GUI), and has been chosen for its ease of use for the computer-based imaging activities which are integrated within the book. Its source code is freely available, so that users have complete freedom to run, copy, distribute, study, change and improve the software (see www.gnu.org/philosophy/free-sw.html). At a more basic level it allows users to collect imaging operations together in macros, which are stored as text files and are easy to write, edit and debug.

However, most of the exercises can be easily duplicated to run in an alternative environment, such as Matlab if the Matlab Toolbox/GUI, DipImage (available as a free download to non-commercial use at www.diplib.org/home2224) is used; without DipImage, the necessary programming in MatLab can be tedious and distract from learning the imaging fundamentals.

The ImageJ homepage contains links to documentation and downloads. ImageJ runs on any computer with a Java 1.1 or later virtual machine, but in order to be able to compile additional "plugins" (optional extras) and manage memory more efficiently, it is recommended that it be downloaded together with the full Java runtime environment. The examples in this book use an expansion of ImageJ version 1.37v with Java 1.5.0 (a total download of about 20 MB). Additional plugins can be downloaded from the ImageJ site or others, and comprise compiled java files (named *.class) which need to be placed in the "Plugins" sub-folder of the ImageJ folder.

It is recommended that you download the latest version of ImageJ bundled with Java 1.5.0 from http://rsb.info.nih.gov/ij/download.html. Once unzipped and installed in a directory called ImageJ, a shortcut will be installed on your desktop and in your Start/All Programs menu. The ImageJ core program (ij.jar) is frequently upgraded. You should visit the ImageJ website (http://rsb.info.nih.gov/ij/) routinely to check for upgrades, download the upgraded *.zip file and use the extracted ij.jar to replace the current ij.jar file. (You can find your current version by opening ImageJ and going to Help, About ImageJ; close ImageJ before replacing the ij.jar file with an upgrade.)

A collection of plugins has been collated, comprising some freely available from the Plugins download site (http://rsb.info.nih.gov/ij/plugins/index.html) and others written specifically for this text. They are available at the book website in folders with names such as Ch.5 Plugins (to facilitate the computer activities in Chapter 5); copy them into the ImageJ folder called "Plugins" on your computer. These additional plugins become available in the Plugins menu when ImageJ is next run. Most of the computer activities require images for processing; these can be found at the book website in folders with names such as Ch.5 Activities, and should be copied to the ImageJ directory in your computer for easy access. After first opening ImageJ, go to Edit, Options, Memory and change the memory allocated to ImageJ to equal 75% of your computer's RAM, which you can find from My Computer, View System Properties, Hardware.

The computer-based activities are referred to within the text and are collected at the end of each chapter. The required images are referred to in bold Courier New font, e.g. `lena`, and the ImageJ menu functions are referred to in bold Arial, e.g. **Image/ Process/Threshold ...** There are also some computer activities which use other resources, including video files and Excel spreadsheets.

Acknowledgements

I would like to thank all my previous students for their feedback on the courses which eventually led to this book; especially Zainab Kawaf, Terry Peters, Jen Eaton, Tom MacGregor, Dolly Thornton, Shahab Lashkari, Kelsey Belden, Mike Ferguson, Aubrey Henderson, Jake King, Sandra Waterbury, James Kang, David Corcoran, Dantha Manikka-Baduge, Feng Lin, Robert Lawson, Janine Lansdown, Jarrod Long, Kimberly Watson, Charles Zilm, Jen Morrison and Dave Bennett. My son Daniel assisted me with many of the illustrations. I am grateful to Diana Gillooly and Catherine Appleton at Cambridge University Press for their support and encouragement throughout the whole process of writing the book, and to various reviewers who have critiqued the manuscript and trialed it with their classes. Special thanks go to my wife Hajijah and family (Adeline, Nadia and Daniel) for their patience, empathy and understanding while I was involved in writing. The book is dedicated to them.

Part I

Introduction to image processing

1 Introduction

Overview

Imaging systems construct an (output) image in response to (input) signals from diverse types of objects. They can be classified in a number of ways, e.g. according to the radiation or field used, the property being investigated, or whether the images are formed directly or indirectly. Medical imaging systems, for example, take input signals which arise from various properties of the body of a patient, such as its attenuation of x-rays or reflection of ultrasound. The resulting images can be continuous, i.e. *analog*, or discrete, i.e. *digital*; the former can be converted into the latter by *digitization*. The challenge is to obtain an output image that is an accurate representation of the input signal, and then to analyze it and extract as much diagnostic information from the image as possible.

Learning objectives

After reading this chapter you will be able to:

- appreciate the breadth and scope of digital image processing;
- classify imaging systems according to different criteria;
- distinguish between analog, sampled and digital images;
- identify the advantages of digital imaging;
- describe the components of a generic digital image processing system;
- outline the operations involved in the various fundamental classes of image processing;
- list examples of digital image processing applications within a variety of fields.

1.1   Imaging systems

Of the five senses – sight, hearing, touch, smell and taste – which humans use to perceive their environment, sight is the most powerful. Receiving and analyzing images forms a large part of the routine cerebral activity of human beings throughout their waking lives. In fact, more than 99% of the activity of the human brain is involved in processing images from the visual cortex. A visual image is rich in information. Confucius said, "A picture is worth a thousand words," and we shall see that that is an underestimate.

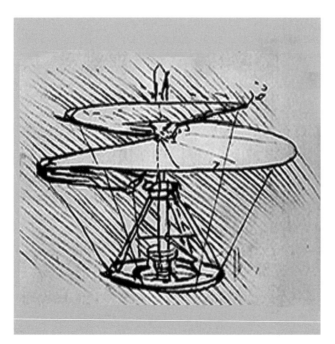

Figure 1.1   Leonardo da Vinci's concept for a helicopter.

On a more sophisticated level, humans generate, record and transmit images. Since the early days of science, researchers have tried to record their observations and even their conceptions pictorially. Leonardo da Vinci was the primary exponent of the visual image of his time: he gave absolute precedence to illustration over the written word (Fig. 1.1).

More recently, technology has tremendously extended the possibilities for visual observation. Photography makes it possible to record images objectively, preserving scenes for later, repeated, and perhaps more careful, examination. Telescopes and microscopes greatly extend the human visual range, permitting the visualization of objects of vastly differing scales. Technology can even compensate for inherent limitations of the human eye. The human eye is receptive to only a very narrow range of frequencies within the electromagnetic spectrum (Fig. 1.2). Nowadays there are sensors capable of detecting electromagnetic radiation outside this narrow range of "visible" frequencies, ranging from γ-rays and x-rays, through ultraviolet and infrared, to radio waves.

Images can be formed from many kinds of objects using differing mechanisms of formation, and, consequently, imaging systems can be classified according to several different criteria. Table 1.1 classifies systems according to the type of radiation or field used to form an image. Electromagnetic radiation is used most often in imaging systems. The radiofrequency band is used in astronomy and in magnetic resonance imaging (MRI). Microwaves are used in radar imaging, since they can penetrate clouds and other atmospheric conditions that interfere with imaging using visible light. A vast number of systems use visible light and infrared radiation, including microscopy, remote sensing and industrial inspection. Ultraviolet radiation is used in fluorescence microscopy, for example, and x-rays are used in medical diagnostic work, in industrial imaging, to detect

Table 1.1 Classification of imaging systems by type of radiation or field used.

Type of radiation or field	Examples
Electromagnetic waves	Radio, microwaves, infrared, visible light, ultraviolet, (soft) x-rays
Other waves	Water, sonar, seismic, ultrasound, gravity
Particles	Neutrons, protons, electrons, heavy ions, (hard) x-rays, γ-rays
Quasistatic fields	Geomagnetic, biomagnetic, bioelectric, electrical impedance

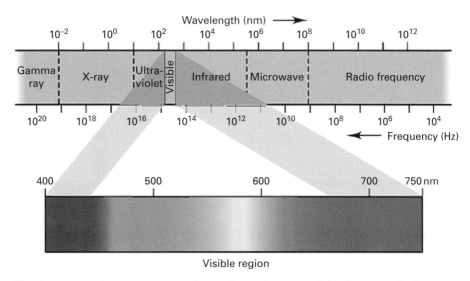

Figure 1.2 The electromagnetic spectrum arranged according to the energy of the photons, or the frequency of the waves. See also color plate.

manufacturing flaws and in astronomy. The more energetic the electromagnetic radiation, such as higher-energy (hard) x-rays and γ-rays, the shorter its wavelength and the better it can reveal small details. We often think of electrons as particles, but they have wave-like properties too. Their wavelength is very much smaller than that of visible light, enabling electron microscopes to "see" much smaller details and achieve much larger magnifications, on the order of 10000 or more, whereas light microscopes have a theoretical limit of about 1000 or so. Low frequency (~100 Hz) sound waves are used in seismic imaging to detect oil and gas deposits and high-frequency (~MHz) ultrasound is used in medical imaging, especially in obstetrics to determine the health of the fetus (Fig. 1.3).

Even static or nearly static (*quasistatic*) fields can be used in imaging. In electric impedance tomographic imaging, electric fields set up within the body, as a result of applying voltages to an array of electrodes on the surface, allow imaging of the internal organs.

Another way of classifying imaging systems is according to the property of the object that is being exploited (Table 1.2). For example, light entering the human visual pathway originates either from a self-luminous object or from light reflected by, or transmitted through, an object. An astronomical image is an emission image, related to the spectral energy distribution of the light emitted by the object over different frequencies. In other

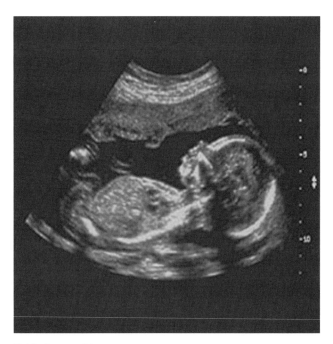

Figure 1.3   Fetal ultrasound image.

cases, the light entering the eye represents the spectral energy distribution of the light reflected from the scene, which is related to the product of the illumination and the optical reflectance of the objects in the scene. For objects that transmit light, the observed spectral energy distribution depends on the product of the illumination and the transmittance of the objects. Radiopharmaceutical substances injected into, or ingested by, the body in nuclear medicine imaging emit γ-rays that characterize the concentration of the source and its location. Radar imaging and medical ultrasound are based on reflectance properties. And x-ray imaging produces radiographs that depend on the transmittance of x-rays through an object. Other properties can also be exploited to produce images. For example, phase-contrast microscopy uses the refractive properties of an object and weather radar uses scattering properties.

Another distinction that can be made is between *direct* and *indirect* imaging systems (Table 1.3). In direct imaging the acquired data is a recognizable image, whereas in indirect imaging a data processing or reconstruction step is required before the image is available for observation.

Direct imaging can be subdivided further, depending on whether the image is acquired as a whole, parallel acquisition, or in parts, serial acquisition. Indirect imaging includes the image stored in the emulsion of a photographic film, which is rendered observable by chemical development of the film; the image consisting of valence electrons stored in the high-energy traps of a photostimulable phosphor image plate as used in computed radiography (CR), rendered observable by stimulating the image plate with laser light and digitizing the resulting image; and tomographic imaging, from the Greek *tomos*, a slice, which requires extensive processing of the raw data to produce a slice image.

Table 1.2 Classification of imaging systems by property of object.

Property	Examples
Source strength	Astronomical imaging, fluorescence microscopy
Concentration	Nuclear medicine, MRI (spin density)
Wave amplitude	Seismology
Field strength	Biomagnetic and geomagnetic imaging
Optical reflectance	Photography, remote sensing
Microwave reflectance	Radar
Acoustic reflectance	Medical ultrasound, sonar
Attenuation	Transmission x-ray, film densitometry
Refractive index	Phase-contrast microscopy
Scattering properties	Medical ultrasound, weather radar
Electric/magnetic properties	Impedance tomography, MRI (magnetization and spin relaxation)
Surface height	Laser ranging, topography

Table 1.3 Classification of imaging systems into direct or indirect systems.

		Examples
Direct imaging	Parallel acquisition	Human eye, electronic (i.e. digital) camera, optical microscope, optical telescope, scintillation camera
	Serial acquisition	Scanning microdensitometer, (confocal) scanning microscope, medical γ-camera
Indirect imaging		Film camera, x-ray CT, SPECT and PET, MRI, holography, synthetic aperture radar (SAR)

Tomographic imaging includes x-ray computed tomography (CT) (Fig. 1.4), emission tomography, such as single-photon emission computed tomography (SPECT) and positron emission tomography (PET), magnetic resonance imaging (MRI) and three-dimensional (3-D) ultrasound.

The disadvantages of indirect imaging are the time delay between capturing the data and obtaining the observable image, and the possible degradation, which may occur during this time, e.g. due to heat, humidity or light leakage affecting the photographic emulsion, or the thermal leakage of electrons out of the traps in an image plate. An advantage of indirect imaging is that the final image is often digital.

1.2 Objects and images

Real objects can be regarded as functions of one or more continuous variables. For example, the position of a star in the sky can be specified by two angles, so that the star is a two-dimensional function. In nuclear medicine the object of interest is the three-dimensional distribution of a radiopharmaceutical substance, i.e. it can be described by a three-dimensional function. If its distribution changes with time, a four-dimensional function would be needed: three spatial dimensions plus time.

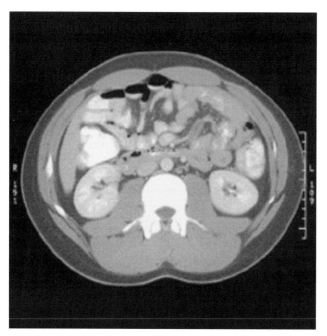

Figure 1.4   Abdominal CT image at the level of the kidneys, reconstructed from several hundred individual one-dimensional projections.

An imaging system senses or responds to an *input signal*, such as reflected or transmitted electromagnetic radiation from an object, and produces an *output signal* or *image*. When this radiation is focused and then sensed by a photographic film, for example, it gives rise to an image that is recognized as *analog*, comprising continuously varying shades or colors. A grayscale photographic image is a two-dimensional function of optical density or brightness with position; if the object can move, the image is an average over the exposure time. A color image is represented by three two-dimensional functions, each corresponding to the density of one of the three color emulsions, red, green and blue, on the film. It might be argued that these images are not continuous (i.e., analog) at the level of the silver halide particles of the photographic emulsion, which are the sensors; but the scale of these is considerably below the level of perception of the human eye.

More recently, with the advent of small solid-state electronic detectors in digital still and video cameras, the option exists to capture the radiation using sensors organized in a two-dimensional array. This sensor array, placed at the focal plane, produces outputs proportional to the integral of the radiation received at each sensor during the exposure time, and these values become the terms in a two-dimensional matrix, which represents the scene; this is called a *sampled* image. It is not yet a digital image. The physical disposition of sensors facilitates the collection of data into an array, but the values themselves are still integrals and hence continuous; they need to be quantized to a discrete scale before the image is a *digital* image. Digital images can be represented by an array of discrete values, which makes them amenable to storage and manipulation within a computer.

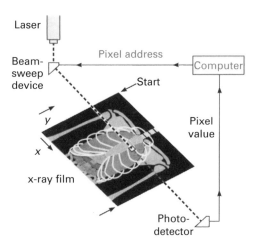

Figure 1.5   Scanning an analog image in a raster fashion. (Adapted from Wolbarst, 1993, p. 207.)

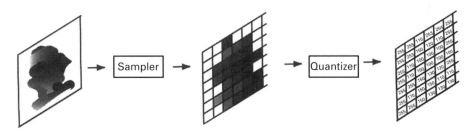

Figure 1.6   The relationship between an analog image and a digitized image.

An imaging system can either be a *continuous-to-continuous system*, responding to a continuous input signal and producing a continuous or analog output image, or it can be a *continuous-to-discrete system*, responding to the continuous input signal by producing a discrete, digital output image. Tomographic images are reconstructed from many, one-dimensional, views or projections collected over the exposure time. X-ray computed tomography (CT) imaging is an example of a continuous-to-discrete imaging system, using computer reconstruction to produce a digital image from a set of projection data collected by discrete sensors.

The advent of computers has opened up vast new possibilities for the quantitative processing and analysis of images, as long as these can be represented by arrays of discrete values, rather than continuous functions. In the case of analog images, they can be converted into digital images by a two-step process known as digitization. This involves scanning the image in a raster fashion (Fig. 1.5), i.e. from top left, in rows, to bottom right. The image is *sampled* (i.e. readings of the amount of light reflected, or transmitted, are taken at equally spaced positions, which defines the size of the resulting pixels), and these readings are *quantized*, i.e. assigned to one of a finite set of pixel values (Fig. 1.6). The image is now digital.

Many digital images contain 256 possible gray levels, running from black to white. This is the number of levels that can be labeled with 8 bits (i.e. 1 byte) in a binary

numbering system. It is convenient to allocate a byte of computer memory to store the brightness (gray) level, and to allocate 0000 0000 to black and 1111 1111 (decimal 255) to white, giving 256 gray levels in total; the resulting images are said to be *8 bits deep*.
Larger units of storage include:

- kilobyte (KB) = decimal 1024 (or 2^{10} bytes);
- megabyte (MB) = 1024 KB (or 2^{20} bytes);
- gigabyte (GB) = 1024 MB (or 2^{30} bytes);
- terabyte (TB) = 1024 GB (or 2^{40} bytes).

A standard CD ROM has about 700 MB of storage; double-sided double-layered DVDs have about 17 GB, while HD-DVDs and Blu-ray disks have about 50 GB; and computer hard disks typically have hundreds of GB of storage.

The ability to process and analyze images is a major advantage in having digital images; they can also be copied an infinite number of times, with appropriate error-checking to ensure perfect copies. Additional advantages include: the ease with which they can be displayed on computer monitors, and their appearance modified at will; the ease with which they can be stored on, for example, CD-ROM or DVD; the ability to send them between computers, via the Internet or via satellite; the option to compress them to save on storage space or reduce communication times. Many of these advantages are particularly relevant to medical imaging. The saving in physical space in not having to store bulky x-ray film is a distinct advantage, and the move towards film-less imaging has saved on chemical processing costs. Increasingly, hospitals are networking their digital imaging systems into either so-called PACS (picture and archiving systems) or RIS/HIS (radiological/ hospital information systems), which include patient diagnoses and billing details along with the images.

1.3   The digital image processing system

A complete digital image processing system (Fig. 1.7) is a collection of hardware (equipment) and software (computer programs) that can:

(i) acquire an image, using appropriate sensors to detect the radiation or field (Table 1.1) and capture the features of interest from the object in the best possible way. If the detected image is continuous, i.e. analog, it will need to be digitized by an *analog-to-digital converter* (ADC);

(ii) store the image, either temporarily in a *working image store* using read/write memory devices known as *random access memory* (RAM) or, more permanently, using magnetic media (e.g. floppy disks or the computer hard disk memory), optical media (e.g. CD-ROMs or DVDs) or semiconductor technology (e.g. flash memory devices);

(iii) manipulate, i.e. process, the image; and

(iv) display the image, ideally on a television or computer monitor, which comprises lines of continuously varying, i.e. analog, intensity. This requires the production of an analog video display signal by a *digital-to-analog converter* (DAC).

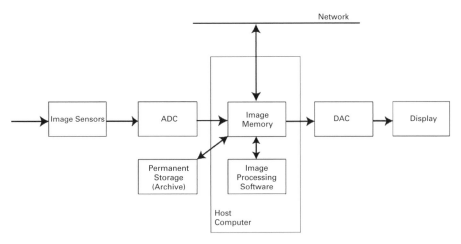

Figure 1.7   A digital image processing system.

Table 1.4 Digital image processing classes and examples of the operations within them.

Classes	Examples of operations
Image enhancement	Brightness adjustment, contrast enhancement, image averaging, convolution, frequency domain filtering, edge enhancement
Image restoration	Photometric correction, inverse filtering
Image analysis	Segmentation, feature extraction, object classification
Image compression	Lossless and lossy compression
Image synthesis	Tomographic imaging, 3-D reconstruction

In this book we shall be interested predominantly in the manipulation or processing operations. These can be grouped, broadly, into five fundamental classes: image enhancement, restoration, analysis, compression and synthesis (Table 1.4). Each class contains certain representative operations.

Image enhancement results in an image which either looks better to an observer, a subjective phenomenon, or which performs better in a subsequent processing class. Enhancement might involve adjusting the brightness of the image, if it were too dark or too bright, or its contrast, if for example it comprised only a few shades of gray, giving it a washed-out appearance. Alternatively, it might involve smoothing an image that contains a lot of *noise* or *speckle*, or sharpening an image so that edges within it are more easily seen.

Images are often significantly degraded in the imaging system, and *image restoration* is used to reverse this degradation. This would include reversing the effects of: uneven illumination, non-linear detectors which produce an output (response) that is not proportional to the input (stimulus), distortion, e.g. "pincushion" and "barrel" distortions caused by poorly focusing lenses or electron optics (Fig. 1.8), movement of the object during acquisition, and unwanted noise (Fig. 1.9). The key to image restoration is to model the degradation and then to use an inverse operation to reverse it.

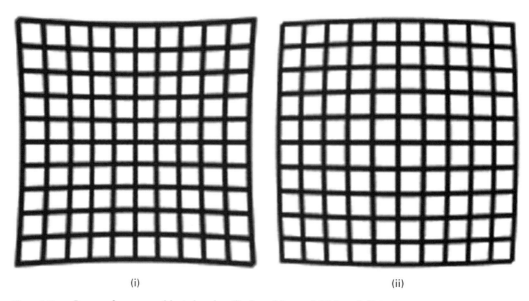

(i)   (ii)

Figure 1.8   Image of a square object showing (i) pincushion and (ii) barrel distortion.

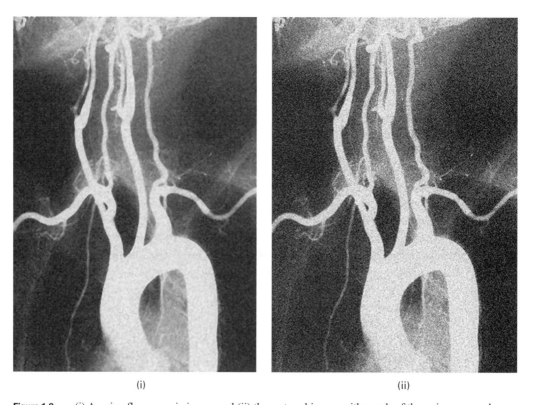

(i)   (ii)

Figure 1.9   (i) A noisy fluoroscopic image and (ii) the restored image with much of the noise removed.

Image analysis involves taking measurements of objects within an image, preferably automatically, and assigning them to groups or classes. Generally, the process begins with isolating the objects of interest from the rest (known as *segmentation* of the image), measuring a number of features such as size, shape and texture, and then classifying the objects into groups according to these features. This permits the categorization of a new object as either belonging to a particular group or not belonging, depending on whether its features fall inside or outside the tolerance of that group, respectively. This latter process is *classification* or *pattern recognition*, and is used for example in classifying lesions as benign or malignant and in recognizing suspicious clusters of microcalcifications in images of the breast.

Image compression reduces the amount of data needed to describe the image. Images require large file sizes, e.g. those comprising 512×512 pixels require about 1/4 MB of space, comparable to a document comprising 40 pages of text. Compression reduces the file size so that the image can be more efficiently stored or transported electronically, via telephony for example, in a shorter time. Compression is possible because images tend to contain redundant or repetitive information. Alternative storage schemes can store the information more effectively, i.e. in smaller files, and decompression algorithms can be used to retrieve the original image data. If all the data are preserved in the compressed file, albeit with different coding, the compression is *lossless*; this is mandatory for medical images. Smaller image files (i.e. greater compression) can be obtained with *lossy* compression techniques, which do not preserve all of the data of the original image, but nevertheless maintain an image of acceptable quality.

Image synthesis creates new images from other images or non-image data. The prime example of this is the reconstruction of axial, or "slice," tomographic images from projection data, as in x-ray computed tomography.

Image processing is not a single-step process. Generally a number of steps will need to be performed one after the other in order to extract the data of interest from the observed scene, and a hierarchy in the processing steps will be evident, e.g. enhancement will precede restoration, which will precede analysis. Often these are performed sequentially, but more sophisticated tasks will require feedback; i.e., advanced processing steps will pass parameters back to preceding steps so that the processing includes a number of iterative loops.

Image processing and computer graphics use the same knowledge base. Image processing manipulates images acquired by certain sensors to obtain information on shape and structure. Computer graphics does the reverse: it attempts to create photo-realistic images from a knowledge of shape and structure. In the future, with the increasing importance of multimedia, we can expect the two areas to move close together. *Visual computing*, the name given to this confluence, will let us interact with and control images by manipulating visual objects.

1.4 Applications of digital image processing

Digital image processing is cross disciplinary in nature. It uses ideas and techniques from optics, solid-state physics, electronics, computer architecture, software design, algebra,

Table 1.5 Examples of image processing applications within various fields.

Field	Examples
Medical diagnostic imaging	Projection radiography and x-ray computed tomography (CT) using transmission of x-rays through the body; digital subtraction angiography (DSA) produces enhanced images of the blood vessels by subtracting "pre-contrast" and "post-contrast" images; and mammography produces images of the soft tissue in the breast
	Nuclear medicine using emission of gamma rays from radiotracers injected into the body; includes planar scintigraphy and emission computed tomography (SPECT and PET)
	Ultrasound imaging using reflection of ultrasonic waves within the body
	Magnetic resonance imaging (MRI) using the precession of spin systems in a large magnetic field; including functional MRI (fMRI)
	Registration of multi-modal images
Biological imaging	Analysis, classification and matching of 3-D genome topology
	Automatic counting and classification of cell types and morphology
	Growth rate measurements using time-lapse image sequences
	Motility assay for motion analysis of motor proteins
Human-machine interface	Gesture and sign language recognition
Forensic medicine and law enforcement	Image enhancement, automated pattern recognition and classification used for fingerprint analysis, face recognition, signature verification
	Databases to organize "mugshots" and evidence
	DNA matching
	Automated reading of license plates
Automation and robotics	Vision systems for automatic part recognition, quality inspection and process monitoring
	Virtual and augmented reality
Document processing	Scanning, archiving, compression and transmission in order to store documents in large, relational, databases
	Optical character recognition (OCR) to convert scanned documents, e.g. bank cheques, into editable text files
Defense/military	Image enhancement and pattern recognition for automatic interpretation of reconnaissance images, e.g. troop movements, missile deployments
	Tracking targets for missile-guidance systems
	Bomb damage assessment
Materials research	Automatic counting and classification of components and impurities using features such as texture
	Surface and structural rendering to create three-dimensional images for heightened perception
Photography/cinematography	Image enhancement, compositing and special effects, such as warping and morphing, and the fabrication of synthetic scenes
	Video archiving and transmission
Publishing	Facilitates desktop publishing with more efficient layout
	Improved color separation and printing
Remote sensing	Land cover analysis of multi-spectral images to analyze crop yields and assess environmental damage
	Weather observation and prediction using images taken in the visible and infrared bands of the spectrum
Communications	File compression
	Teleconferencing, image phones
Space exploration	Terrain rendering, based on satellite and space rover imagery
Astronomy	Image enhancement and restoration, e.g. of distorted images from the Hubble telescope
	Automatic detection of solar flares and other cosmic phenomena

statistics, graph theory and more, and applies them to images from every field of the natural sciences and the technical disciplines. Knowledge of the application area, not only knowledge of image processing techniques, is required to obtain the best solution to a particular problem.

The applications are many and constantly increasing. Table 1.5 shows numerous examples but is not exhaustive. They illustrate that image processing enables complex phenomena to be investigated, which could not be adequately accessed using conventional measurements. Although the techniques for processing and analyzing images are universal, we will be applying them mainly to medical images obtained from medical imaging systems or *modalities*. This application provides ways to look inside the human body and diagnose disease non-invasively without having to cut the body open through surgery, or put something into it such as an optical fiber or endoscope.

Exercises

1.1 List four advantages of digital images over analog images.

1.2 What property of the object is exploited in creating the following images:
- medical ultrasound images,
- CT images,
- MRI images,
- nuclear medicine images,
- impedance tomography images?

1.3 To what class of image processing operations do the following examples belong:
- tomographic reconstruction,
- removing distortion,
- pattern recognition,
- edge enhancement,
- noise removal,
- brightness adjustment?

1.4 Distinguish between direct and indirect imaging systems, giving examples to illustrate each system.

1.5 How many images, each with 512×512 pixels and each pixel requiring one byte of storage, can be stored on (i) a 3 1/2" floppy disk with a capacity of 1.4 MB, (ii) a standard CD ROM with a capacity of 700 MB, (iii) a DVD-ROM with a capacity of 4.7 GB?

1.6 How many different shades of gray can be present in an image that is (i) 8 bits deep, (ii) 12 bits deep, (iii) 16 bits deep?

1.7 Explain the differences between spatial resolution and brightness (gray scale) resolution in a digitized image.

2   Imaging systems

Overview

Analogies are often drawn between the human visual pathway and computer imaging systems, so it is important to realize both the utility and the limitations of this approach. Since computers can process only digital images, they must be manipulated in order to render them readable; this process is called *digitization*. It is important to understand the steps in this process and their implications for the quality of the resulting image.

Learning objectives

After reading this chapter you will be able to:

- describe the human visual pathway and outline its characteristics;
- compare the performance of the human visual pathway with that of film and semi-conductor sensors;
- explain the two processes involved in digitizing an image;
- recognize the problem of undersampling;
- identify the characteristics of a digital image;
- outline the factors affecting the quality of a digital image;
- interpret how the point spread function (PSF) and the modulation transfer function (MTF) characterize an imaging system;
- describe the sources of noise in an imaging system;
- measure the signal-to-noise ratio of an image;
- distinguish between true color and indexed color images;
- identify an imaging application which uses pseudocolor.

2.1   The human visual pathway

In order to design efficient image processing systems it is important to have an understanding of the *human visual pathway*, which comprises the eye, its associated nerves and portions of the brain.

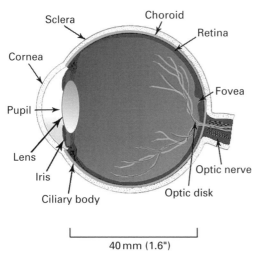

Figure 2.1   Cross-section through a typical human eye.

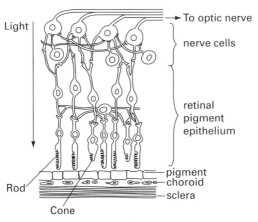

Figure 2.2   Structure of the photoreceptors of the human eye.

The eye is almost spherical in shape, with an average diameter of about 40 mm (Fig. 2.1). It converts information entering through the pupil as visible light into electrical impulses, which are transmitted along the *optic nerve* to the brain, for interpretation. Visible light is refracted by the cornea and enters the pupil, after which it is again refracted, by the lens, to form an inverted image on the innermost membrane of the eye, the *retina*. The retina is composed of several layers, and one of these, the *retinal pigment epithelium*, contains the *photoreceptors* that sense the light and convert it to electrical impulses which are taken by the optic nerve to the brain. There are two types of photoreceptor, *rods* and *cones* (Fig. 2.2). The rods are more numerous, with about 100 million distributed throughout the entire layer; they are more sensitive to light than the cones. There are fewer cones, about 6–7 million, and they are highly concentrated, approximately $180\,000\,\text{mm}^{-2}$, in a circular region near the center of the retina,

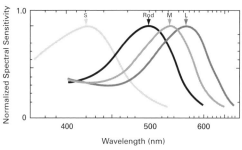

Figure 2.3   Spectral sensitivity of the rods and cones. (Note that each curve has been normalized to the same peak height.)

about 1.5 mm in diameter: the *fovea*. Complicated cross-linking of cells facilitates some basic processing even before the information leaves the retina. There is a region, devoid of photoreceptors, where the optic nerve leaves the retina: it is known as the *optic disk* and accounts for the *blind spot* in the visual field.

Rods are sensitive to blue-green light, with peak sensitivity at a wavelength of around 498 nm, but they cannot detect color, only light intensity. Several rods are connected to a single nerve, and this makes them unable to discern fine detail. They can function in situations of low light intensity and are vital for night vision. There are three types of *cones*, which together permit color vision: their sensitivity overlaps with L-cones (red or Long-wavelength), having peak sensitivity around 564 nm, M-cones (green or Medium wavelength), with peak sensitivity around 533 nm, and S-cones (blue or Short wavelength), with peak sensitivity around 437 nm (Fig. 2.3).

2.1.1   Brightness response of the eye

The rods in the retina respond to low intensity levels (*scotopic* or dim-light vision) and the cones to higher intensity levels (*photopic* or bright-light vision); between them they can adapt to a huge range of light intensities, on the order of 10^{10}, known as the *dynamic range*. Their combined sensitivity produces a logarithmic response curve (Fig. 2.4), with the perceived brightness varying roughly as the log of the light intensity incident on the eye, measured in milli-lambert (mL).

Although the eye has a huge dynamic range, it cannot simultaneously distinguish all these intensity levels; instead, it adapts to regions within the total dynamic range by a process known as brightness adaptation or *accommodation*. For example, when the eye is adapted to a brightness level of B_1 (Fig. 2.4), the range of subjective brightness levels that it can perceive is given by the short dashed curve in the figure.

The human visual response is limited to detecting brightness changes of about 2–3%, so that typically it can distinguish only around 25–30 brightness levels in a scene. Thus, if the range between black and white were divided into more than 30 equal levels of brightness, the eye would be unable to distinguish between adjacent levels. Human vision does not measure absolute brightness, but relies on local comparisons to determine if a region or an object is brighter than another. Its sensitivity to percentage changes in

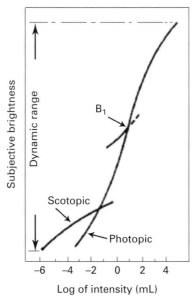

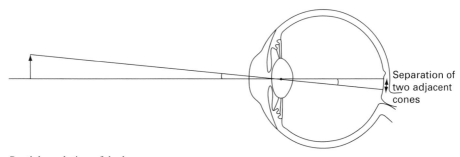

Figure 2.4   Response of the eye to light intensity. (Courtesy of NASA.)

Figure 2.5   Spatial resolution of the human eye.

brightness, rather than absolute changes, is a direct consequence of its logarithmic response to light intensity.

2.1.2   Spatial resolution of the eye

The eye cannot distinguish two objects as separate unless the light from them falls on two different cones; i.e., objects can just be differentiated if they subtend an angle at the eye which is related to the angle subtended within the eye by two adjacent cones (Fig. 2.5). Diffraction effects and lens aberrations, together with limits in neural processing, further limit the resolution of the human visual pathway. In practice, objects can be detected only if they subtend an angle of about 1 minute of arc, and this value is taken as the *visual acuity* or *spatial resolution* of a normal eye.

The human visual system is extremely powerful at recognizing objects. Not all of the information from the rods and cones is used directly: lateral neural connections are used to enhance edges or boundaries; hierarchical filter techniques select information based on local orientation and texture; and scenes are interpreted in terms of familiar shapes and structures. The visual system is not, however, well suited to measure accurately intensities, distances and areas, which can be done relatively easily with computer visioning systems.

2.2 Photographic film

In imaging systems, incoming signals emitted from, transmitted through or reflected from a three-dimensional (3-D) object are mapped onto a two-dimensional (2-D) surface, and different physical attributes of the object are represented by different shades of gray or color in the image. Many imaging systems act like a camera, which is itself modeled on the human eye. The incoming radiation is focused onto a film, which detects the radiation, taking the place of the retina, and stores the resulting image. Photographic film has been the principal medium for acquiring and storing medical images for more than a century, although more recently it is being replaced by other sensors which can be integrated into digital imaging systems.

Radiographic film is a specialized form of photographic film comprising a thin sheet of inert plastic, the base, coated on both sides with emulsion. The film emulsion contains sub-micron sized microcrystals of silver halide in a gelatin base. The microcrystals are the photodetectors: they are activated when exposed to x-rays or light and store a "latent image," which is not evident until the film is developed. The development process reduces the microcrystals to a dark silver deposit, the activated crystals being reduced at a much faster rate. The non-activated crystals are then removed by fixation with a thiosulfate solution, which binds tightly to them to form a soluble complex that is easily washed off the film base.

Radiographic film is relatively sensitive to x-ray photons, and is usually sandwiched between two fluorescent *intensifying screens* within a film cassette. The intensifying screens fluoresce on exposure to x-ray photons, producing many more visible light photons which then interact efficiently with the film. The intensifying screens produce an amplifying effect, and consequently the x-ray exposure can be reduced, resulting in a smaller patient dose, and adequate film darkening still obtained.

2.2.1 Response of film to light

Optical density is a measure of the amount of light transmitted through an object, and therefore it determines the brightness of the object. If the light intensity incident on it is I_0 and the light intensity transmitted through it is I_T, then the transmittance of the object is I_T/I_0 and its *optical density* is given by

$$OD = \log_{10}(1/T) = \log(I_0/I_T) \tag{2.1}$$

For instance, if the object is totally transparent and 100% of the incident light passes through it, its optical density is 0; if 10% of the incident light passes through it, its optical

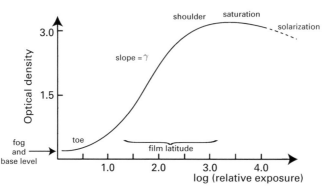

Figure 2.6   Characteristic response curve for film.

density is 1; if 1% of the light passes through it, its optical density is 2; and if 0.1% of the light passes through, its optical density is 3. Note that the optical density is a relative measure; it is a number only and has no units. Objects which pass less light have higher optical densities and appear darker with the same amount of illuminating light. The logarithmic scale is useful to approximate the logarithmic response of the human eye to light intensity.

Figure 2.6 shows the characteristic response of a film emulsion to light: optical density, OD, is plotted against the logarithm of the exposure. The higher the exposure (to light or x-rays), the darker the film becomes. The exposure is the total amount of incident radiation, and is expressed as the product of its intensity and the exposure time, for exposure times from milliseconds to seconds. At exposure times outside this range, the emulsion is less sensitive to the total incident light, an effect known as *reciprocity failure*. Film darkens slowly with time, even without exposure to light or x-rays. The combination of this effect, and the optical density of the film base itself, comprises the *fog and base level*, which results in a residual optical density of about 0.20 in the absence of exposure and gives a non-linear *toe* to the graph.

Over a relatively long range, known as the film *latitude*, the optical density has an approximately linear relationship with exposure (Fig. 2.6), and this is the normal working range of the emulsion. For many x-ray films, it corresponds to a range of optical densities from about 0.25 to about 2.25. The gradient of this region is called the *gamma* (γ) of the film, and represents the *contrast* of the film, i.e. the change in optical density caused by a change in exposure. Typically, an x-ray film has a γ value of around 2.0, measured at an optical density of around 1.2–1.25, the center of its approximately linear range. The *speed* of a film is a measure of the ease with which useful optical density is reached; it is defined as the inverse of the exposure that achieves an optical density value of 1.0 above the fog and base level. Thus a high-speed film requires little exposure to reach this level of darkening, whereas a low-speed film requires more exposure to reach the same level. Beyond the linear region, there is a *shoulder* before *saturation*, which corresponds to all the microcrystals being activated, and then a region of *solarization*, not normally reached, where increased exposure actually results in a reduction of optical density.

The images captured on film are continuous-tone images and eventually need to be digitized, using a film scanner or a digital camera, before they can be manipulated by a computer. Photographic film is able to distinguish about 4000 measurable intensity variations between the darkest and brightest recorded levels, corresponding to an optical density range of about 3.6 ($\log_{10} 4000$). X-ray film emulsion contains a higher concentration of silver halide, and so can capture larger optical density differences, up to an optical density of about 4.2. Photographic prints, on the other hand, can reproduce only about 20 different intensity levels.

2.2.2   Spatial resolution of film

The characteristic curve represents the sensitivity of the film emulsion to electromagnetic radiation, but provides no information about the spatial resolution of the film, i.e. its ability to differentiate two objects that are close together. This may be illustrated as follows.

(i) Consider how an image of a point in an object is obtained. No imaging system is perfect, so the point is inevitably blurred to some degree during the imaging process; the better the imaging system, the less the blurring. The image of a point object is called the *point spread function*, PSF. Since all objects can be considered to comprised a series of points, the point spread function of an imaging system provides a complete, quantitative description of its resolution and directly characterizes the image degradation within the system, apart from effects due to noise. In projection radiography it can be obtained, conveniently and directly, from a pinhole radiograph of the x-ray source.

Figure 2.7(i) shows the two-dimensional point spread function of a typical x-ray projection radiography system, obtained directly using a pinhole camera to obtain the image of the focal spot in the image plane. Figure 2.7(ii) shows the film density plotted vertically: for suitable film and exposure conditions, it is directly proportional to the x-ray intensity of the source. The bimodal shape is a consequence of the shape of the helical filament which heats the cathode in the x-ray tube, causing x-rays to be emitted.

The width of the point spread function characterizes the blurring of the imaging system and corresponds to its spatial resolution; i.e., two small objects (points) within this distance are blurred to such an extent that they cannot be resolved as two separate entities. The width of the point spread function depends on the quality of the system, which comprises the source of the illumination, the focusing elements and the detectors. Each of these components contributes to the overall blurring, i.e. each has its own characteristic point spread function, and the overall system point spread function is a combination of the component point spread functions. For a linear system comprising three components, each with its characteristic point spread function, i.e. PSF_1, PSF_2 and PSF_3, the system point spread function is given by

$$PSF = PSF_1{}^* PSF_2{}^* PSF_3 \qquad (2.2)$$

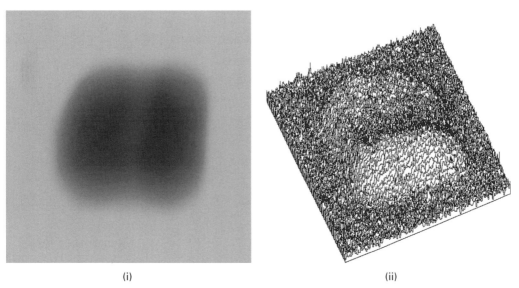

(i)   (ii)

Figure 2.7   (i) The two-dimensional point spread function from a typical x-ray tube (GE Advantx RFX) and (ii) its functional plot, with the film density plotted vertically.

where the * indicates a process known as *convolution*. The point spread function of film, often used as the final detection stage in analog radiographic systems, depends to a large extent on the concentration and size of the light-sensitive particles in the film emulsion: if they are made larger to increase the sensitivity, or speed, of the film, then the point spread function is wider, i.e. the spatial resolution is poorer.

(ii) Alternatively, consider the ability of an imaging system to form an accurate image of a sinusoidal pattern. The pattern is characterized by its repeat distance or wavelength, or equivalently, by its spatial frequency, f, which is the inverse of the repeat distance, or wavelength, of the pattern. Thus, spatial frequency has dimensions of length^{-1}, and its units are variously given as mm^{-1}, cycles mm^{-1} or, especially in medical imaging, lp mm^{-1} where lp indicates a line-pair, i.e. a pair of lines, one black and one white.

Consider a film emulsion exposed to a spatially sinusoidal pattern (Fig. 2.8) of light intensity, given by

$$\log\ E = \log\ E_0 + A \sin(2\pi f x) \tag{2.3a}$$

where E_0 falls around the center of the linear portion of the characteristic curve and A is small enough to keep the response within the linear portion. The resulting optical density of the developed film depends on the contrast of the film and is expected to take the following form:

$$D(x) = D_0 + \gamma\ A \sin(2\pi f x) \tag{2.3b}$$

where $D(x)$ fluctuates about a central value D_0 (Fig. 2.9(i)) and γ is the slope of the characteristic curve, i.e. the *gamma* or contrast of the film.

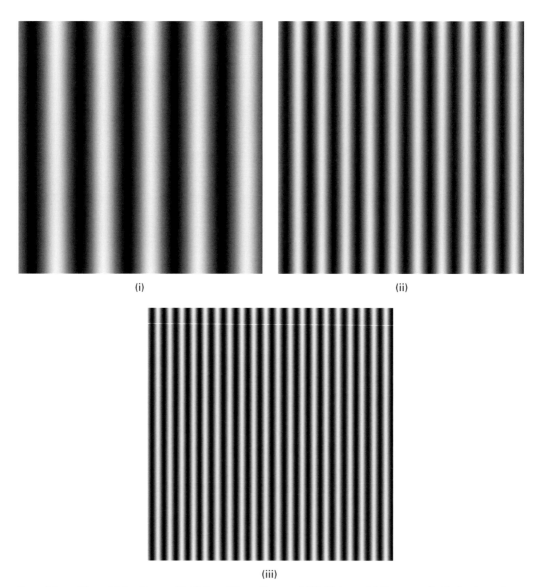

(i)   (ii)

(iii)

Figure 2.8   Sinusoidal patterns with (i) low, (ii) medium and (iii) high spatial frequency in the horizontal direction.

However, at high spatial frequencies, i.e. small repeat distances in the pattern, limitations within the film emulsion, such as microcrystal size, and scatter of the radiation reduce the emulsion's ability to detect the high-frequency variations and the observed density is then given by

$$D(x) = D_0 + \gamma \, M(f)A \, \sin(2\pi f x) \quad \text{with } 0 \leq M(f) \leq 1 \qquad (2.4)$$

where $M(f)$ is known as the *modulation transfer function*, MTF, and represents the loss of image contrast as a function of spatial frequency (Fig. 2.9(ii)).

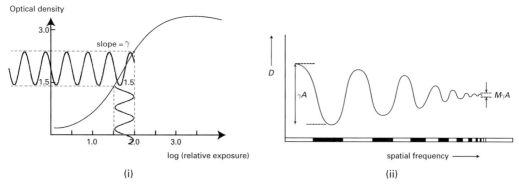

Figure 2.9 (i) The optical density produced from a sinusoidal pattern of exposure, for a film with a characteristic slope of γ. (ii) The observed optical density profile from a pattern of increasing spatial frequencies, showing the reduced response at higher spatial frequencies.

The modulation transfer function of an imaging system depends on the modulation transfer function of the components that comprise it. For a system comprising three components, each with its characteristic modulation transfer function, MTF_1, MTF_2 and MTF_3, the system modulation transfer function is given by their product:

$$MTF = MTF_1 \times MTF_2 \times MTF_3 \tag{2.5}$$

which is a much simpler operation than convolution. The spatial frequency at which the system modulation transfer function falls to 0.1 is often taken as its *spatial frequency, f_L*. It is effectively the highest spatial frequency that the imaging system can reasonably record, and is known as the *limiting spatial resolution* of the system. Analog radiographic systems often use a fluorescent screen in combination with film as the detector, in order to increase the blackening of the film. The modulation transfer functions associated with blur due to the finite size of the radiation-sensitive particles in the screen/film, patient movement and the finite size of the x-ray source (*focal spot* size) in a typical system are plotted in Figure 2.10, along with the composite, total system modulation transfer function, which is equal to their product. The modulation transfer functions become smaller at high spatial frequencies, representing the poorer quality images obtained from smaller objects. The resolution of this imaging system is about 2 cycles mm^{-1}. The inverse of the limiting frequency gives the limiting, i.e. the smallest, repeat wavelength that can be resolved by the system. Since a wavelength is composed of two parts, the upper portion and the lower portion, its length represents twice the size of the smallest resolvable object.

Worked example

What is the spatial resolution of a film that has a limiting spatial frequency of 70 cycles mm^{-1}?

This spatial frequency corresponds to a wavelength of 0.014 mm or 14 µm. The smallest object that can be resolved is half of this, i.e. 7 µm.

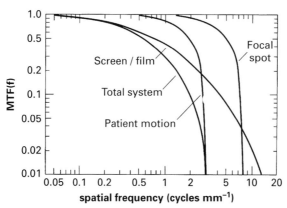

Figure 2.10   The modulation transfer function, MTF, of a radiographic imaging system as the product of the modulation transfer functions of its component parts. (Note the logarithmic scaling of this plot.) (After Wolbarst, 1993, p. 214.)

The point spread function and the modulation transfer function both contain equivalent information on the spatial resolution of an imaging system, the former in terms of the smallest distance that the system can resolve and the latter in terms of the highest frequency that the system can properly record.

2.3   Other sensors

There are other radiation sensors besides photographic film. X-ray and γ-ray photons can be detected by converting them to visible light photons using a scintillator, and then converting the light into an electric signal using a semiconductor photodiode. Such detection systems include the photostimulable phosphors used in the image plates of computed radiography, image intensifier tubes as used in fluoroscopy, and ionization chambers and scintillation detectors used in computed tomography (CT) scanners. The semiconductor photodiodes are based on silicon technology, which limits their size because of the difficulty and expense involved in manufacturing large crystals free of defects. More recently, detectors have been developed using amorphous selenium, which can be readily manufactured into large flat panels, to convert x-ray photons directly into electric charge. Elimination of the intermediate visible light stage results in higher-resolution images with less noise.

The output from semiconductor detectors is linear with incoming intensity, rather than logarithmic, as with film and human vision. This results in a much smaller dynamic range than that of the human visual system, and images of scenes that have a high dynamic range appear inferior to what is seen directly. Some imaging systems use a non-linear amplifier, after the semiconductor detector array, to produce a logarithmic output. This converts the signal intensity, I, from the detector into an output gray level, O, according to

$$O = I^{\gamma}$$

(2.6)

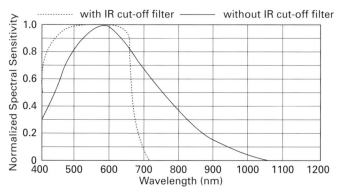

Figure 2.11 Spectral sensitivity of a typical semiconductor sensor. (Dashed line shows response with an infrared blocking filter.)

where the exponent is called the *gamma value*, and is typically about 0.4. With such a conversion, the logarithmic response of the human visual system can be approximated.

Semiconductor sensors have a very different sensitivity to the wavelength of electromagnetic radiation than the eye or photographic film (Fig. 2.11). They cover a much broader range, extending far into the infrared, and require some adjustment to make them useful at mimicking human vision. Most of them incorporate an infrared blocking filter to prevent infrared radiation from reaching the sensor.

2.4 Digitizing an image

We have discussed some of the advantages of digital images, including easy storage and post-processing. If an image is analog, for example a film radiograph, it can be *digitized* to obtain a digital image; the same considerations apply in mapping a real object directly to a digital image. There are two steps involved: *spatial quantization* and *intensity quantization*. The term *quantization* means that a variable is not allowed to take any value, but can only take certain allowable (*quantized*) values; for example, only integer values but not the non-integer values between them.

2.4.1 Spatial quantization

Digitization is conveniently explained in terms of a single-sensor, flat-bed scanner. Laser light is swept across the original analog image in a *raster* pattern, and the reflected light (if the image is a photographic print) or transmitted light (if it is a photographic negative or an x-ray film) is detected by the photodiode. The photodiode records values at equally spaced positions along the raster, and these values are saved as a two-dimensional array. This recording is called *sampling* or *spatial quantization*. The more frequently the samples are taken, the more accurately the "scene" will be captured; this results in more readings and therefore more storage space in a computer. The rate at which samples are

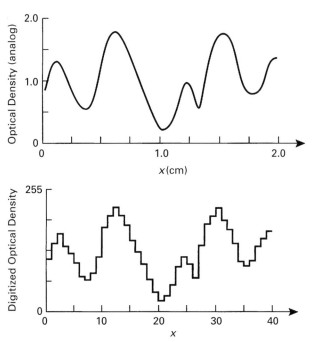

Figure 2.12   Digitization of a one-dimensional profile. (Analog) profile through a section of film (top); after digitization (bottom), comprising spatial and intensity quantization. (After Wolbarst, 1993, p. 304.)

taken is the *sampling rate* or *sampling frequency*, f_s, and is expressed as the number of samples taken per unit distance, in units of samples per centimeter or dots (samples) per inch, (dpi). The distance between samples, d, is the inverse of the sampling frequency. The sampled values can be considered as samples of the continuous profile, although in practice they are not quite sampled points but have some finite physical size, albeit small, depending on the sensor size and imperfections in the optics. These values are stored until a new sample, whose position is determined by a chosen mechanical increment, is taken. The process is thus one of "sample and hold," and the recorded profile has a step-like appearance (Fig. 2.12), approximating the continuous profile it is sensing.

Usually the sampling frequency is the same in both directions, and the small, square, area around each position, with sides equal to the distance between samples, d, make up a single pixel in the digitized image. The sampling frequency determines the distance between samples, and this distance becomes the linear *pixel size*.

Each pixel represents not a point in the image, but rather an elementary cell of the grid with its own individual brightness; the image has become *spatially quantized*. Distance along the x and y directions is no longer continuous; instead it proceeds in discrete increments, each given by the size of a pixel. With large pixel sizes, not only is the spatial resolution poor, since there is no detail within a pixel, but the gray-level discontinuities at the edges of the pixels (*pixelation*) become distracting. With small pixels the spatial resolution improves, until there is the impression of a spatially continuous image; this occurs when the pixels are smaller than the spatial resolution of the human visual system at that particular observation distance.

How small should the distance between samples be, in order to capture accurately the detail in the analog image during digitization for later reconstruction of the analog image? Or, in the case of a two-dimensional sensor array, how small should the detectors be, in order to capture the detail from the input signal? All images contain a mixture of details, some at a fine scale and some at a coarse scale. The French mathematician Fourier recognized that any repetitive pattern can be made up from a number of sinusoidal patterns of differing spatial frequencies. The high frequencies contain the information about the small details and sharp edges in an image, while the low frequencies contain the information on larger features within the image. In order to capture adequately the fine detail information, the image needs to be sampled at a sampling frequency, f_s, that is *at least twice* that of the highest frequency (f_{max}) contained in it; this is known as the *Nyquist–Shannon sampling theorem*:

$$f_s \geq 2 \times f_{max} \tag{2.7a}$$

This is necessary because at least two samples per cycle of a sine wave are needed in order to capture both halves of the oscillation (Fig. 2.13). If fewer than two samples per cycle are sampled, reconstruction results in a wave of lower frequency (Fig. 2.13 (i)); at least two samples per cycle are required to reconstruct the original wave with its proper frequency (Fig. 2.13 (ii)).

The *Nyquist frequency*, f_N, is one-half of the sampling frequency, f_s; thus, the Nyquist–Shannon sampling theorem can be expressed as:

$$f_N \geq f_{max} \tag{2.7b}$$

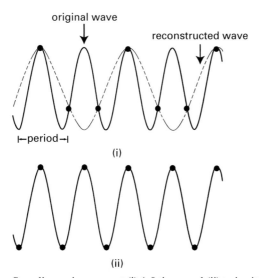

Figure 2.13   Sampling a sine wave at (i) 1.5 times and (ii) twice its frequency.

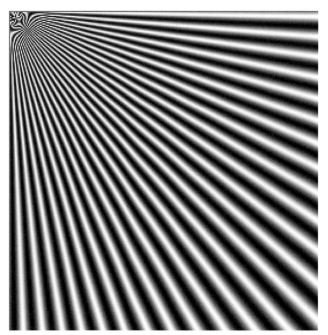

Figure 2.14   Some high spatial frequencies at the top left of the image are not reproduced properly, instead being aliased and appearing at a lower frequency.

If a sampled image contains frequencies above the Nyquist frequency, they are *under-sampled* and appear as lower frequencies in the image reconstructed from these samples. This is known as *aliasing*, and the false, lower frequency, or *aliasing frequency* (f_{alias}), appears as far below the Nyquist frequency as it actually was above it, i.e. the frequency which is too high to be properly sampled is "folded back" around the sampling frequency until it appears in the image at a frequency less than f_N:

$$f_{alias} = f_N - (f - f_N) \qquad (2.8)$$

For example, if the sampling frequency is $10\,\text{mm}^{-1}$, i.e. 10 samples taken per millimeter, then the Nyquist frequency, f_N, is $5\,\text{mm}^{-1}$. A spatial frequency of $7\,\text{mm}^{-1}$ cannot be sampled properly, because it is above f_N; instead, it appears aliased at $3\,\text{mm}^{-1}$. Very high frequencies are repeatedly folded back around multiples of the sampling frequency until the aliased frequency appears at a frequency less than f_N.

In a complex image, comprising a range of spatial frequencies, high-frequency detail is not captured properly, and appears aliased at lower frequencies in the sampled image if the sampling frequency is not high enough to capture the high frequencies (Fig. 2.14).

Interestingly, telecommunications pioneer Harry Nyquist's name is itself an alias. His family name was Jonsson, but Harry's father, Lars, changed it, because another Lars Jonsson lived just down the road, and mail delivery became a real problem!

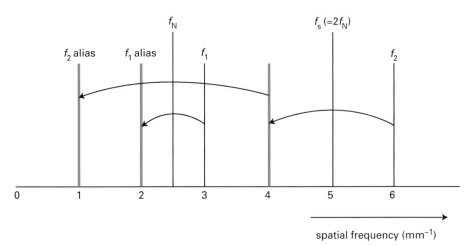

Figure 2.15 The aliasing of higher frequencies by mirroring around multiples of the Nyquist frequency.

Worked example

In a system with $200\,\mu m$ pixels, the sampling frequency is $5\,mm^{-1}$, and the highest (spatial) frequency possible, the Nyquist frequency, is $2.5\,mm^{-1}$. Any frequency higher than that in the pre-sampled image appears at a lower frequency in the sampled image: its actual position is mirrored around the Nyquist frequency or multiples thereof until it appears at a frequency less than the Nyquist frequency (Fig. 2.15). For example, a frequency of $3\,mm^{-1}$ in the pre-sampled image appears as a frequency of $2\,mm^{-1}$ in the sampled image, i.e. it masquerades, or "takes the alias of," another frequency. A frequency of $6\,mm^{-1}$ in the pre-sampled image appears as a frequency of $1\,mm^{-1}$ in the sampled image; mirrored about $5\,mm^{-1}$ (twice the Nyquist frequency) it would appear at $4\,mm^{-1}$, which is then mirrored about $2.5\,mm^{-1}$ to give $1\,mm^{-1}$.

The sampling theorem can be expressed equivalently in terms of distances rather than spatial frequencies; the sampling distance, d (the pixel size), must be less than, or equal to, half of the inverse of the maximum spatial frequency in the image, f_{max}. Thus, it must be less than, or equal to, half of the size of the smallest detail in the image (L_{min}) in order to digitize the image accurately. That is,

$$d \leq 1/(2 \times f_{max}) \tag{2.9a}$$

or

$$d \leq L_{min}/2 \tag{2.9b}$$

Worked example

A chest radiograph is 14 inches by 17 inches ($36\,cm \times 43\,cm$). If we want to preserve all the detail in the image, to a spatial resolution of 5 cycles mm^{-1}, how many pixels would be required?

To preserve the spatial resolution of 5 cycles mm^{-1}, we need to sample 10 pixels mm^{-1} (i.e. 2 pixels per cycle) resulting in pixels of size 0.1 mm. This would require 3600×4300 pixels to cover the radiograph. If each pixel is 8 bits deep (i.e. 1 byte per pixel) this would require a file of size 14.8 MB; if we required more gray levels, and used 16 bits per pixel, the file size would be twice as big.

In practice, almost all digital systems are undersampled to some degree in order to save on design constraints, e.g. size of detectors or size of image file. A slightly coarser pixel size than optimum is chosen, whereby the pre-sampled modulation transfer function extends a little beyond the Nyquist frequency. This allows the majority of the frequency content to be recorded with adequate fidelity but permits a degree of aliasing at the higher frequencies.

The worst aliasing artifacts occur when fine repetitive patterns are undersampled; these can result in distracting Moiré patterns in the digitized image. Smoothing the analog image, so as to remove higher spatial frequency components, prior to digitization can reduce the effect, but the only effective strategy is to re-sample at a higher sampling frequency. If the analog image is not available, the digital image can be smoothed (Fig. 2.16), but re-sampling is the preferred option.

2.4.2   Intensity quantization

The discrete pixels formed around the sampled locations comprise the *spatially quantized* image, but the values within the pixels are still the sampled values measured from the original analog (i.e. continuous) image. In order to form a digital image, these values need to be assigned to a finite set of discrete values. This is the second step in the process of digitizing an analog image, and is known as *intensity* (or *brightness*) *quantization*.

Many digital images are *8 bits deep*, i.e. they allocate 8 bits to each pixel, resulting in 256 possible gray levels spanning black to white. In general, allocating n bits per pixel gives 2^n shades of gray. (Using 12 bits per pixel gives 4096 more finely spaced gray levels.) Each sampled value needs to be placed on the nearest available gray level. This gives rise to an approximation error known as the *quantization error*, whose effect is minimized by the use of greater numbers of finely spaced gray levels but at the cost of larger image files.

The result of digitization, i.e. spatial and brightness quantization, is an n-dimensional array of numbers (a matrix), representing a digital image. Each number represents image brightness within a small discrete area (a pixel) in a two-dimensional ($M \times M$ pixels) grid representing a two-dimensional image, or within a small discrete volume (a *voxel*) in a three-dimensional ($M \times M \times M$ voxels) grid representing a three-dimensional image. The

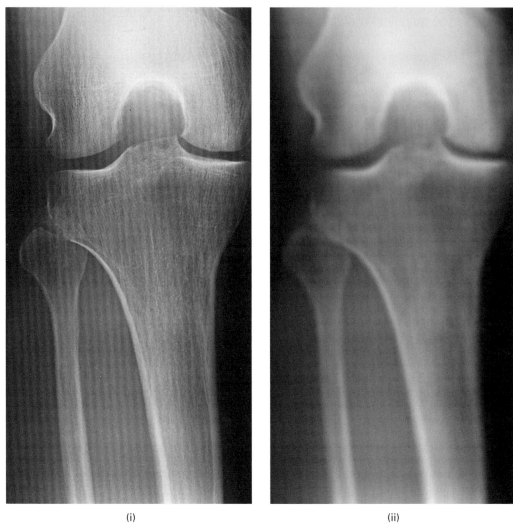

(i)   (ii)

Figure 2.16   (i) A Moiré pattern in a computed radiography image and (ii) the result of smoothing it. The preferred option would be to re-scan the image at a higher sampling frequency.

length of a side of the pixel, or voxel, can be related to real distance in a scene by dividing the field of view (FoV) of the scene, that is the real distance spanned in the scene and represented in the digital image, by the number of pixels along that side of the image:

$$\text{pixel size (or voxel size)} = \text{FoV}/M \qquad (2.10)$$

When the image is to be displayed, on a computer monitor for example, the brightness level at any location is generally taken as being directly proportional to the value stored in the corresponding pixel.

2.5   The quality of a digital image

Any imaging system must be judged on the quality of the images it produces. For medical imaging systems the images must be diagnostically useful, that is capable of leading to the detection and identification of an abnormality and its interpretation so as to determine its cause, and obtained at an acceptable dose to the patient. An image is a spatial pattern of intensities. Fundamentally, the quality of a digital image depends on the size of the pixels, relative to the size of the image, and the number of available values of gray tone that are accessible to describe the intensity range between black and white: image quality is highest for small pixels and a large number of available gray tones.

2.5.1   Spatial resolution and pixel size

Spatial resolution is a measure of the ability of the image to show fine detail. It can be reported as the minimum separation of small features in the object that can just barely be distinguished as separate in the image. The spatial resolution of a digital image depends on the resolution of the imaging system that produced it, characterized by its point spread function, PSF, or equivalently by its modulation transfer function, MTF, and the size of the pixels used to represent the digitized image. This latter is determined, either by the sampling frequency used in digitization or by the size and separation of the detectors in a two-dimensional detector array. Figure 2.17 shows an image and the effect of increasing pixel sizes after acquisition. The larger the pixel sizes, the less detail can be seen. In fact the pixel size determines the smallest detail which can be seen, since pixels are shaded a uniform gray and there is no detail within them. Increasing the pixel size reduces the spatial resolution, since it reduces the ability to see fine detail within the image. Activity 2.1 explores this relationship.

The point spread function of an imaging system is the image that results from a point object, and thus its width determines the size of the smallest observable detail in an analog image. Figure 2.18 shows the point spread function of a two-dimensional digital imaging system, with different-sized pixel grids superimposed on it. The smaller the pixels of the grid the more detail can potentially be displayed. Taking into account the sampling theorem we might choose the pixels to be about half the width of the point spread function to adequately sample it (Fig. 2.18 (i)). There is nothing to be gained from using much smaller pixels than this, since there is no additional detail within the point spread function (Fig. 2.18 (ii)); at best it may produce a cosmetically more appealing image with less evident pixelation, but at the cost of a larger file size. On the other hand, using a larger pixel size would be detrimental to image quality, since the point spread function would spread to occupy a single large pixel (Fig. 2.18 (iii)).

There is an argument for reducing the pixel size a little further than one-half of the width of the point spread function, since the point spread function of the underlying, analog, imaging system does not have a brick-wall shape. If the point spread function is taken as Gaussian in shape, which is appropriate for most systems, and its width is taken as the full width at half maximum height (FWHM) of its point spread function, then the

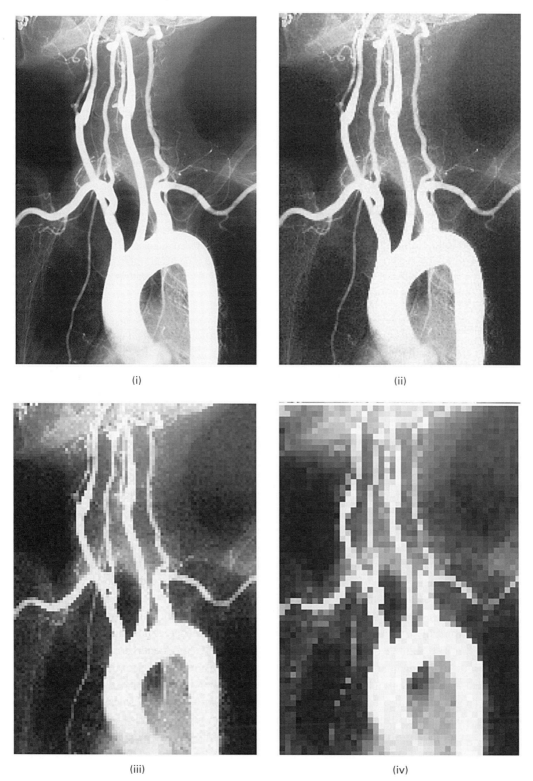

Figure 2.17 (i) Image using original pixels and with pixels which are (ii) 2×2 times larger, (iii) 4×4 times larger and (iv) 8×8 times larger.

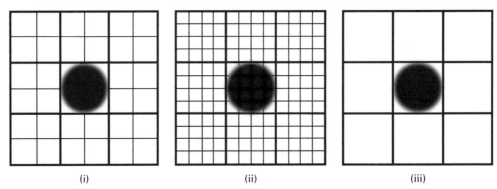

(i)   (ii)   (iii)

Figure 2.18   Grids of various sizes superimposed on the point spread function image. (i) The optimal pixel size. (ii) Smaller pixels offer little advantage since there is no detail within the point spread function. (iii) Larger pixels are not recommended since the analog point spread function would spread (not shown) to occupy a single pixel.

sampling distance, i.e. pixel size, should be about one-third of the FWHM to avoid significant loss of spatial resolution, thus:

$$d \leq \mathrm{FWHM}/3 \qquad (2.11)$$

This represents a somewhat tighter restriction on pixel size than Equation (2.9b), and is widely used as the rule-of-thumb in nuclear medicine imaging.

2.5.2   Brightness resolution

Different features in an image are displayed as different shades of gray. In medical images these differences are determined in part by the properties of the tissues, such as their thickness, density and chemical composition, and by aspects of the imaging process that are controllable, such as the energy of the x-ray photons. It is crucial to be able to distinguish parts of the body that differ anatomically or physiologically only a little from each other. This requires a sufficient number of different gray values so parts which we want to be able to distinguish are assigned different gray values.

The number of gray values available in an image depends on the number of bits used during quantization: using n bits per pixel results in 2^n shades of gray. Digitization with an 8-bit analog-to-digital converter, resulting in 256 possible shades of gray, is more than adequate for most visual purposes, since our visual system can distinguish only about 30 shades of gray, and most computer monitors have been manufactured to reproduce 256 gray levels. Images displayed with an insufficient number of shades of gray, i.e. fewer than about 32, suffer from *false contouring* or *posterization*, an effect mimicking topographic contours, which is most noticeable in areas of constant gray level (Fig. 2.19). Activity 2.2 explores the relationship between pixel depth and false contouring.

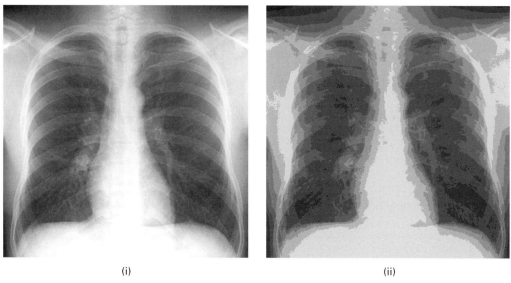

(i)   (ii)

Figure 2.19   An image displayed using (i) 64 and (ii) 8 shades of gray, with significant false contouring (posterization) visible in the latter image.

Some images require higher brightness resolution if quantitative analysis of image properties are to be made accurately. For example, the pixels in x-ray CT images have 12-bit depth and therefore can have 4096 (2^{12}) possible values.

2.5.3   Noise content

Noise is the unwanted, random (stochastic) fluctuations in an image. The principal sources of noise in a digital imaging system are *photon* (or *quantum*) *noise*, which arises from the discrete nature of electromagnetic radiation and its interactions with matter, and *electronic noise* in detectors or amplifiers. If a film-screen cassette is used to acquire the image, individual grains within the film and fluorescent screen produce random variations in the film density: the noise contribution from the screen (*structure mottle*) is larger than that from the film (*film granularity*). The process of digitization is also responsible for adding noise (quantization noise) to an image. Photon (or quantum) noise usually obeys the *Poisson distribution function*, and electronic noise is almost always Gaussian.

These unwanted stochastic variations can be quantified most easily in a region of the image that is expected to have a constant brightness. The *noise power* (P_N) can be taken as the variance, i.e. the square of the standard deviation, of the pixel values in such a region. To understand its significance, the noise should be compared to the average power or intensity of the signal (P_S), which is given by the average value of the pixels in the image. The *signal-to-noise ratio* (SNR or S/N) is the ratio of the intensity of the signal to the noise power; it is often expressed in decibels (dB) by taking ten times the logarithm, to the base 10, of the ratio. Thus:

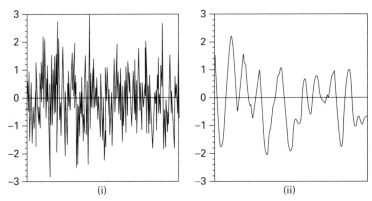

Figure 2.20   One-dimensional profiles with the same noise variance but differing correlation distances.

$$\mathrm{SNR(in\ dB)} = 10\log_{10}(P_\mathrm{S}/P_\mathrm{N}) \qquad (2.12)$$

This describes the noise adequately if it is spatially uncorrelated, that is the amount of noise at one position in the object is not related to the amount of noise at any other position. Figure 2.20 shows one-dimensional profiles with the same variance but greatly differing appearances. The noise in Figure 2.20 (i) is almost spatially uncorrelated or, to be more precise, it is correlated only over a very short distance; while the noise in Figure 2.20 (ii) is correlated over a longer distance, such that values are similar for positions which are close to each other. The extent of spatial correlation can be characterized by the autocorrelation function. Examples of noise that exhibit different characteristic correlations include Gaussian noise and uniform noise, and the colorfully named "white" noise, "pink" noise and "brown" noise.

The noise produced within an imaging system is a combination of several noise sources, and it may not be possible to identify them separately. The image produced by a uniform gray scene, which should result in a uniform brightness, has a distribution of gray tones around an average value; the width of the distribution is a measure of the noise content of the image.

In medical x-ray and γ-ray imaging systems, the number of photons emitted per unit time from the source varies and so too do its interactions with the patient's body. The result of both these factors is that the image has a spatial and temporal randomness. This source of noise, often referred to as *quantum noise*, is a fundamental and unavoidable noise source in medical imaging. In a good medical imaging system, quantum noise, which is unavoidable, is the dominant source of random fluctuation. Quantum noise is characterized by Poisson statistics, which is used to describe independent counting events, especially when the events are comparatively infrequent. An important characteristic of the Poisson distribution is that the standard deviation in the number of counts is numerically equal to the square root of the mean of the counts (SD = $\sqrt{N}$, where N is the number of photons carrying the signal). The relative width of the distribution decreases as the mean grows larger; thus,

$$\text{relative variation} = \sqrt{N}/N = 1/\sqrt{N} \tag{2.13a}$$

or, conversely, the signal-to-noise ratio is given by

$$\text{SNR} = N/\sqrt{N} = \sqrt{N} \tag{2.13b}$$

since N is a measure of the signal strength. The signal-to-noise ratio increases as the mean gets larger: thus, the greater the number of x-ray or γ-ray photons that can be detected, the higher the image signal-to-noise ratio and the less noisy it appears.

The presence of noise in an image affects the ability to detect small objects of low *contrast*, i.e. with a brightness level only marginally different from their surroundings (Fig. 2.21). Reducing the relative noise in the final image, equivalent to increasing its signal-to-noise ratio, requires an increase in the number of photons detected. This can be achieved by increasing the intensity of the x-ray beam, or γ-ray source, or by increasing the exposure time; it can also be achieved by averaging several images. However, in each case, the patient is exposed to a higher dose of ionizing radiation. A more acceptable option is to improve the *quantum efficiency* of the detectors, i.e. the probability that the incoming photon interacts with, and thus is detected by, the detectors. Alternatively, with a digital system, the pixel size can be increased by combining several of the original pixels to form new, larger pixels, which then contain larger values, resulting in a higher signal-to-noise ratio. However, in this case, the improvement in signal-to-noise ratio is obtained at the expense of poorer spatial resolution; this is a useful strategy for detecting large objects of low contrast in an image, but does not help in the detection of small objects. This illustrates a fundamental trade-off between image quality and dose; i.e., for any imaging procedure using ionizing radiation it is necessary to compromise on exposure in order to obtain an adequate image without posing undue risk to the patient. It also demonstrates that there is a trade-off between the different parameters of image quality, namely spatial resolution, contrast and noise.

The situation can be complicated since different characteristics may be more important in different diagnostic situations. When looking for hairline cracks, spatial resolution is of paramount importance, and the huge contrast between bone and soft tissue could be sacrificed for it. In the search for soft tissue lesions of the brain using computed tomography (CT), contrast is of primary importance and noise needs to be minimized

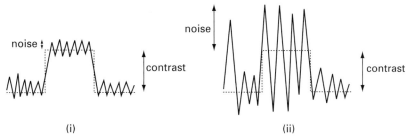

(i)   (ii)

Figure 2.21 Profiles to show the effect of noise on detectabilty. (i) A low contrast object with relatively low noise is detectable. (ii) A low contrast object with high levels of noise is not detectable.

even by sacrificing some spatial resolution. Fluoroscopic examinations tend to be lengthy, so doses need to be kept as low as possible, even though this results in high noise and makes it difficult to visualize small blood vessels even when they are filled with a contrast agent to increase their contrast relative to the surrounding tissue.

During image digitization, the process of intensity quantization potentially adds noise to the digitized image since it involves an approximation in placing a sampled value on one of the finite number of available levels, of which there are 2^n in an n-bit deep image. It is important to choose an appropriate image depth, by using an appropriate analog-to-digital converter (ADC), such that this source of noise remains insignificant compared to the quantum noise of the system and does not contribute any further image degradation.

2.6   Color images

The human visual pathway uses three types of cones, *trichromacy*, to discern and discriminate many thousands of different colors, whereas it can only distinguish about thirty different levels of brightness. This expands our ability to recognize and identify objects in a scene. While photographs replicate the colors seen by our eye, diagnostic medical images do not record color, only brightness; the brightness indicating, for example, the attenuation of x-rays or the scattering of ultrasound. Under some circumstances, it may be advantageous to add color to an image in order to better discern features in the image; the added color is false color, or *pseudocolor*, added to improve our visualization of the image, not to attempt to replicate the true colors of the features in the image.

There are different systems or models used to characterize and specify true color. Each comprises a coordinate system, within which each color is represented by a point. The *RGB* (red, green, blue) model is widely used in acquiring, processing and displaying digital images, for example with color video cameras and color monitors, although it is not the only model. Most colors can be created by mixing the three *primary* colors, taken to be red, green and blue by analogy with the response of the cones of the human retina. The RGB color space is a unit cube, with each axis representing one of the primary colors (Fig. 2.22). The origin is the absence of all colors and represents black, while the opposite vertex is a mix of all three primary colors and represents white. The other vertices represent the *secondary* colors cyan, magenta and yellow, each resulting from adding two primary colors (Activity 2.3).

In this model, all other colors are points within the cube specified by three components, each specifying the amount of primary color needed to add together to obtain the required color. Each of these components is usually specified by a single byte (giving a range of 0 to 255). Bright red would be (255, 0, 0), and bright yellow would be (255, 255, 0). Since red, green and blue can be chosen independently, this gives a total of 256^3 (16×2^{20}, or 16M) possible colors. The image file can be organized into three separate images or planes, one for each primary color. Since each pixel is represented by 3 bytes, the image file has a depth of 24 bits and is about three times larger than a grayscale image file with the same number of pixels. These images are referred to as 24-bit or "true color" images.

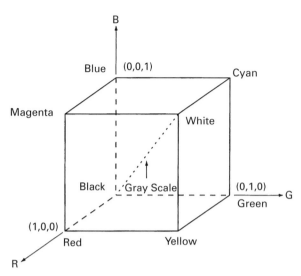

Figure 2.22   Schematic of red–green–blue (RGB) color space.

Although the RGB model seems to match the physiology of the eye with its cones sensitive to three different colors, application of processing methods to RGB pictures frequently causes unwanted results. Some grayscale image processing algorithms can be used directly for RGB images, by applying them separately to each of the three color planes; some cannot be used directly; and for some algorithms there is a computational advantage to processing in a different color space. Edge enhancement, for example, is more efficiently applied in a color space that separates *lightness*, or pixel intensity, from *chrominance*, color information. Chrominance is determined by the *hue*, the frequency of the dominant color, and the *saturation*, the purity of the color, i.e. the amount of white light mixed in with a spectral color. For example, white light mixed in with red (saturated) gives pink (less saturated). In such a color space, e.g. *HSV* (hue, saturation, value) or *HSB* (hue, saturation, brightness), only the value/brightness component (i.e. intensity) needs to be processed for edge-enhancement and for spatial smoothing. Applying sharpening and smoothing algorithms in RGB space can cause color shifts. The eye is particularly sensitive to changes in hue or color and finds even small color shifts such as caused by sharpening or smoothing algorithms in RGB space noticeable, and frequently objectionable, while it tolerates changes in intensity or saturation much more readily. Linear transformations applied to each of the RGB planes are usually acceptable, but non-linear operations such as histogram equalization (Section 5.2.2) and median filtering (Section 6.4.1) should generally not be attempted. If non-linear operations are required, then the RGB image should be converted to an HSV or HSB image, and the operations applied to just the value or brightness plane, and possibly to the saturation plane. The hue plane should almost always be left alone.

There are standard algorithms and transforms to convert RGB values into other color spaces, and then to return the results of the various image processing algorithms

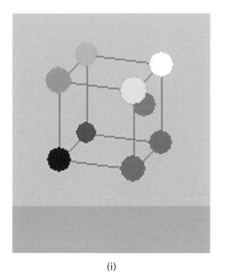

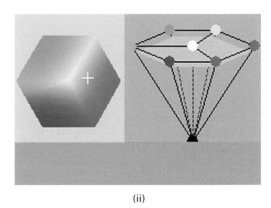

(i)   (ii)

Figure 2.23   (i) A color (bottom) and its position in RGB space, shown by the gray ball at red = 240, green = 160, blue = 140 and (ii) the same color (bottom) and its position in HSV space, with hue = 0.02, saturation = 0.40 and value = 0.93; in the hexagonal cone, the hue is the angle from the red axis, the distance to the center is the saturation, and the position up the vertical axis is the value. See also color plate.

to RGB space, prior to display. Figure 2.23 shows a color both in RGB space and in HSV space. Activities 2.4 and 2.5 involve changing between RGB and other color spaces.

An alternative to these systems is the storage of the image as indexed color, using a palette of only 256 colors optimized for the particular image (Fig. 2.24). Each pixel contains a pixel value described by a single byte. These values are used as indices or addresses into a color look-up table, LUT, or palette, which stores the 256 usable colors. Since each pixel is described by a single byte the file size of an indexed color image is similar to that of a grayscale image, apart from the space required to store the color palette, typically 256 bytes. These images are often referred to as 8-bit color images.

It is possible to colorize grayscale images by applying a color look-up table rather than a grayscale look-up table (Activity 2.7). The 256 pixel values are used as addresses in a color palette to get colors which are used to paint the pixels on the monitor, rather than using shades of gray. The resulting colors are false, in that they have been added arbitrarily and bear no relationship to the true colors of the original objects, but nevertheless they can lead to a clearer visualization of structures in the image. Pseudocolor is added to Doppler ultrasound images to colorize blood flow in shades of red if it coming towards the sensor or blue if it is moving away from it; the faster the flow the brighter the false color used.

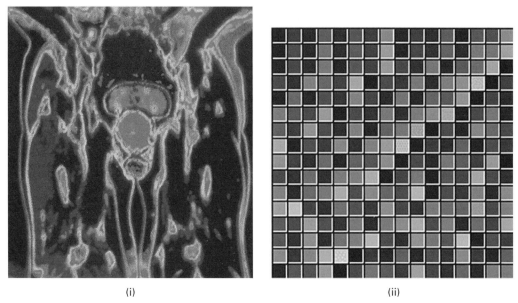

(i)   (ii)

Figure 2.24   (i) An indexed color image and (ii) its color palette, comprising 256 colors with indices running from 0 at top left to 255 at bottom right. See also color plate.

Computer-based activities

Activity 2.1 Spatial resolution

Open the image **Xray** in the program ImageJ (see the Preface). The size of this image is 320×240 pixels.

In **Plugins/Ch.2 Plugins/Spatial resolution**, choose "160×120 pixels" from the dialog box and click "OK," and "OK" again in the next box. Does the image change? To get the original image back, go to **File** on the toolbar, and click **Revert** or **Edit/Undo**: you will need to do this often. Try the other "Spatial resolution" settings. Which images show *pixelation*, i.e. in which images do the pixel boundaries become noticeable? Why does this happen? And under what circumstances does it happen?

Activity 2.2 Brightness resolution

Start ImageJ and open the image **Xray**.

Go to **Plugins/Ch.2 Plugins/Brightness resolution**. Go down the "Menu": 7, 6, 5, 4, 3, 2, 1 bit, restoring the original image before each new choice, using **File/Revert**. At what stage do you see a noticeable degradation, false contouring, of the image? Can you explain this degradation, and why it occurs where it does?

How many gray levels are there when you select (a) 1 bit per pixel (the resulting image is known as a *binary* (or *binarized*) image) or (b) 2 bits per pixel? What is the connection between the number of bits per pixel and the number of gray (brightness) levels?

Activity 2.3 RGB color space

Open the folder **Colors** and click on **TabbedcolorBox.html** (courtesy: Phillip Dukes, University of Texas at Brownsville); choose "Mixing Lights." The three squares contain the primary colors for color addition: red (R), green (G) and blue (B). The squares can be moved (drag and drop) using the mouse; the overlap areas show the result of adding the colors. Move the three squares so that they overlap to some degree. What is the result of (i) R + G, (ii) G + B, (iii) B + R, (iv) R + G + B?

Activity 2.4 Color spaces and conversions

Open the folder **Color conversions** and click on **CSC.html** (courtesy: Eugene Vishnevsky, Spectronic Instruments Inc.); you may have to manually allow blocked content if your Web browser restricts the running of scripts. Choose "RGB": the RGB frame contains the wire-frame RGB cube with colored vertices. The gray ball represents the current position. Move the Red, Green and Blue sliders and watch the current position in RGB space and the resulting color in the bottom window. The two windows shown above the current color represent the blue-magenta-red-black and green-yellow-red-black sides of the RGB cube, and the current color can be changed by using the mouse to drag the current position within them.

Select the HSV model to see the current color in terms of its hue, saturation and value (intensity). The HSV color space is defined inside a hexcone (six-sided pyramid turned upside down). The vertical position defines value/brightness, the angular position gives the hue (color), and the radial position gives the saturation. As the hue is diluted with white light, and moves to the central axis of the hexcone, the saturation decreases. Saturation ranges from 0 to 1, and specifies the relative position from the vertical axis to the side of the hexcone. The colored hexagon on the left is a horizontal slice of the hexcone, shown on the right as a light-gray plane. The white cross indicates the current H and S values.

The frames are synchronized, to show each color's representation in different color spaces simultaneously.

Activity 2.5 RGB and HSB stacks

Open the image `prostate`, which is an RGB image, in ImageJ. Choose **Image/ Type/RGB Stack** to see the individual RGB planes: pull the slider at the bottom to move from Red to Green to Blue. Alternatively you can go to **Image/Stacks** and use **Next Slice** and **Previous Slice** to navigate between the planes. Go to **Make Montage** to see all three images side-by-side.

Open the original image `prostate` again, and choose **Image/Type/HSB Stack** and then **Make Montage** to see the image split into Hue, Saturation and Brightness planes. Compare this with the original image and the HSB montage.

Activity 2.6 Indexed color and color LUTs

Open the image `prostate` in ImageJ, make a duplicate (**Image/Duplicate...**) and click on **Image/Type/8 bit Color** to change it from an RGB to an indexed color image. Did you notice much of a change? Compare it with the original image. With the indexed color as the current image, go to **Image/Color/Edit LUT** to see the 256 colors used in this image as a 16×16 LUT or palette, with the colors indexed to the pixel values of the image. Pixel value = 0 is at the top left and value 255 is at the bottom right. Click **Invert** to see the effect of inverting the order, and **Invert** again to return to the original LUT. Go to **Image/Color/ShowLUT** to see the LUT as a set of colors from left to right, and their relationship to various mixtures of RG and B (click **List** to see this more clearly). Save the indexed color version as prostate1.tif and compare its file size with the RGB **prostate** file. What do you find?

Activity 2.7 Pseudocolor

Open **arteriogram**, a grayscale image of the blood vessels in the neck and upper chest. Go to **Image/Color/Edit LUT** to see its grayscale LUT. Make a duplicate image, and add pseudocolor to it using **Image/Lookup Tables**. There are a number of built-in tables to use: choose **Spectrum**. Then go to **Image/Color/Show LUT** to see the LUT as a band of colors, and to see how it was obtained from a combination of R, G and B. Go to **Image/Color/Edit LUT** to see the 256 colors used in the image as a palette running from 0 to 255. Look at some of the other LUTs, including **Fire**. Note that the pixel values are not changed, just used as addresses within different color look-up tables. Do you think false color is effective at enhancing the appearance of the image?

Exercises

2.1 If the concentration of cones in the human fovea is $180\,000$ mm^{-2}, how far apart are they? What angle is subtended at the lens by adjacent cones?

2.2 The total MTF of an imaging system at 2 lpmm^{-1} is 0.25. Assuming three serial components contribute to system blurring, and that two are identical with an MTF value of 0.75 each at 2 lpmm^{-1}, calculate the MTF value of the third component at that frequency.

2.3 Figure E2.1 shows the MTF curves for four different imaging systems, A–D. Which is the best overall system? Which is the best for imaging small details, less than 0.125 mm in size?

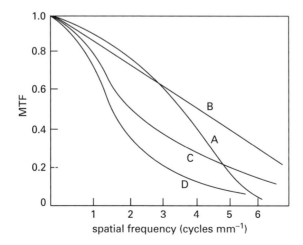

Figure E2.1

2.4 What is the size of the smallest object that the imaging system, whose MTF is shown in Figure 2.12, can resolve?

2.5 Figure 2.12 shows the digitization of an analog profile. What is the size of the resulting pixels? To what sampling frequency (in dpi) does this correspond?

2.6 If a particular x-ray film has an optical density range of 4.2, how many bits should a digitizer have in order to quantize the gray levels, without loss of quality?

2.7 High-definition television (HDTV) in the United States has adopted a standard of 1125 lines per frame (of which 1080 are active) and an aspect ratio of 16:9. If these images were captured as digital images, to what size of digital image ($M \times N$) would they correspond? These images are transmitted 30 times a second; how much memory would be required to store a 2-hour HDTV program as a series of uncompressed images?

2.8 A laser beam, 100 μm in diameter, is used to digitize a 35 cm × 42 cm radiograph. If each pixel is to have dimensions comparable to that of the laser beam, of how many pixels is the digitized image composed?

2.9 The FWHM of the PSF of a certain CT imaging system is 2 mm. How small should the pixels be? If the field of view (FoV) is 25 cm, how many pixels are there along each side of the image?

2.10 Consider two different x-ray films: a fast film, A, comprising larger, coarser silver bromide crystals, and a slow film, B, with smaller, finer crystals. Why is film A faster, and what advantage does that confer? Which of the two films produces the sharper image?

2.11 You are looking at a red light reflected off a wall. The lighting configuration that would give rise to this sensation is
  (i) a red light source is reflected off a black wall;
  (ii) a blue light source is reflected off a red wall;
  (iii) a yellow light source is reflected off a magenta wall;
  (iv) a magenta light source is reflected off of a cyan wall.
You may like to experiment further with the applet in Colors (Activity 2.3) to assist with this question; try both "Mixing Lights" (color addition) and "Mixing Pigments" (color subtraction).

2.12 Which of the three colors in RGB space below is the most saturated? (Use the Color conversions applet of Activity 2.4.)
  (i) (0.3, 0.5, 0.2);
  (ii) (0.7, 0.9, 0.7);
  (iii) (0, 0.2, 0);
  (iv) (0.5, 0.5, 0.1).

3 Medical images obtained with ionizing radiation

Overview

The introduction of advanced imaging modalities has significantly improved the diagnostic information available to physicians. Computer technology has enabled tomographic and three-dimensional reconstruction of images, illustrating both anatomical features (using x-rays) and physiological functioning (using γ-rays emitted from ingested or injected radioactive tracers), free from overlying structures. Since both x-rays and γ-rays are forms of ionizing radiation, they must be used prudently in order to minimize damage to the body and its genetic material.

Learning objectives

After reading this chapter you will be able to:

- explain the basis of imaging using x-rays and γ-rays;
- outline the physical factors involved in imaging modalities using ionizing radiation;
- identify the factors that affect image quality in imaging systems that use ionizing radiation;
- explain the advantages of computed radiography over film radiography;
- describe the specific challenges in mammography and explain how they are addressed;
- describe the imaging pathway in fluoroscopy;
- explain the advantages and limitations of digital subtraction angiography;
- distinguish planar imaging from topographic imaging;
- reconstruct a simple x-ray tomographic image using backprojection;
- explain how the production of a tomographic image in single-photon emission tomography (SPECT) differs from that in x-ray computed tomography (CT);
- identify the organs and tissues most sensitive to damage by ionizing radiation.

3.1 Medical imaging modalities

Medical imaging systems detect different physical signals arising from a patient and produce images. An imaging *modality* is an imaging system which uses a particular technique. Some of these modalities use *ionizing* radiation, radiation with sufficient energy to ionize atoms and molecules within the body, and others use *non-ionizing* radiation. Ionizing radiation in medical imaging comprises x-rays and γ-rays, both of which need to be used prudently to avoid causing serious damage to the body and to its genetic material. Non-ionizing radiation, on the other hand, does not have the potential to damage the body directly and the risks associated with its use are considered to be very low. Examples of such radiation are ultrasound, i.e. high-frequency sound, and radio frequency waves.

The modalities which use ionizing radiation, and the issues involved, have been grouped in this chapter, while the modalities which use non-ionizing radiation are dealt with in the next chapter. Our treatment of the imaging modalities is not exhaustive, and concentrates on the images and the issues encountered in obtaining them rather than the technical details of the imaging equipment.

3.2   Images from x-rays

X-ray imaging has been used in clinical diagnosis almost from the time of Roentgen's discovery of x-rays. X-rays are generated in an x-ray tube, which consists of an evacuated tube with a cathode and an anode (Fig. 3.1(i)). Heating a tungsten filament within the cathode releases electrons by thermal excitation. The filament is located within a depression or cup having sharp contoured edges which electrostatically focus the electron beam (Fig. 3.1(ii)). Increasingly negative voltages applied to the cathode cup can focus the electrons into a narrow beam or even switch off the beam entirely. The electrons are accelerated towards the positive (50–120 kV) anode, where they strike an embedded tungsten target, producing x-rays. The tube is evacuated so that the electrons pass to the anode in a straight path, and are not scattered by other particles in the tube. The majority of x-ray tubes, apart from those in low output dental and small mobile x-ray units, employ rotating anodes so that the electrons strike a larger area around the rim of the anode and do not over-heat the target. The region on the target from which x-rays are produced is called the *focal spot*, and its diameter is known as the *focal spot size*.

The electrons acquire a large kinetic energy during their acceleration in the electric field. When an electron is accelerated through an electric potential of 60 kV, for example, it acquires an energy of 60 keV, where the electron-volt (eV) is a small unit of energy ($1 \, \text{eV} = 1.6 \times 10^{-19}$ J). The electrons lose this energy when they are decelerated at the target. About 99% of the energy lost by the electrons goes into heat and the remaining 1% is converted into x-rays. The maximum energy of each x-ray photon produced in these collisions is 60 keV; many have less energy, if the electron does not come to a complete stop. Usually most of the x-rays produced are part of a continuous spectrum (*bremmstrahlung* x-rays) with energies up to the energy of the accelerated electrons (Fig. 3.2(i)), although there are some x-rays (*characteristic* x-rays) with discrete energies produced as a result of electrons being ejected from the innermost (K) shell of the atoms of the target, and other electrons falling into the vacancies left behind, giving up their excess energy in forming a characteristic x-ray (Fig. 3.2(ii)).

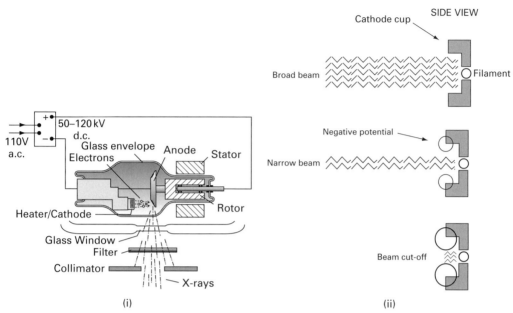

Figure 3.1 (i) A standard x-ray tube; (ii) focusing the electron beam using a negative voltage to the cathode cup. (Part (ii) after Dowsett *et al.*, 2006, p. 76. Reproduced by permission of Edward Arnold (Publishers) Ltd.)

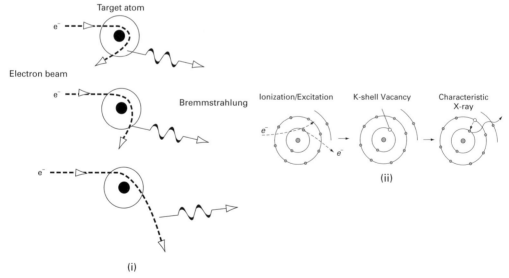

Figure 3.2 Production of (i) bremstrahlung x-rays, when electrons are deflected by a heavy nucleus, and (ii) characteristic x-rays, resulting from the excess energy of an electron falling into the vacancy caused by an ejected inner shell electron. (Part (ii) after Wolbarst (1993), p. 57.)

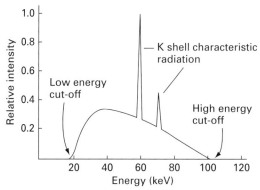

Figure 3.3 Spectrum of x-rays from an x-ray tube, with a tungsten target, operating at 100 kVp. The high-energy cut-off is determined by the electron energy, which in turn is determined by the kVp across the tube; the low-energy cut-off is determined by the thickness of an aluminum window on the tube, which stops very low energy x-rays. Characteristic K-shell radiation is shown superimposed on the bremmstrahlung spectrum. (Copyright (1999). From *Physics for Diagnostic Radiology*, 2nd Edition, by Dendy & Heaton. Reproduced by permission of Taylor and Francis Group, LLC, a division of Informa plc.)

Characteristic x-rays are characteristic of the target material, since they depend on the energy level differences of the atoms of the target. In regular radiography, using a tungsten target, most of the x-ray energy produced is *bremmstrahlung* radiation (Fig. 3.3); whereas in mammography, using a molybdenum target, most of the x-rays produced are (molybdenum) characteristic x-rays, with precise energies.

The high voltage to the anode is switched on for only a fraction of a second to produce a pulse of x-rays, which exit through a glass window in the metal housing of the x-ray tube. The x-rays are filtered by a thin sheet of aluminum to remove low-energy x-rays which would be unable to penetrate body parts. If these were not filtered out, they would be absorbed by the body and increase the dose to the patient.

The radiographer can control the exposure in two ways. Changing the voltage (kV) across the tube changes the *energy* of the electrons, and hence the maximum energy of the x-ray photons and their penetrating ability. Changing the filament current (mA) changes the *number* of electrons produced, and therefore the number of x-ray photons, i.e. the intensity of the x-ray beam.

X-rays and visible light are both part of the electromagnetic spectrum (Fig. 1.2), and, as such, have both wave and particle properties. As particles, the energy of a single photon, E, is given by

$$E = hf \tag{3.1}$$

where h is Planck's constant (6.626×10^{-34} J s) and f is the frequency of the corresponding wave. For a 60 keV x-ray photon, the frequency of the x-ray wave is 1.45×10^{19} Hz.

All waves obey the following relationship:

$$f\lambda = c \tag{3.2}$$

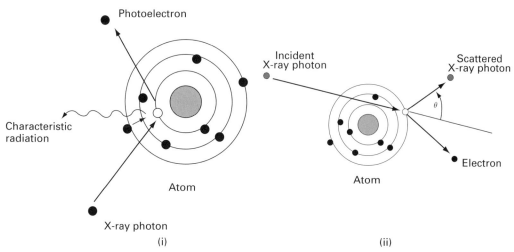

Figure 3.4   (i) X-ray interaction with the body by photoelectric absorption; the x-ray photon gives up most of its energy to liberate a K-shell electron, with any excess given to the (photo) electron as kinetic energy. (ii) Compton scattering, where only part of the x-ray photon energy is used to liberate an electron from an outer shell and the photon changes direction.

where λ and c are the wavelength and speed of the wave, respectively. For electromagnetic waves in air the speed is 3×10^8 m s^{-1}. Thus, a 60 keV x-ray photon has a wavelength of about 0.02 nm. By comparison, the wavelength of visible light varies between about 400 nm (red) and about 750 nm (blue), corresponding to photon energies of 3–6 eV. X-ray photons have much greater energy than visible light photons, which is why they can penetrate the body and cause damage if they are absorbed.

X-rays interact with the body either by (*photoelectric*) absorption (Fig. 3.3(i)), where the x-ray photon is absorbed in the course of liberating an electron from the inner shell of an atom, or by (*Compton*) scattering (Fig. 3.3(ii)), where only part of the x-ray photon energy is used to liberate an electron from an outer shell and the photon changes direction (Fig. 3.4). The former contributes to *radiation dose* (absorbed energy per unit mass) and consequently to the risk of biological damage to the patient; the latter results in a loss of image quality.

The consequence of these interactions is that the intensity of the beam, which is proportional to the number of x-ray photons in it, is reduced. Different tissues affect the beam by differing amounts, depending on their thickness (t) and the *attenuation coefficient* (μ) of the material. The intensity, I, of an x-ray beam after passing through a material of thickness, t, is related exponentially to its initial intensity, I_0, by

$$I = I_0 e^{-\mu t} \tag{3.3}$$

Photoelectric absorption depends on the effective atomic number of the material, Z_{eff}, and the x-ray energy, E, roughly as Z_{eff}^3/E^3; and Compton scattering depends on the electron density of the material, ρ_{elect}, which varies roughly as Z_{eff}, and the x-ray energy,

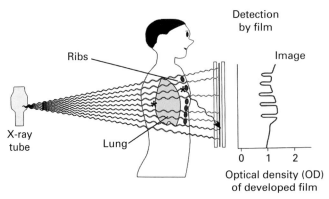

Detection
by film

Image

Ribs

X-ray
tube

Lung

0   1   2
Optical density (OD)
of developed film

Figure 3.5 Basic components of x-ray imaging. Fewer x-rays pass through the ribs, due to their high attenuation, resulting in less blackening of the film, i.e. the ribs appear whiter. (After Wolbarst (1993), p. 16.)

as ρ_{elect}/E. Thus materials such as bone have a higher value of attenuation coefficient and attenuate x-rays more than soft tissues, as a consequence of their larger Z_{eff}, and (photoelectric) absorption is the dominant interaction. Materials with a high effective atomic number, such as iodine ($Z_{\text{eff}} = 53$) or barium ($Z_{\text{eff}} = 56$), can be used to increase attenuation. They can be injected or swallowed to change the attenuation of soft tissues filled with the material compared to other soft tissues, and are known as *contrast agents*. For higher-energy x-rays, the overall attenuation is smaller with very much smaller photoelectric absorption and Compton scattering becoming dominant.

In *projection* or *planar* x-ray radiography the image is a simple two-dimensional projection or *shadowgram* of a three-dimensional object, the part of the patient in the field of view (Fig. 3.5); x-ray film is the detector. Projection radiography includes

- *film-screen radiography*, including chest radiography, abdominal radiography, angiography (studies of blood vessels) and mammography (Activity 3.1 has examples of the resulting radiographs and their visualization);
- *fluoroscopy*, in which images are produced in real time using an image intensifier tube to detect the x-rays;
- *computed radiography*, in which a re-usable imaging plate containing storage phosphors replaces the film as the detector;
- *digital radiography*, which uses semiconductor sensors.

Images of the human body can be acquired or displayed in three main orientations (Fig. 3.6). The *coronal* plane divides the body into front and back. This is the orientation displayed in the common posterior–anterior (PA) chest radiograph, where the x-rays enter from the patient's back (posterior) and are collected by a film placed at his front (anterior). The acquired image is a superposition of many coronal images at different depths within the body. The *sagittal* plane is a side view, dividing the body into right and left, and the *transverse* plane, sometimes referred to as the *axial* or transaxial plane, is a plane perpendicular to the long axis of the body, dividing it into top and bottom planes.

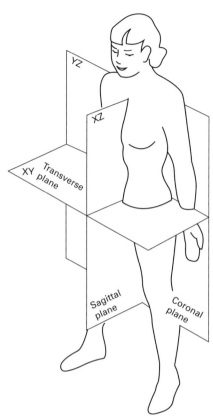

Figure 3.6 The three main imaging orientations for the human body: the coronal, sagittal and transverse planes. (After NASA RP-1024, *Anthropometric Source Book.*)

3.2.1   Plain (film–screen) radiography

A typical normal posterior–anterior (PA) chest radiograph is shown in Figure 3.7(i). The exposure settings for chest radiographs are chosen so that the visualization of the lungs is favored: the heart can also be seen, with the left ventricle and the aortic arch giving rise to more prominent shadows on the left side of the patient's spine. The radiograph is always viewed so that you seem to be facing the patient, so that the patient's left is on the right hand side of the image. Figure 3.7(ii) shows a patient with tuberculosis, with patchy opacities noticeable in the upper parts of the lungs. Activity 3.2 is an exercise in measuring the average width of a rib from a chest radiograph.

Unsharpness

In order to obtain as sharp an image as possible, the x-ray machine should produce a narrow beam of x-rays, while the patient should be close to the detectors and far away from the x-ray tube (Fig. 3.8).

From the geometry of the image formation (e.g. the similar triangles ABP and CDP), the blurring effect due to geometric unsharpness, U_G (equal to CD) is given by

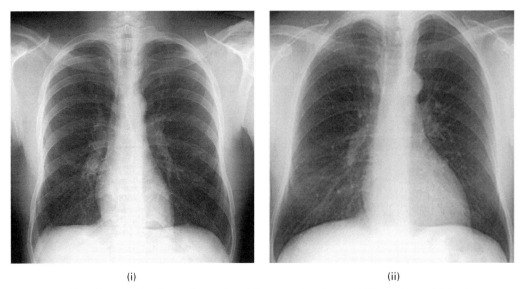

(i)   (ii)

Figure 3.7   Posterior–anterior chest radiographs of (i) a normal patient and (ii) a patient suffering from tuberculosis.

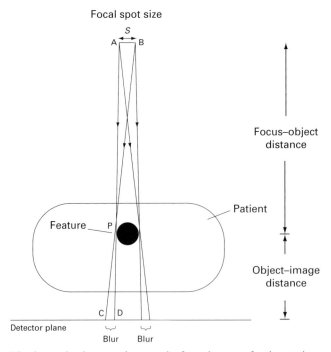

Figure 3.8   Blurring at the detector plane results from the x-ray focal spot size and placement of the patient. The closer the patient is to the detectors, the smaller the blurring.

$$U_G = \frac{\text{focal spot size(s)} \times \text{object–image distance}}{\text{focus–object distance}} \tag{3.4}$$

In order to minimize blurring and to keep the image as sharp as possible, the focal spot size of the x-ray generator should be small and the patient placed close to the detector to keep the object–image distance small and the focus–object distance large.

The sensitivity of photographic film to x-rays is so low that it would require a large number of x-ray photons, and hence a large dose of radiation to the patient, to produce an image. Only about 2% of incoming x-ray photons are captured by film and result in an image; the percentage of detected photons, or probability that a single photon is detected, is called the *quantum efficiency* (QE). In order to circumvent this problem, a fluorescent intensifying screen containing phosphor particles is used to convert x-rays into visible light, to which the film is more sensitive. Moreover, each x-ray photon is converted into thousands of visible light photons, which is possible because x-ray photons have much greater energy than light photons. Generally, two screens are used, either side of a double-emulsion film, so that most of the light produced is utilized (Fig. 3.9). The overall effect is to increase the quantum efficiency of the film-screen combination to about 25% permitting a consequent reduction in the x-ray photon numbers, which minimizes the x-ray dose to the patient. Shorter exposure times reduce the image unsharpness that occurs because of patient motion, U_M, which may be a combination of voluntary and involuntary motion.

The thicker screen absorbs more of the x-rays, and this improves the signal-to-noise ratio, SNR, of the image. However, the light photons produced within the screen diverge before they reach the film, resulting in an additional contribution to the overall unsharpness, which becomes more significant with thicker screens (Fig. 3.10). In addition, faster screens comprising large phosphor particles, which are more sensitive to incoming x-rays, contribute more to unsharpness (Fig. 3.11). The contribution of all the effects contributing to unsharpness as a result of the detector is known as the detector unsharpness, U_D.

The total blurring or unsharpness of a system comprising a combination of contributing sources is given by the full width at half maximum, FWHM, of its total point spread function, PSF, which is obtained by convolving the contributing point spread functions (Equation (2.2)). Rather than using convolution, which is a somewhat complicated operation, the contributions can be added in quadrature, i.e. as the square root of the squares, to a close approximation, i.e.

$$U_{TOT} \approx \sqrt{(U_G^2 + U_M^2 + U_D^2 + U_I^2)} \tag{3.5}$$

where U_G, U_M, U_D and U_I are, respectively, the contributions to unsharpness from the geometric positioning effect, the effect of patient motion, the effect of the detector, and what is known as the intrinsic unsharpness, which is determined by the shape of the object being imaged. In such a situation the contribution with the largest unsharpness dominates. The total unsharpness of the system is essentially its spatial resolution, the size of the smallest detectable feature or the minimum resolvable separation of features in

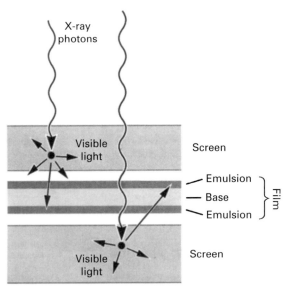

Figure 3.9   Film-screen combination, comprising two fluorescent screens either side of a film to increase sensitivity.

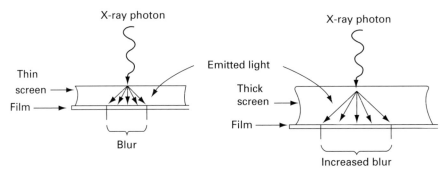

Figure 3.10   Increase in the unsharpness of the image due to light spreading within the screen. The thicker screen results in more unsharpness.

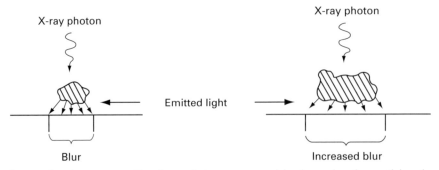

Figure 3.11   Increased unsharpness resulting from a fast screen, comprising large phosphor particles, shown at right, compared with a reduced unsharpness resulting from a slow screen, which comprises small phosphor particles, shown at left.

Table 3.1 Typical spatial resolution of medical imaging modalities.

Modality	Spatial resolution (mm)
Film-screen radiography	~0.05
Computed radiography	0.1–0.2
Computed tomography (CT)	0.25–0.5
Fluoroscopy	~0.5
Magnetic resonance imaging (MRI)	0.5–1.0
Ultrasound	1.0–5.0
Nuclear medicine (NM)	3.0–10.0

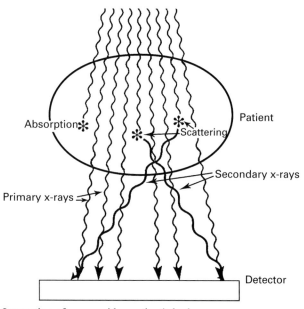

Figure 3.12   Interaction of x-rays with a patient's body.

the object. Typical values for the spatial resolution of various medical imaging systems are given in Table 3.1.

Contrast

X-rays interact with a patient's body in various ways (Fig. 3.12). They can penetrate the body, moving in a straight line from source to detector; these are the *primary* x-rays that produce a faithful shadowgram. Some x-rays are absorbed within the body by the photoelectric effect; these x-rays do not contribute to producing an image, and instead increase the dose, and therefore the risk, to the patient. Others undergo (Compton) *scattering* within the patient, producing scattered or *secondary* x-rays, some of which reach the detector; they produce random blackening over the film. If the *subject contrast* is defined as $\log_{10} (I_1/I_2)$, where I_1, I_2 are the transmitted x-ray intensities

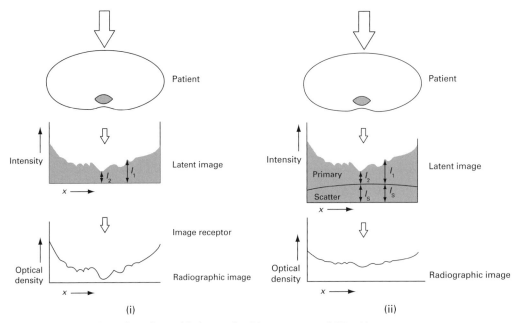

Figure 3.13   Formation of a radiographic image (i) without scatter and (ii) with scatter.

passing through the soft tissue and bone, respectively (Fig. 3.13(i)), the effect of scatter is to produce a roughly constant background intensity, I_S, superimposed on the real image and consequently to reduce the contrast to $\log_{10}((I_1 + I_S)/(I_2 + I_S))$ (Fig. 3.13(ii)). This ratio of the contrast in the presence of scatter to the contrast if there was no scatter is termed the *scatter degradation factor*, SDF; it is a value less than unity, with smaller values indicating a greater reduction in contrast due to scatter. The scatter degradation factor is related to the ratio of the total scattered to primary radiation intensities, S/P, by

$$SDF = P/(P + S) = (1 + S/P)^{-1} \qquad (3.6)$$

The amount of scatter increases with the volume of the body part irradiated (i.e. both a larger field of view, FoV, and a larger thickness result in additional scattering) and with increasing kVp (since the ratio of Compton scattering to photoelectric events increases with kVp). Mammography uses lower-energy x-rays and compression of the breast (to decrease the overall tissue thickness) to reduce the scatter-to-primary ratio (to ~0.4–1.5), resulting in a higher scatter degradation factor (of 0.71–0.4) and less degradation of the subject contrast by scatter.

Another way of minimizing scatter degradation is to place an anti-scatter grid between the patient and the detector (Fig. 3.14(i)). This grid consists of thin strips of lead foil interspersed with highly transmissive interspace material, such as aluminum or carbon fiber, as a support, with the strips oriented parallel to the direction of the primary radiation. Most of the primary x-rays pass between the lead strips, whereas

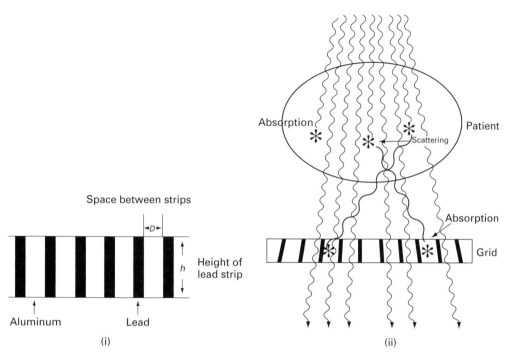

Figure 3.14 (i) A parallel grid, shown end on; the lead strips are of height h and separated by a distance D. (ii) A focused grid matches the divergence of the x-ray beam to allow more primary x-rays to pass through. (After Wolbarst, 1993, p. 175.)

the scattered x-rays enter the grid at an oblique angle and are absorbed by the lead strips. The *grid ratio*, h/D, where h is the height of the lead strips and D is their separation, determines that angle and is the primary determinant of the effectiveness of a grid in removing scattered radiation. Grid ratios vary between about 6:1 and 16:1 in routine radiographic systems, with less scattered radiation reaching the image receptor for large grid ratios. Since scatter depends on the thickness of the body part, lower grid ratios, or no grid at all, can be used with thin body parts (e.g. extremities, such as the hand or foot) but larger grid ratios are used for thick body parts (e.g. abdomen or chest). In mammographic systems the grid ratio can be as low as 2:1. The simple linear grid has now been largely replaced by the focused linear grid, where the lead strips are progressively angled on moving away from the central axis (Fig. 3.14(ii)). This eliminates the problem of "cut-off" at the periphery of the grid but requires careful placement of the grid so that the angles of the strips match the divergence of the x-rays. In order that the lead strips do not cast a shadow on the image, the grid is usually placed in a special holder ("*Bucky*") which moves the grid during the exposure to blur this effect.

There is a price to be paid for using grids to reduce scatter in order to preserve contrast in the image. Some primary radiation strikes the lead strips head-on and is absorbed. In order to compensate for this loss, the x-ray tube current needs to be increased somewhat, which increases the radiation dose to the patient. This is part of a general underlying

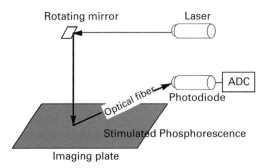

Figure 3.15   Reading of an imaging plate in computed radiography.

principle: the better the quality of image required, the more radiation is needed. In x-ray imaging, a compromise between patient radiation dose and image quality must be sought.

3.2.2   Computed radiography

Computed radiography (CR) is fast superseding plain (film-screen) radiography. It uses a *photostimulable phosphor plate* (PSP) or *imaging plate* (IP) to replace the standard intensifying screen/x-ray film combination in a cassette. The imaging plate comprises a screen coated with a storage phosphor. When the imaging plate is exposed to x-rays, electrons absorbed by the phosphor are excited to higher energy levels and are trapped there, typically for several days, resulting in a latent (or hidden) image. Reading the latent image in the imaging plate involves scanning the plate in a raster pattern with a well-focused laser beam. The laser light stimulates the release of the trapped electrons, accompanied by the release of blue light, which is converted to a voltage by a photomultiplier; the voltage signal is digitized and stored in a computer (Fig. 3.15). This process avoids the chemical processing required with traditional film, and, after scanning, the imaging plate can be erased by exposure to intense visible light, for subsequent re-use.

The imaging plate has a further advantage over film-screen because its response to x-rays is linear, unlike the sigmoidal response of film (Fig. 3.16). With film the exposure needs to be adjusted so that all objects of interest fall on the approximately linear part of the curve, in order to avoid under- or over-exposure; this is very difficult when, for example, imaging bone and soft tissue together. The linear response of the imaging plate results in a much wider useful exposure range with the exposure being much less critical. Since the images are now stored digitally, they can be manipulated at will to adjust, for example, their brightness and/or contrast. In theory, a reduction in the exposure, and hence dose to the patient, is possible; however, reduced exposure of the imaging plate would result in a lower signal-to-noise ratio, so that in practice similar exposure factors to film-screen systems are generally used.

The spatial resolution of computed radiography depends on the sampling rate at read-out, which depends on the optics. For typical sampling rates of 5–10 mm^{-1}, the spatial

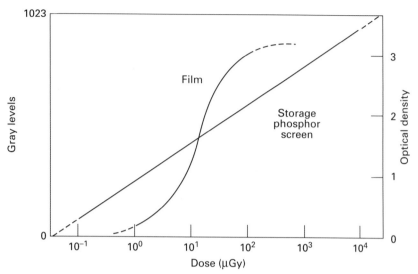

Figure 3.16 Response curves of film and imaging plates (1024 gray levels are shown, corresponding to a 12-bit system).

resolution is 2.5–5.0 lp mm^{-1}. Although not as high as film-screen radiography, this is certainly adequate for most diagnostic radiography.

3.2.3 Mammography

X-ray mammography is one of the most challenging areas in medical imaging. It is used to distinguish subtle differences in tissue type and detect very small objects, while minimizing the absorbed dose to the breast. Since the various tissues comprising the breast are radiologically similar, the dynamic range of mammograms is low. Special x-ray tubes capable of operating at low tube voltages ($\sim$25–30 kV) are used, because the attenuation of x-rays by matter is greater and predominantly by photoelectric absorption at small x-ray energies, resulting in a larger difference in attenuation between similar soft tissues and, therefore, better subject contrast. However, the choice of x-ray energy is a compromise: too low an energy results in insufficient penetration with more of the photons being absorbed in the breast, resulting in a higher dose to the patient. Most modern x-ray units use molybdenum targets, instead of the usual tungsten targets, to obtain an x-ray output with the majority of photons in the 15–20 keV range.

In order to detect microcalcifications, with diameters that can be less than 0.1 mm, the spatial resolution of the imaging system needs to be optimized. The target within the x-ray tube is angled so as to produce a small focal spot size (0.1–0.3 mm), and large focal spot-to-film distances (45–80 cm) reduce the effects of geometric unsharpness. Compression of the breast, normally to about 4 cm in thickness, reduces x-ray scatter and ensures a more uniform exposure. Immobilization allows a shorter exposure time which minimizes motion blurring. In film mammography, single-emulsion film, without an intensifier screen, is used to minimize the detector contribution to unsharpness, even

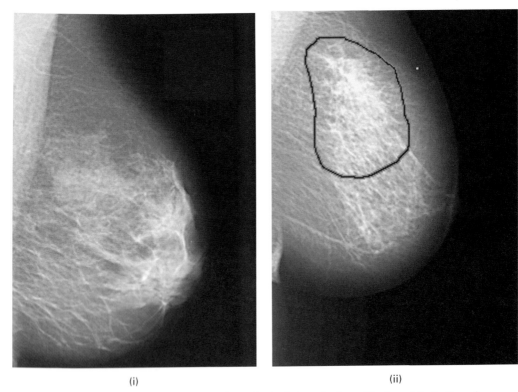

(i)   (ii)

Figure 3.17   (i) Normal breast. (ii) Dense opacity and spiculations (in the outlined area) indicative of a malignant lesion.

though this necessitates the use of higher x-ray doses: in digital mammography, the film is replaced by semiconductor sensors.

Currently, most mammograms are visually examined by humans in search of subtle and complicated indicators of breast cancer (Fig. 3.17). Clusters of microcalcifications, tiny calcium deposits, are diagnostic of early stage breast cancer. Ill-defined masses with strands of tissue (*spiculations*) radiating out from them, and producing a stellate appearance, are a diagnostic feature of malignancy. Reading mammograms can be a tedious and time-consuming task: computer-assisted diagnosis software is able to highlight suspicious areas in digital mammograms automatically for checking by a human expert.

Other imaging approaches, which obviate the need for ionizing radiation, have been used to diagnose early breast cancer. The most notable of these are ultrasound, magnetic resonance imaging (MRI), electrical impedance tomography and thermography. Ultrasound has been shown to complement x-ray mammography, since it is capable of differentiating solid tumors from cystic lesions. Magnetic resonance imaging is useful in imaging dense breast tissue, which is often found in younger women. Electrical impedance scanning devices are being used to detect breast tumors, which have much lower electrical impedance than normal breast tissue. Pre-cancerous and cancerous masses need an abundant supply of nutrients to maintain their growth. In order to provide this they increase circulation to their cells and create new blood vessels; this process results in an

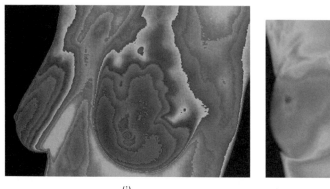 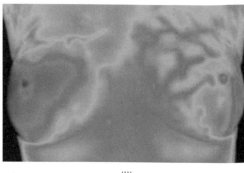

(i)   (ii)

Figure 3.18 Breast thermograms of (i) normal breasts and (ii) breasts showing a suspicious difference in temperatures. See also color plate.

increase in regional surface temperatures of the breast. Breast thermography uses ultra-sensitive infrared cameras to produce high-resolution images of these temperature and vascular changes (Fig. 3.18).

3.2.4 Fluoroscopy and digital subtraction angiography

X-ray fluoroscopy is a continuous or *dynamic* imaging technique, where moving images of the patient can be seen in real time. The resultant x-ray dose can be very high, since the procedure can last for tens of minutes. In an attempt to limit the dose, a lower x-ray tube current is used. As a result of the reduced numbers of x-ray photons per unit time, the signal-to-noise ratios of the images are inherently low.

The film detector is replaced by an image intensifier (II) tube (Fig. 3.19). Incoming x-ray photons strike a fluorescent tube producing visible photons, which liberate (photo) electrons at a photocathode; these electrons are focused and accelerated towards an output fluorescent screen, where they produce visible photons. The number of light photons produced within the tube is amplified, typically by a factor of several thousand. This is known as the *brightness gain* of the II tube, and results in images bright enough to be captured by a video camera and displayed on a monitor, even when relatively low x-ray intensities are used. In digital fluoroscopy the video signal is digitized and the image stored in a computer.

The spatial resolution of fluoroscopic images is determined by the size of the detectors at the input (fluorescent) screen, which are small needle-shaped crystals of cesium iodide typically about 0.1 mm in diameter. This corresponds to a spatial frequency of about 5 line-pairs (lp) mm^{-1}, which is inferior to that of x-ray film-screen radiography. The combination of factors leading to loss of spatial resolution is best seen in the frequency domain using modulation transfer functions, MTFs (Fig. 3.20). The total modulation transfer function is the product of the component modulation transfer functions (Equation (2.5)). The modulation transfer function of the monitor is the smallest and reduces the total modulation transfer function of the fluoroscopic imaging system to give

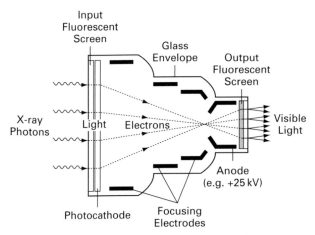

Figure 3.19   Image intensifier tube. (After Wolbarst, 1993, p. 233.)

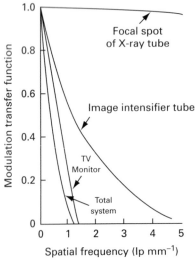

Figure 3.20   The modulation transfer function of a fluoroscopic system in terms of its individual components: the MTF = 0.1 level is marked in gray. (After Wolbarst, 1993, p. 236.)

a limiting spatial frequency, measured at MTF = 0.1, of about 1 lp mm^{-1}. Thus the smallest detectable object is 0.5 mm.

Solid-state flat-panel detectors are an alternative to image intensifiers. They offer increased sensitivity to x-rays, and therefore have the potential to reduce patient radiation dose. Their temporal resolution is better than that of image intensifiers, reducing motion blurring. Flat-panel detectors have a linear response over a very wide latitude of x-ray intensity, and can therefore deliver images of greater contrast. Their spatial resolution is similar to that of image intensifier tubes, and they are free of the pin-cushion distortion and uneven illumination (vignetting) that plagues image intensifiers. However, flat-panel detectors are considerably

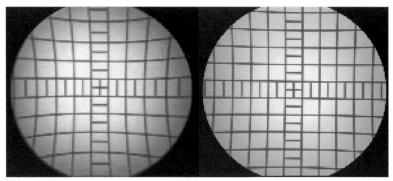

Figure 3.21 Schematic digital x-ray fluoroscopic imaging system as used for digital subtraction angiography. (After Wolbarst, 1993, p. 312.)

more expensive than image intensifier tubes, so that their uptake is primarily in specialties that require high-speed imaging, e.g. vascular imaging and cardiac catheterization.

The contrast of the fluoroscopic image is limited by x-ray scatter in the patient, which can be minimized by using smaller fields of view to limit the volume involved and by using anti-scatter grids. If the fluoroscopic images are digitized, or if a CCD video camera is used, then contrast can be adjusted within the computer system.

The acquisition of digital fluoroscopic images can be combined with injection of contrast material and real-time subtraction of pre- and post-contrast images to perform examinations that are generally referred to as *digital subtraction angiography*, DSA (Fig. 3.21). The result is an image of only the contrast material-filled vessels (Fig. 3.22). Since the images were formed by detection of x-rays that had been attenuated exponentially in the body, subtraction of pre- and post-contrast images must take this exponential attenuation into account by subtracting, pixel by pixel, the logarithm of the respective images: hence the log amplifier in Figure 3.21.

The process of subtracting two images has the unfortunate consequence of producing a noisier subtracted image. Consider subtracting two corresponding pixels: one from the *mask* (pre-contrast) image, resulting from a signal of 10 000 ($\pm$100) photons, and one from the *live* (post-contrast) image, resulting from a signal of 9900 ($\pm$100) photons. The subtracted image has a pixel value corresponding to 100 ± 141 photons, i.e. the pixels are subtracted, but the noise adds as the square root of the sum of the squares of the amplitudes. The initial two images with signal-to-noise ratios of 100 and 99, respectively, result in a subtracted image with a signal-to-noise ratio of only 0.7! In the normal course of events this would be unacceptable. However, subtracted angiographic images, although noisy, are useful because they make the small differences between the two original images, pre- and post-contrast, very noticeable or conspicuous and the small contrast-laden vessels are easily seen. They are said to have high *conspicuity*, rather like the spot-the-difference pictures in popular magazines.

Frame averaging can be used to decrease displayed image noise. The current image or frame can be averaged with one or more previous frames, since averaging reduces random, uncorrelated noise according to the square root of the number of frames

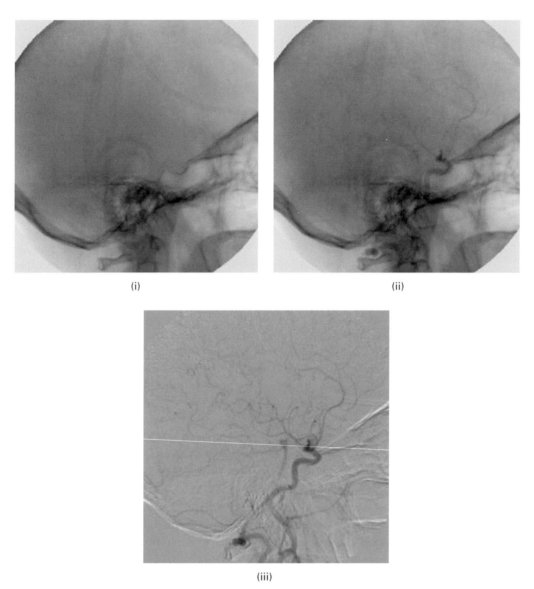

(i)   (ii)

(iii)

Figure 3.22   (i) Mask or pre-contrast image; (ii) live or post-contrast images; (iii) the subtracted image (live-mask), clearly showing the blood vessels.

averaged. Frame averaging may work well for static images, at the cost of increased radiation exposure to the patient, but the increased image lag may be unacceptable for producing images of a dynamic process. The signal-to-noise ratio is also directly proportional to the concentration of the contrast medium, but increasing its concentration involves increased risk to the patient also.

The patient should be immobile between the acquisition of the mask and live images, otherwise the images will not be registered properly and motion artifacts, in the form of whitish streaks, will be visible in the subtracted image. The solution is to shift the mask

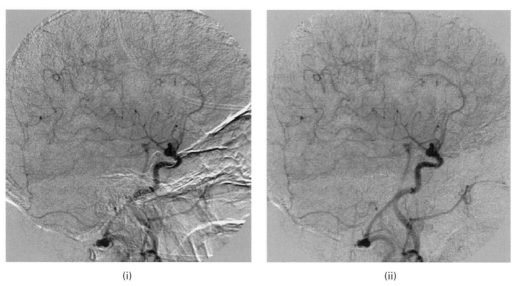

(i)   (ii)

Figure 3.23   (i) Motion artifacts appearing as white streaks in the image. (ii) Minimization of motion artifacts by pixel-shifting.

image by a few pixels, to obviate the motion, before subtraction (Fig. 3.23). This *pixel-shifting* tends to be a trial-and-error process, involving a combination of shifts in different directions and by differing amounts. Motion artifacts can be a significant problem in cardiac studies, resulting from the involuntary motion of the soft tissues.

3.2.5   Computed tomography

Conventional radiographic procedures, those which we have described so far, produce *planar* images that are projections of three-dimensional objects onto two-dimensional planes. This results in a considerable loss of information. The superpositioning of over-lying organs complicates their identification, unequal magnification effects cause distortion, and x-ray scattering can result in poor dynamic range. Tomographic imaging, of which x-ray computed tomography (CT) is an example, is a technique that was developed for producing transverse images, by scanning a slice of tissue from multiple directions using a narrow fan-shaped beam. The data from each direction comprise a one-dimensional *projection* of the object, and a transverse image can be retrospectively reconstructed from multiple projections. The body can be compared to a loaf of sliced bread, and a transverse image can be produced as if it were a selected slice viewed face-on (Fig. 3.24). The slice thickness can be reduced to 1 mm or so, so that very little superpositioning occurs. Indeed, if many transverse images are obtained, the data can be presented as an image in any plane, or even as a three-dimensional composite image.

A computed tomography (CT) scanner looks like a big, square doughnut. The patient is placed within the aperture of the rotating frame or *gantry* (Fig. 3.25(i)). The geometry of scanning has been changing with time, with each major step forward being called a

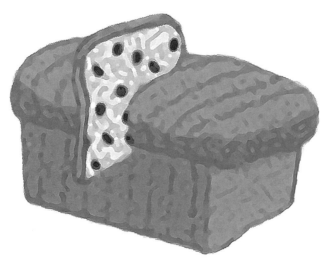

Figure 3.24   The body as a loaf of sliced bread; a transverse image is a slice of bread viewed end on.

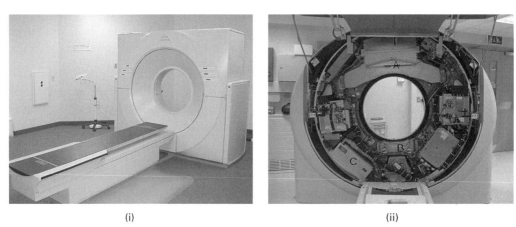

(i)   (ii)

Figure 3.25   (i) Outside view of third-generation CT scanner showing the patient table and gantry aperture. (ii) When the cover is removed, the x-ray tube and the arc of detectors can be seen. The gantry holding the x-ray tube and detector rotate around the patient as the data are gathered.

new *generation*. In the *third-generation* scanners, an x-ray tube mounted on the gantry revolves around the patient, a tightly collimated fan-beam of x-rays enters the patient, and an arc of detectors on the opposite side, and rotating synchronously with the x-ray tube, records the intensity of emerging radiation (Fig. 3.25(ii)). The x-ray tube is always on, and readings from the detectors are taken about a thousand times during the rotation.

The *first-generation* CT scanner, used for scans of the head, illustrates many of the principles of the method, and is easier to visualize (Fig. 3.26). A tightly collimated beam minimizes scatter and radiation dose to adjacent tissue. The beam is swept linearly across the patient's head, and a single detector, moving synchronously with it, measures the transmitted radiation at regular intervals; this is known as a *scan*. The tube is turned off,

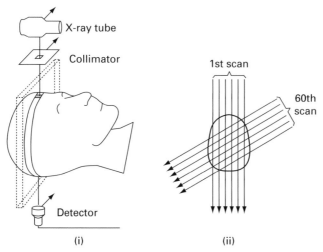

Figure 3.26 Operation of a first-generation CT scanner. (i) Translate motion comprising a single scan. (ii) Different scans are taken after a rotation of the beam and detector. (After Wolbarst, 1993, p. 322.)

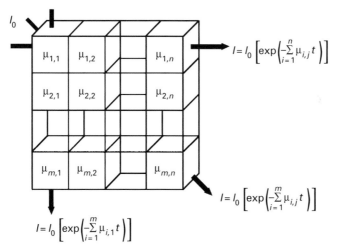

Figure 3.27 Matrix of voxels comprising the patient, with x-rays shown entering and leaving at differing angles.

the gantry rotated by a small angle ($\sim 1°$), and another scan performed. This is repeated to give scans covering 180°. The sampling interval and the angle of rotation determine the pixel size in the reconstructed transverse image, and the collimator width determines the slice thickness. The motion is known as *translate-rotate*.

A transverse slice of the body is schematically divided into many small volume elements or *voxels* (Fig. 3.27). They are displayed on a monitor as an array of pixels, where the third dimension, the slice thickness, has been flattened. Using the first-generation scanning as the model, the measured x-ray intensity depends on the sum of the attenuation coefficients ($\mu_{i,j}$) for each of the voxels in that particular path. Substituting the sum of the attenuation coefficients along a line of voxels ($\mu_{i,j}$) into Equation (3.3) and taking the natural logarithm gives the *ray sum*, p, along this particular path:

$$p = -\ln(I_0/I) = \Sigma\mu_{i,j}t \tag{3.7}$$

The reference intensity, I_0, is measured for each detector in a calibration step. A complete set of ray sums at a particular gantry angle comprises a *projection* or *profile*. Measurements of the x-ray beam intensity after penetrating the patient, I, are recorded; since the output of the x-ray tube, I_0, and the size of the voxels, t, are known, the sum of the attenuation coefficients ($\sum \mu_{i,j}$) along particular paths can be calculated. These values are calculated for many different directions. The task of x-ray computed tomography image reconstruction is to solve for the individual attenuation coefficients of each voxel, and to assign a value depending on the attenuation coefficients to each pixel in a two-dimensional array which then describes the transverse image.

Several correction factors need to be implemented prior to the calculation. The x-ray beam is not mono-energetic and attenuation is known to depend on x-ray energy. The effective energy of the x-ray beam increases as it passes through the patient due to the greater attenuation of lower-energy x-rays, an effect known as *beam hardening*. This results in the effective attenuation coefficients of a voxel containing a particular material decreasing with its distance into the patient; correction algorithms typically estimate the distance traveled by the x-rays to each voxel. A further complication is that x-ray beams at an angle to the voxel grid traverse different path lengths through different voxels.

The individual attenuation coefficients for each voxel can be obtained exactly, by using simultaneous equations, essentially by matrix inversion. However, for a matrix size of 512×512, at least 262144 simultaneous equations would be needed to ensure that they were independent, and more would be required to account for noise and patient motion. Matrix inversion is being used in industrial applications where limited rotation angles are possible. In medical imaging a number of alternative algorithms, such as

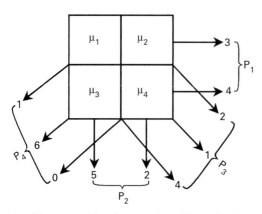

Figure 3.28   An object comprising four voxels and its projections.

backprojection, filtered backprojection and direct Fourier reconstruction, are routinely used. They will be considered in detail in a later chapter (Chapter 7).

The idea behind backprojection (i.e. the linear superposition of backprojections) is straightforward. Projections are acquired at a number of different directions. Taking each projection in turn, the values in the projection are projected back through the matrix, giving each voxel the full value rather than attempting to split it between the different voxels along the path. Values are added from the different directions. In a final stage they are adjusted to obtain the correct attenuation values, which are then scaled to give gray values for displaying the reconstructed image.

Figure 3.28 shows a simple example of an object comprising four voxels, with projections acquired for four different directions. Taking each projection in turn, the values in the projection are back projected, giving each voxel the full value. For example, back projecting P_1 gives

3	3
4	4

Back projecting P_2, and adding to the values already in the pixel positions, gives

8	5
9	6

Repeating this procedure for P_3, and adding to the values already in the pixel positions, gives

9	7
13	7

and back projecting P_4, and adding to the values already in the pixel positions, gives

10	13
19	7

These values are too high since we have not attempted to split projection values between voxels, and have added together the values from different projections. To counter these effects, the sum of the values in any of the projections (7, in this example) should be subtracted from every voxel to give

3	6
12	0

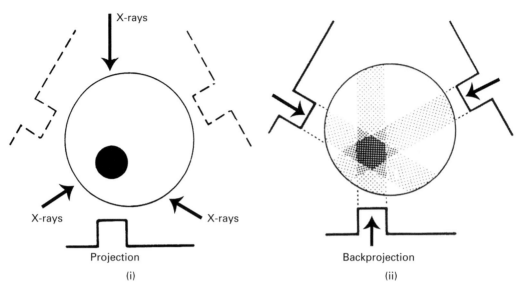

Figure 3.29   A schematic representation of backprojection. Three projections are (i) collected and then (ii) back projected. (After Wolbarst, 1993.)

The values should then be normalized by dividing by the highest common factor (3, in this example), which gives

1	2
4	0

These are indeed the attenuation values which result in the measured projection values of Figure 3.28.

Backprojection can be considered schematically (Fig. 3.29). Several scans are taken from different directions, each providing information on the total attenuation along that path. These are then back projected, giving the total attenuation to all voxels in the path. Note however that there is a typical *star artifact* around the image; the more scans, at many varying angles, which are collected, the less noticeable is this blurring. This is a limitation of the algorithm since projections at an angle to the image grid intersect incomplete pixels. To minimize this effect, *filtered backprojection* is required; this involves filtering the projections prior to back projecting them.

The problem of reconstructing a two-dimensional (transverse) image from a series of one-dimensional projections is common to a number of imaging modalities. The radiation can be transmitted through the object such as in x-ray computed tomography or emitted from internal radiation sources as in nuclear medicine scans (SPECT and PET); or the radiation involved can be non-ionizing radiofrequency pulses, as used in magnetic resonance imaging, MRI.

Table 3.2 CT numbers of various tissues.

Tissue	CT number (HU)
Bone	1000 +
Hemorrhage	60–110
Liver	50–80
Muscle	44–59
Blood	42–58
Gray matter	32–44
White matter	24–36
Heart	$\sim$24
Cerebrospinal fluid	0–22
Water	0
Fat	-20 to -100
Lung	-300
Air	-1000

From Webster (1988).

With x-ray computed tomography, instead of using the attenuation coefficients, $\mu_{i,j}$, directly as the gray values of the pixels in the reconstructed image, CT numbers or Hounsfield units (HU) are used. These are defined relative to the attenuation of water as follows:

$$CT \text{ number (or HU)} = 1000^* \frac{(\mu - \mu_{H_2O})}{\mu_{H_2O}} \tag{3.8}$$

This definition minimizes the dependence of the reconstructed image on the energy of the x-ray beam used and produces unit-less pixel values, which are essentially integral. Using this equation the CT number of water, which constitutes 80–90% of soft tissue, is conveniently defined as zero, and that of air as -1000. Other materials have either positive CT numbers, if they attenuate x-rays more than water does, or negative CT numbers if they are less attenuating than water. Table 3.2 shows the typical CT numbers of various tissues. Very dense bone has a CT number of $\sim$3000, so that the range of CT numbers is from -1000 to $\sim$3000. This range, of about 4000, requires 12-bit pixels to describe them adequately, since that provides 4096 levels ($2^{12} = 4096$).

A range of 4096 pixel values in a computed tomography image is useful for quantitative processing. However, all of these values cannot be displayed separately on a computer monitor, which can only display 256 shades of gray. This mismatch requires either that blocks of 16 (i.e. 4096/256) CT numbers be displayed with the same shade of gray, in which case values within each group cannot be distinguished in the image, or that only a restricted range or *window* of CT numbers be visualized and used to span the range from black to white (Fig. 3.30). In this latter case, the range of CT numbers is known as the *window width*, WW, and the middle of the range is known as the *window level*, WL.

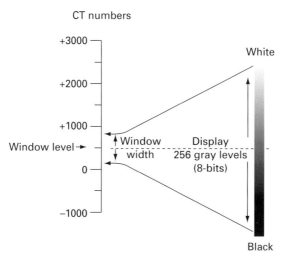

Figure 3.30   Windowing: a range of CT numbers is chosen to span the range of 256 shades of gray (from black to white) on a display monitor. The width of this range is the window width, and the mid-point is the window level.

For example, for visualizing brain tissue it would be appropriate to choose a window level at 40 HU and a window width of 128. Thus the window would span CT numbers from −24 to 103 HU. These 128 CT numbers would be mapped to the 256 available gray levels on the monitor, such that every other gray level would be used by a particular CT number. This results in an image of greater contrast than if blocks of CT numbers were displayed with the same shade of gray, but only objects with CT numbers falling within the window width are properly displayed: values below the bottom of the window, i.e. < −24 HU, appear black, and those above the top of the window, > 103 HU, appear white. Even greater contrast can be obtained if the window width is reduced further. Such windowing can be easily implemented with an appropriate display look-up table, LUT (Chapter 5).

The spatial resolution in a computed tomography image depends mainly on the size of the focal spot of the x-ray tube, the size of the detector element and the collimation, and the shape of the reconstruction filter. It can be equivalently described in terms of the smallest sized object that can be seen in the image, which is given by the width (FWHM) of the point spread function, or by the highest spatial frequency which can be properly imaged, in which case the modulation transfer function is used. Typically, the in-plane resolution of a CT image is about 0.5 mm, corresponding to about 1 lp mm^{-1}. This is not as good as film-screen radiography ($\sim$0.05 mm or $\sim$10 lp mm^{-1}) or mammography ($\sim$0.025 mm or $\sim$20 lp mm^{-1}). However, the small slice thickness ($\sim$0.5 mm) used in computed tomography imaging results in a clear image, free of the superpositioning of structures present in projection radiography.

The main contributor to CT image noise is quantum noise as a result of the statistical nature of x-ray emission. The random fluctuation in the number of detected x-ray quanta per pixel, N, is given approximately by $\sqrt{N}$, so that the signal-to-noise ratio increases

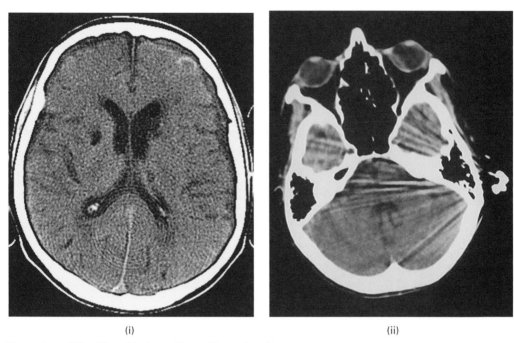

(i)   (ii)

Figure 3.31   CT artifacts: (i) ring artifacts; (ii) streak artifacts.

as $\sqrt{N}$. Increasing the number of emitted quanta or the scan time would increase the dose to the patient; more useful would be to increase the quantum efficiency of the detectors. If the voxel size is increased, then signal-to-noise ratio would improve but at the expense of reduced spatial resolution, either in-plane or axially. Using a reconstruction algorithm that incorporates smoothing would also improve the signal-to-noise ratio at the expense of spatial resolution.

Because CT images are digital their contrast can be easily manipulated by the display look-up table used after image reconstruction. This makes noise the major limitation in detecting low-contrast details. Typically computed tomography can distinguish differences of $\leq 0.5\%$, i.e. $\leq 5\,\mathrm{HU}$, which is better than film-screen radiography which needs about a 10% difference.

If the patient moves during the acquisition time, characteristic streaks appear in the image. Ring artifacts occur if the detectors are poorly calibrated or if several fail (Fig. 3.31(i)). Beam-hardening artifacts can occur if the necessary pre-processing corrections were not accurate. Partial volume effects result when voxels are partially filled by highly attenuating materials; the weighted average attenuation can be close to the full value for that material, resulting in narrow, highly attenuating objects, such as the bony skull, appearing wider than they should be. Streak artifacts (Fig. 3.31(ii)) are common around metal objects, such as dental fillings, and are due to a combination of effects including partial voluming, scatter and incomplete beam-hardening correction.

In conventional CT scanners only a single slice is acquired at a time, with the patient table stationary. The gantry would spin $360°$ in one direction and enough readings would

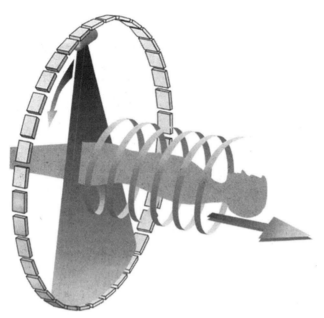

Figure 3.32   Schematic to illustrate spiral CT.

be acquired to reconstruct a single slice; then it would spin 360° back in the other direction to make a second slice. In between each slice, the gantry would come to a complete stop and reverse directions while the patient table would be moved forward by an increment equal to the slice thickness. In the 1980s an innovation known as the slip ring was developed that allowed electric power to be transferred onto a continuously rotating gantry, so that scanners could rotate continuously without having to slow down to stop and start again. This resulted in *spiral* or *helical* computed tomography, where data are acquired while the patient is moved continuously through the scanner (Fig. 3.32). The trajectory of the x-ray beam, through the patient, traces out a helix: hence the name. The backprojection reconstruction algorithm has to be modified to accommodate the helical shape of the resulting section. The efficiency of spiral CT can be increased by incorporating multiple detector arrays in the direction of the patient motion: so-called *multi-slice* spiral CT. Multiple slices of data can be collected in ~100 ms, and images in any plane, or volumetric (three-dimensional) images, can be reconstructed in less than a second. The faster acquisition times result in significantly reduced motion artifacts.

CT imaging is the primary digital technique for imaging the chest, lungs, abdomen and bones due to its ability to combine fast data acquisition and high resolution, and is ideally suited to three-dimensional reconstruction. It is particularly useful in the detection of pulmonary (i.e. lung) disease, because the lungs are difficult to image using ultrasound and MRI. It is often used to diagnose diffuse diseases of the lung such as emphysema, which involves a sticky build-up of mucus in the lungs, and cystic fibrosis, which leads to irreversible dilation of the airways (Fig. 3.33).

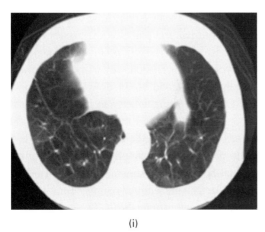
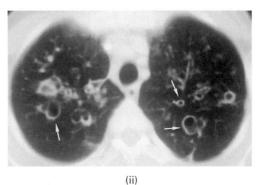

(i)   (ii)

Figure 3.33   CT image of a patient with (i) emphysema, showing damage to both lungs, and (ii) cystic fibrosis, showing dilated airways and the presence of small, opaque areas filled with mucus (arrows).

Activity 3.3 uses a "stack" of images of a brain showing hydrocephalus, in which excessive accumulation of cerebrospinal fluid CSF results in an abnormal dilation of the ventricles (spaces) in the brain, causing potentially harmful pressure on the brain tissues. The user can move through the stack to identify the slices which show enlarged ventricles.

3.3   Images from γ-rays

Nuclear medicine (NM) imaging uses the γ-rays emitted from radioactive isotopes attached to pharmaceutical tracers that are specific to certain physiological, metabolic and pathological activities, e.g. cerebral perfusion, myocardial perfusion, cancer. These radio-labeled pharmaceutical tracers are ingested or injected into the body where they are circulated and/or metabolized. The γ-rays which they emit during radioactive decay pass out of the body and are collected by detectors (*gamma cameras*) placed around the patient; these measure the distribution of the tracer within the body, and produce images which show the *functional* or metabolic activity in the relevant organs.

The ideal radioisotope should release only monochromatic, i.e. single-energy, γ-rays and not α and β particles; γ-ray photons with energy in the range of about 70–500 keV are ideal since they are able to penetrate out of the body and be detected. The half-life of the radioisotope, $T_{1/2}$, i.e. the time taken for half of it to decay, should be several hours, allowing time for uptake and distribution of the radiopharmaceutical tracer and subsequent imaging, while ensuring that the radioisotope does not continue emitting radiation for longer than necessary, since that would increase the dose of radiation to the patient. By far the most widely used radioisotope in nuclear medicine imaging is the metastable, excited form of technicium-99 (^{99m}Tc), which emits 140 keV γ-rays and has a half-life of 6 hours.

The essential characteristic of the pharmaceutical tracer is that it be organ specific, preferably with a differential uptake between normal and pathological tissues. ^{99m}Tc-labeled sestamibi, a large synthetic molecule which is passively absorbed through cell membranes, is the agent of choice for myocardial perfusion. As it moves through the heart muscle, it is absorbed by areas that have good blood flow. Areas of poor absorption indicate that the blood flow is reduced, *ischemia*, which may be due to arterial blockage.

There are three basic imaging modalities in nuclear medicine. Projection studies, called *planar scintigraphy*, are analogous to projection radiography; all depth information is lost. A single gamma camera, or a dual-head gamma camera to take anterior and posterior images simultaneously, is used to detect the emitted γ-rays. Tomographic imaging, called *single-photon emission computed tomography* (SPECT), uses a rotating gamma camera to obtain projection images from multiple angles, which are used to reconstruct cross-sectional images. And *positron emission tomography* (PET) detects pairs of 511 keV gamma photons, emitted when positrons are annihilated.

3.3.1   Planar scintigraphy

γ-rays are emitted in all directions and pass through the body much like x-rays. In order to locate the source of the γ-rays, a collimator is placed between the patient and the detector (Fig. 3.34). The detector, the *gamma camera*, comprises a single, large scintillation crystal to convert the γ-rays into light photons; the most commonly used scintillation crystal is sodium iodide, doped with thallium, NaI (Tl). The light photons are subsequently detected by a hexagonal array of photomultiplier tubes (PMTs), which convert the light into an electrical signal and amplify it. For every 7–10 light photons incident on the photocathode of the photomultiplier tube, a single electron is released by the photoelectric effect. It is accelerated and produces 3–4 secondary electrons by collision with electrodes, known as dynodes; the process is repeated and, after 10–14 successive stages, about 10^6–10^8 electrons reach the output anode. This current pulse is amplified to provide a voltage pulse with a peak voltage, its *pulse height*, which depends on the energy of the γ-photon.

The collimator is a 2.5–5 cm thick slab of lead of the same cross-sectional size as the scintillation crystal, and with a geometric array of holes in it. Its purpose is only to allow γ-photons incident on it almost perpendicularly to pass through; photons from other directions are absorbed by the lead, as with secondary radiation grids in radiography. However, unlike in radiography, the source of the photons in nuclear medicine is not known; they come from a spatial distribution rather than a point source. The purpose of the collimator is to impose spatial information on them.

When a γ-photon interacts with the scintillation crystal, thousands of light photons are produced and pass through the collimator to be detected by the photomultiplier tubes. The gamma camera determines the position and energy of the original γ-photon interaction from the weighted average of the positions and outputs of several photomultiplier tubes (Fig. 3.35). The position (x, y) and the energy (z, proportional to the pulse height) of each interaction in the crystal is recorded and used to form an image of the distribution of

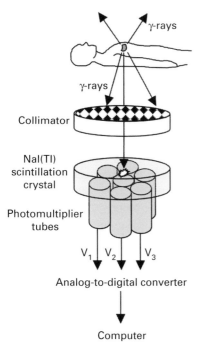

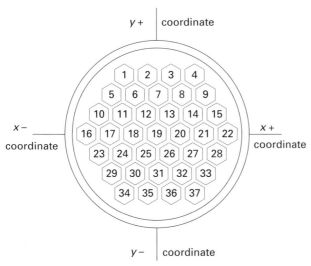

Figure 3.34 Schematic diagram for obtaining a planar nuclear medicine image, using a gamma camera. (After Webb, 2003, p. 58.)

Figure 3.35 Position encoding within the gamma camera.

radioactivity. The collimator only allows γ-photons traveling in a certain range of directions to interact with the scintillation crystal, so that the site of origin of the radioactive event in the patient can be found. However, (Compton) scattering within the patient results in some scattered γ-photons entering the field of view and degrading the

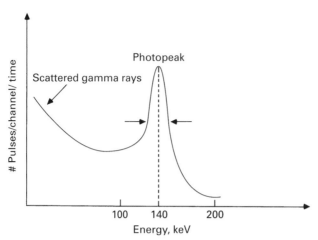

Figure 3.36   Pulse height spectrum for ^{99m}Tc, showing a 14% energy resolution.

contrast of the image. These scattered photons have less energy than the direct photons, and can be removed by only counting those pulses which fall within an energy *window* around the known energy of the γ-photons emitted by the particular radioactive source (Fig. 3.36). In an ideal detector the *photopeak* would correspond to this energy, but in practice it is broadened by the statistical nature of the light emission and the finite energy resolution of the pulse height analyzer. Typically the energy resolution, defined as (FWHM/energy of emitted photon × 100) is 8–14%.

Planar scintigraphy images (and SPECT images (Section 3.3.2)) have poor spatial resolution (~4 mm) and signal-to-noise ratio, but are very sensitive, being able to detect tiny amounts of radioactivity. The poor spatial resolution results in images comprising a few pixels, typically 64 × 64 for a field of view of 25 cm. The spatial resolution is related to (i) the intrinsic resolution of the gamma camera, as a result of imprecision in determining the positions (x, y) and the degree of scattering within the patient, (ii) the collimator resolution, due to its geometry, which is generally the dominating factor, and (iii) the use of filtering after data acquisition, particularly in SPECT. Since factors (i) and (ii) depend on the depth of the targeted organ within the body, the spatial resolution of the imaging system depends on the depth, becoming worse for deeper organs. The signal-to-noise ratio of the images depends on the square root of the number of detected γ-ray photons, and is larger for less deep organs.

Whole-body bone scans, using ^{99m}Tc-methylenediphosphonate (MDP) or a similar agent, can be used to detect bone tumors and soft-tissue tumors in which bone remodeling is taking place. Such agents bind to the metabolically active bone mineral hydroxyapatite, whose formation is often increased at, or near, the site of a tumor (Fig. 3 37). The patient bed is slowly translated past a gamma camera. The spine is more visible in the posterior image, on the right, due to reduced attenuation. This patient shows increased uptake of the radiotracer around the right knee.

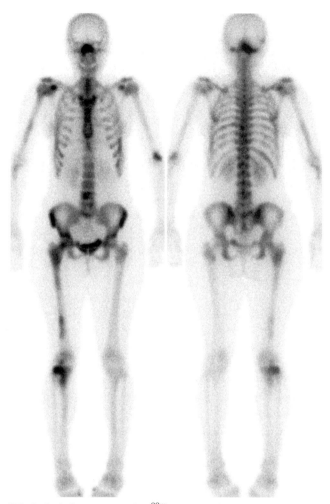

Figure 3.37 Whole-body bone scan, using ^{99m}Tc-MDP. The anterior view is on the left, and the posterior view is on the right. Increased uptake of the tracer around the right knee indicates the presence of a tumor.

3.3.2   SPECT imaging

In single-photon emission computed tomography, SPECT, a rotating gamma camera, with one, two or three detector heads, rotates around and as closely as possible to the patient because spatial resolution decreases with the distance from the collimator. Sensitivity increases and acquisition time decreases with more detector heads.

The different acquired projections are used to reconstruct cross-sectional or three-dimensional images by filtered backprojection. Reconstruction computations are more complicated than with x-ray computed tomography because the detected signals depend upon both the spatial distribution of the radioisotopes and the attenuation properties of the voxels. As with x-ray computed tomography imaging, the main advantage of SPECT

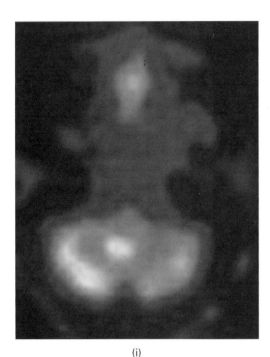

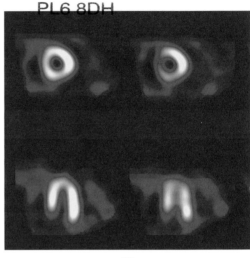

(i)   (ii)

Figure 3.38   SPECT images showing (i) a brain tumor (in white), using ^{99m}Tc-GH (glucoheptinate), and (ii) thinning of the cardiac wall (reduced intensity), using ^{99m}Tc-sestamibi. See also color plate.

over planar imaging is the absence of superpositioning of overlying and underlying signals. A time-sequence of sequential SPECT images of the heart can easily be viewed as an animated sequence (Activity 3.4).

SPECT studies of the brain are used to diagnose a large range of diseases that cause altered blood perfusion (Fig. 3.38(i)). SPECT scans can be used to measure cardiac wall thickness (Fig. 3.38(ii)). Pseudocolor is often added to the images to increase clarity.

3.3.3   PET imaging

Positron emission tomography, PET, is the most recent nuclear medicine imaging technique: in common with the others, it measures physiological function (e.g. perfusion, metabolism), rather than gross anatomy. A small, positron-emitting radioisotope with a short half-life (such as carbon-11, ^{11}C (about 20 min), nitrogen-13, ^{13}N (about 10 min), oxygen-15, ^{15}O (about 2 min), and fluorine-18, ^{18}F (about 110 min)) is incorporated into a metabolically active molecule (such as glucose, water or ammonia), and injected into the patient. Such labeled compounds are known as *radiotracers*. When a positron, i.e. a positively charged electron, is emitted within a patient, it travels up to several millimeters while losing its kinetic energy. When the slowly moving positron encounters an electron, they spontaneously disappear and their rest masses are converted into two 511 keV *annihilation* (gamma ray) *photons*, which propagate away from the annihilation site in

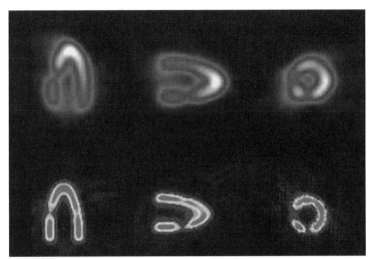

Figure 3.39   A realistic heart phantom imaged along three axes by SPECT with ^{99m}Tc (top row) and PET with 18F-fluorodeoxyglucose (bottom row). See also color plate.

opposite directions. The patient is surrounded by multiple rings of gamma photon detectors, so that no detector rotation is required.

Positron emission tomography, PET, is distinct from single-photon emission computed tomography, SPECT, in that two γ-ray photons are produced at the same time. The output of detectors on opposite sides of the PET scanner is analyzed by a *coincidence detector*, which only counts events that are simultaneous to within a user-set time window (∼2–20 ns); this ensures that only the 511 keV photons are counted. Simultaneous triggering reveals the line of sight of the two photons, and the original positron-emitting radiopharmaceutical must be somewhere along that line. The intersection of many such lines delineates the distribution of the pharmaceutical.

PET images (Fig. 3.39) have higher signal-to-noise ratio and better spatial resolution (∼2 mm) than planar scintigraphy and SPECT images. However, PET systems are much more expensive. Cyclotrons are required to produce the short-lived positron-emitting isotopes, due to their short half-lives. Few hospitals and universities are capable of maintaining such systems, and most clinical PET is supported by third-party suppliers of radiotracers which can supply many sites simultaneously. This limitation restricts clinical PET primarily to the use of radiotracers labeled with fluorine-18 ($T_{1/2} \approx 110$ minutes), which can be transported a reasonable distance before use, or to rubidium-82 ($T_{1/2} \approx 75$ seconds), which can be created in a portable generator and is used for myocardial perfusion studies.

To facilitate the process of correlating structural and functional information, scanners that combine x-ray CT and radionuclide imaging, either SPECT or PET, have been developed. These dual-modality systems use separate detectors for x-ray and radio-nuclide imaging, with the detectors integrated on a common gantry. Because the two scans can be performed in immediate sequence during the same session, with the patient not changing position between the two types of scans, the two sets of images are more precisely registered. In the *fused image* the radionuclide distribution can be displayed in color on a gray-scale CT image to co-register the anatomical and physiological features and thereby improve evaluation of disease.

3.4   Dose and risk

X-ray and γ-ray photons have sufficient energy to ionize atoms and molecules within the body, causing serious and lasting biological damage. The absorbed dose, D, is equal to the radiation energy absorbed per unit mass of body; it is measured in units of grays (Gy), where 1 gray is the dose when 1 joule of energy is absorbed per kilogram of irradiated material. However, the absorbed dose gives little indication of the risk to the patient; the biological damage caused also depends on the type of radiation. To take this into account, the absorbed dose is multiplied by a radiation weighting factor to give the *equivalent dose* in sieverts (Sv). The quality factors range from 1 for x-rays to 20 for alpha-particles.

The damage caused also depends on the irradiated organ. The *effective dose* to the patient is the sum of the doses delivered to the specific organs, weighted by a tissue weighting factor, which characterizes the relative radiosensitivity of that organ, with respect to cancer and genetic risks. Table 3.3 shows the radiosensitivity, or tissue weighting factors, of various organs; the most radiosensitive organs are those that involve rapid cell division, such as the gonads.

Typical effective dose equivalents for various diagnostic x-ray procedures are given in Table 3.4; note the high doses for CT scans due to the large number of individual scans taken in each procedure.

More than 80% of the annual effective dose ($\sim$3 mSv) to an individual comes from natural background radiation, a combination of cosmic rays and radionuclides in the body and in the environment. Medical exposure, the majority of it from diagnostic radiology, contributes a further 15% or so. Since background radiation is unavoidable and therefore considered an acceptable dose, radiation doses can be rated according to the time required to obtain the same effective dose from background radiation; this is known as the Background Equivalent Radiation Time (BERT). For example, a chest radiograph with a dose equivalent of 30 μSv would have a Background Equivalent Radiation Time of about 3.5 days (one-hundredth of a year), i.e. we get the same radiation dose from a chest radiograph as we would accumulate from background radiation in 3.5 days; thus the dose from a single chest radiograph would be considered fairly insignificant. A whole-body x-ray CT scan of 10 mSv, obtained within a few minutes, has a Background Equivalent Radiation Time of 3.3 years and is not insignificant!

Much of the data on cancer induction and genetic damage caused by radiation has been obtained after high exposures, for example on people exposed to the atomic bomb explosions in Japan, to fallout from nuclear weapons' tests and during radiation accidents. The risks for low doses, such as diagnostic doses, in radiology, are more difficult to assess. However, to err on the side of safety, it is assumed that the relationship between risk, or effect, and dose is "linear, no-threshold," with a gradient (risk/dose) of 5×10^{-5} mSv^{-1} for fatal cancer, and values of 0.8×10^{-5} mSv^{-1} for non-fatal cancer, and 1.3×10^{-5} mSv^{-1} for hereditary effects (International Commission on Radiological

Table 3.3 Relative radiosensitivity of the organs of the human body.

Organ/tissue	Relative radiosensitivity
Gonads	0.20
Bone marrow (red)	0.12
Colon	0.12
Lung	0.12
Stomach	0.12
Bladder	0.12
Breast	0.05
Liver	0.05
Esophagus	0.05
Thyroid	0.05
Skin	0.01
Bone surface	0.01
Other organs	0.05

Based on the International Commission on Radiological Protection (1991).

Table 3.4 Typical effective dose equivalents for various diagnostic procedures.

Examination	Range (μSv)
Dental x-ray	10–20
Chest	10–50
Skull	100–200
Pelvis	700–1400
Abdomen	600–1700
Mammogram (each image)	1000–2000
Lumbar Spine	1300–2700
Barium meal	1900–4800
IVU (intra-venous urography)	2500–5100
Head CT scan	2000–4000
Body CT scan	5000–15 000
Nuclear medicine	2000–10 000

Protection (ICRP), 1991)). Using the figure for fatal cancer, if 100 000 people were to receive uniform whole-body doses of 1 mSv each, then about five of them would die prematurely of radiation-induced cancer.

When a medical exposure is made, there should always be the expectation that some benefit will come of it, and that the dose to everyone involved, patient and staff, should be **as l**ow **as r**easonably **a**chievable, the so-called ALARA principle. Minimizing exposure time, maximizing the distance from the radiation source, and establishing proper shielding, e.g. using leaded walls and lead-glass windows, and wearing lead aprons, are the primary ways to limit radiation exposure, both to the patient and to medical personnel.

Computer-based activities

Activity 3.1 Radiographs

Open `chest1` in ImageJ, which is a radiograph of the chest. Adjust the brightness and contrast of the image and note which structures become more visible. This patient complained of pain in the left chest and shortness of breath. Are there any visible features which might explain these symptoms?

Open `barium`, which is an image of the colon filled with a barium-containing contrast material to increase the contrast. This patient complained of pain in the lower left quadrant of the abdomen; are there any features of the colon that might explain these symptoms?

Open `arteriogram`, which is an image showing the blood vessels of the neck and upper chest. Apply psuedocolor to see whether the vessels can be better visualized.

Activity 3.2 Measurement of size

Open the image `x-ray` in ImageJ. Choose the straight line selection from the Tools bar, and draw a line perpendicular to several ribs. Draw a profile (**Analyze/ Profile**) along that line; the lighter ribs appear higher on a (sloping) background. Move the cursor horizontally within the profile image to get an average value of the width of a rib (in inches). Try to reduce the slope of the background using **Process/ Subtract Background** and an appropriate value for the "rolling ball radius" to make the measurement of the width of the ribs easier.

Activity 3.3 X-ray CT image stacks

Open the file `Hydro022`, a stack of images of a brain showing hydrocephalus, in ImageJ. Manually move through the stack, and then go to **Image/Stacks/Start Animation** to move through the images automatically. The images are shown at reduced size; you can see them at full size, and read the annotation, if you set **Edit, Options** and click **Open images at 100%** prior to opening. An alternative is to use **Image/Stacks/Make Montage** after opening and specify the magnification.

In CT images, the white matter of the brain, which appears centrally in the hemispheres, appears slightly less dense (i.e. blacker) than the peripheral gray matter, because the white matter contains more fatty tissue. The cerebrospinal fluid (CSF) in the ventricles appears even blacker. In hydrocephalus the cerebrospinal fluid builds up often due to an obstruction in the normal circulation, enlarging the ventricles. Which figures in the stack show the enlarged ventricles? (Note the numbers at top left of the window.) Use **Z Project**, with **Average Intensity**, to see through all the slices at once.

The standard treatment for hydrocephalus is surgery, to divert and drain excess cerebrospinal fluid through a surgically implanted shunt. Open the image stack

Shunt022. Which images show the shunt? How effective has the treatment been in this case?

Activity 3.4 SPECT images of the heart

Start **ezDicom**, then **File/Open Dicom** and open the file **NM0001**. (The file can also be opened in ImageJ, but with limited functionality.) Use the **Video** icon to animate the sequence; after viewing the animated sequence, move Video to O (still) and use the slider to view the images sequentially. How many images (frames) are there? What is the size, in pixels, of each frame? Check the details by looking at the DICOM header.

Exercises

3.1 What determines the highest energy of x-ray photons emitted from an x-ray tube? What determines the energy spectrum of the x-ray photons? Why are low-energy x-ray photons removed from the x-ray beam before they reach the human body?

3.2 Why is it preferable to use a screen, rather than let the x-ray photons strike the film directly? Can you think of any disadvantage to using a screen?

3.3 An x-ray photon with energy of 60 keV produces visible light photons of wavelength 420 nm in an intensifying screen. If the energy conversion efficiency is 20%, how many visible light photons are produced for each incident x-ray photon? ($1 \text{eV} = 1.6 \times 10^{-19}$ J; Planck's constant, $h = 6.63 \times 10^{-34}$ J s.)

3.4 Which, bone or soft tissue, is imaged as a darker shade of gray on the radiograph? Why?

3.5 What is (i) an advantage and (ii) a disadvantage of using two intensifying screens, one either side of a film, compared with using only a single intensifying screen?

3.6 If 80% of x-ray photons of a certain energy pass through a slab of material, what percentage passes through a slab of the material which is twice as thick as the original slab?

3.7 The linear attenuation coefficient of a phosphor used for detection of x-rays is 550 cm^{-1} for an x-ray energy of 150 keV. What percentages of x-rays are detected by phosphor layers of 100, 250 and 500 µm thickness, respectively? What are the effects on spatial resolution?

3.8 Why are barium and iodine salts used to improve the contrast of certain images? What is their particular property that is so useful? In what procedures are they typically used?

3.9 In a typical chest x-ray set-up, how close should the patient be to the film to obtain the sharpest image possible? Should the patient face the x-ray tube or not? (Consider which organs are of most interest.)

3.10 In a certain exposure, the contribution to the unsharpness due to geometric positioning (U_G) is 0.25 mm, the detector unsharpness (U_D) is 0.2 mm, the motion unsharpness (U_M) is 0.5 mm and the intrinsic unsharpness (U_I) is 0.15 mm. What is the resolution of the system? How could it be improved?

3.11 For the following changes in an x-ray imaging system indicate the effect on subject contrast (i.e. increase, decrease or no effect):
- increase in patient thickness,
- increase in kVp,
- reduction in quantum efficiency of the detector,
- reduction in field of view,
- use of a high atomic number contrast medium.

3.12 Comment on how compression of the breast in mammography affects (i) the spatial resolution, (ii) the contrast and (iii) the signal-to-noise ratio of the image.

3.13 (i) List three ways in which the contrast is maximized in mammography, with a short explanation of the principles behind each. (ii) List two factors that help achieve high spatial resolution in mammography. (iii) Why should noise be minimized in mammograms? How can it be minimized?

3.14 In digital subtraction angiography (DSA), what is the effect of doubling the x-ray intensity on the signal-to-noise ratio of the image? What would be the effect of doubling the dose of contrast agent on the signal-to-noise ratio of the image?

3.15 How could the contrast of a displayed x-ray computed tomography image be increased? Explain.

3.16 What are the factors which determine the in-plane (x–y) spatial resolution of a computed tomography scanner? What is the effect of choosing thinner slices?

3.17 If the standard deviation of pixel values in the CT image of a uniform phantom is 5 HU, what percentage of pixels have values more than 5 HU above the mean value?

3.18 In a nuclear medicine scan using ^{99m}Tc, the signal-to-noise ratio for a 30-minute scan was 50:1 using a certain injected radiation dose immediately prior to imaging.
 (i) If the injected dose were doubled, what would the signal-to-noise ratio be for a 30-minute scan?
 (ii) If the dose were kept the same, but the scan time doubled, what would be the signal-to-noise ratio of the acquired image?

3.19 In a SPECT brain scan, each image is formed from, typically, 500 000 counts. Myocardial SPECT has a lower number of counts, typically 100 000 per image. If the brain images were to be collected on a 128×128 matrix, what matrix size would be appropriate for the myocardial image to achieve a similar signal-to-noise ratio?

3.20 In a 128×128 SPECT image, how many total counts are necessary for a signal-to-noise ratio of 50?

3.21 What is the typical dose from (i) a mammogram, (ii) a head CT scan? What is the Background Equivalent Radiation Time for each? What are the corresponding risks of getting cancer?

3.22 If one million people were to receive a uniform exposure of 1 mSv each, how many fatal cancers would this likely induce, assuming the linear, no-threshold dose-exposure relationship? How many of these will be stomach cancers given the organ weighting factors in Table E3.1?

Table E3.1 Tissue weighting factors.

Organ or tissue	W_T
Gonads	0.20
Red bone marrow	0.12
Colon	0.12
Lung	0.12
Stomach	0.12
Bladder	0.05
Breast	0.05
Liver	0.05
Esophagus	0.05
Thyroid	0.05
Skin	0.01
Bone surface	0.01
Remainder	0.05

Based on the International Commission on Radiological Protection (1991).

3.23 In 1980 (!), the collective dose to patients from diagnostic medical x-ray examinations in the United States was 92 000 Sv. How many fatalities from radiogenic cancers would be expected to result from these procedures?

4   Medical images obtained with non-ionizing radiation

Overview

Diagnostic medical ultrasound uses high-frequency sound and a simple pulse–echo technique. When an ultrasound beam is swept across a volume of interest, a cross-sectional image can be formed from a mapping of echo intensities. Current medical ultrasound imaging systems are based on envelope detection, and therefore only display intensity information. Despite this shortcoming, ultrasound imaging has become an important and widely accepted modality for non-invasive imaging of the human body because of its ability to produce real-time images, its low cost and its low risk to the patient. Magnetic resonance imaging (MRI) uses the phenomenon of nuclear magnetic resonance (NMR): unpaired nucleons, such as protons, orientate themselves in a magnetic field, and radiofrequency pulses can be used to change the balance of the orientations. When the system returns to equilibrium it produces signals that can be used to produce an image, which is characterized by its high contrast for soft tissues. MRI images map function, as well as structure. Digital images from any imaging modality can be compared or combined, after image registration, using a networking system.

Learning objectives

After reading this chapter you will be able to:

- explain the basis of imaging using non-ionizing radiation, specifically ultrasound and radiofrequency (RF) radiation with a strong magnetic field;
- outline the physical factors involved in these imaging modalities;
- describe the factors which determine the speed of ultrasound waves in a material;
- explain the purpose of time gain compensation and describe how it is implemented;
- summarize the steps involved in the reconstruction of B-mode ultrasound images;
- identify the factors that affect image quality and artifacts in ultrasound imaging;
- describe the phenomenon of nuclear magnetic resonance (NMR);
- explain how MRI images can be constructed from NMR spectra;
- describe the use of magnetic field gradients to add spatial information to MRI images;
- summarize the changes that occur to the spins using the spin echo pulse sequence;
- identify the factors that affect image quality and artifacts in MRI imaging;

- describe how functional information can be obtained from MRI imaging;
- summarize the advantages of a picture, archiving and communications system (PACS);
- outline the factors involved in the co-registration of images from different modalities.

4.1 Ultrasound imaging

Ultrasonic imaging uses high-frequency (~1–10 MHz) sound waves and their echoes to produce images that can demonstrate organ movement in real time. Unlike electromagnetic waves, such as x-rays and γ-rays, ultrasound is non-ionizing and, as such, is considered safe at the intensities used in clinical imaging systems. Ultrasound images are constructed by calculating the time taken for ultrasound pulses to travel into the body and return, after reflection off a tissue surface.

Ultrasound pulses, generally 1–5 μs long, are generated from an ultrasound transducer comprising a piezoelectric crystal, such as lead zirconate titanate (PZT), sandwiched between a pair of electrodes. A small sinusoidal voltage applied to the crystal causes it to resonate, producing sound waves as its surfaces move backwards and forwards; the crystal also detects ultrasound waves by producing a varying electrical signal. A typical pulse, just over 1 μs in duration with a frequency of 5 MHz, contains 5 cycles of the wave (Fig. 4.1). Pulses might be separated by perhaps 1 ms, resulting in a *pulse repetition rate* of 1000 Hz; they travel through soft tissue at a speed of about 1540 m s^{-1} compared with the speed of sound in air of about 330 m s^{-1}.

Worked example

A standing wave can be established in a piezoelectric crystal when its wavelength is twice the thickness of the crystal. Each face of the crystal is oscillating with maximum amplitude and the center is at rest; this corresponds to the first harmonic. (Higher harmonics are also produced, but the first harmonic predominates.) What thickness of crystal is required to generate a 1.5 MHz ultrasound wave?

The resonance condition is that

$$\lambda_{\text{res}} = 2t \tag{4.1}$$

where t is the required crystal thickness and λ_{res} is related to the frequency, f, and the velocity, v, of the ultrasound wave in the crystal, by the basic equation for waves, namely

$$v = f\lambda \tag{4.2}$$

Using $v = 4000$ m s^{-1} for the speed of sound in PZT and $f = 1.5$ MHz gives a value for the wavelength of 2.7 mm; thus, the required crystal thickness is 1.3(5) mm.

There are also some resonant frequencies produced at the odd harmonics, namely 4.5, 7.5, 10.5 MHz etc.

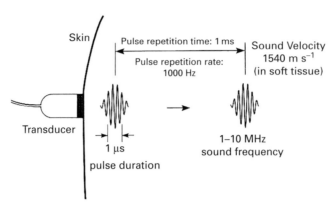

Figure 4.1   Schematic diagram of a typical clinical ultrasound beam. (After Wolbarst, 1993, p. 408.)

Sound waves are *longitudinal* waves, i.e. the particles of the material move back and forth in the same direction that the wave is traveling. The speed of sound in a material, v, is characteristic of that material and depends on the density of the material, ρ, and its compressibility, K. The easier it is to compress a material, the higher is its compressibility. Thus:

$$v = \frac{1}{\sqrt{K\rho}} \tag{4.3}$$

We can compare bone with soft tissue. Although bone has a larger density, it has a much smaller compressibility than soft tissue. The product $K\rho$ is smaller for bone than soft tissue, resulting in a larger velocity for sound waves through bone.

A pulse of ultrasound, which is what is often used in medical ultrasound rather than a continuous wave, actually comprises a range of frequencies: the shorter the pulse the larger the range of frequencies comprising it. Luckily, the velocity of sound in a medium is nearly independent of frequency or wavelength, otherwise the pulse would spread out as it traveled leading to pulse blurring. This behavior is different from that of light: the speed of light in a medium depends on wavelength, which is why prisms split sunlight into its constituent colors.

When an ultrasound wave encounters a tissue surface, separating tissues with different acoustical properties, a fraction of the wave is backscattered and detected by the transducer on its return. Generally, only those waves that reflect back through about 180° can contribute to an ultrasound image. By measuring the delay between pulse transmission and pulse reception, and knowing the speed of propagation, the depth of the feature can be calculated. For example, if the time delay is 160 μs and the pulse is passing through soft tissue with a speed of $1540\,\mathrm{m\,s^{-1}}$, the round-trip path is 24.6 cm and the tissue depth is 12.3 cm.

The intensity of the echo is used to determine the brightness of the image at the reflecting tissue surface (Fig. 4.2). The intensity *reflection coefficient*, R, at a boundary

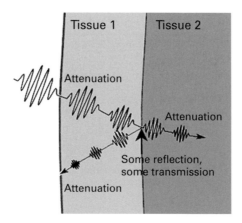

Figure 4.2   The returning echo pulse suffers continuous attenuation along its path, and an abrupt change in intensity on reflection at the interface. (After Wolbarst, 1993, p. 408.)

which is smooth compared to the ultrasound wavelength and perpendicular to the direction of wave propagation, is given by

$$R = \frac{(Z_1 - Z_2)^2}{(Z_1 + Z_2)^2} \tag{4.4}$$

where Z_1, Z_2 are the *acoustic impedances* of the materials to either side of the surface. Acoustic impedance is a constant for a specific material (Table 4.1) and is analogous to electrical impedance: as impedance increases it inhibits velocity (current) for a given pressure (voltage). Acoustic impedance is given by

$$Z = \rho v = \sqrt{\frac{\rho}{K}} \tag{4.5}$$

The SI unit of acoustic impedance is the rayl (kg m^{-2} s^{-1}).

There is little reflection if the materials are acoustically similar and a lot of reflection when there is a mis-match of acoustic impedances. For example, at an interface between soft tissue and bone a very large reflected signal or echo results, comprising about 40% of the incident intensity. This greatly attenuates the transmitted beam and makes the imaging of structures deeper-lying than bone extremely difficult. At a soft tissue/gas interface, around 99% of the beam intensity is reflected, making it impossible to scan distal structures deeper than the lungs or gas-containing bowel.

Even when the beam is traveling through biological tissue, it loses intensity continuously as a result of scattering and absorption (Fig. 4.2). Although the mechanisms are complicated, the overall effect is that the beam energy decreases more or less exponentially as it penetrates the tissue, similar to the attenuation of x-ray intensity. Thus, the ultrasound beam intensity, I, decreases with propagation distance, x, from its starting value at $x = 0$, I_0, according to

$$I(x) = I_0 e^{(-\mu x)} \tag{4.6}$$

Table 4.1 Acoustic properties of various materials.

Material	Speed of sound, v (m s^{-1})	Acoustic impedance $Z = \rho c$ (10^6 kg m^{-2} s^{-1})	Attenuation coefficient at 1 MHz (dB cm^{-1})
Blood	1575 ± 11	1.62 ± 0.02	0.15 ± 0.04
Bone	3180–3500	4.8–7.8	14.2–25.2
Brain	1565 ± 10	1.54 ± 0.05	0.75 ± 0.17
Breast	1430–1570		0.3–0.6
Fat	1450	1.38	0.63
Peritoneal	1490		2.1
Subcutaneous	1478 ± 9		0.6
Heart	1571 ± 19	1.64	2.0 ± 0.4
Liver	1604 ± 14	1.63–1.75	1.2
Lung			40
Muscle	1581	1.70	0.96 ± 0.35
Soft tissue (mean)	1540	1.63	1
Air	331	0.0004	45
Castor oil	1500	1.4	0.95
PZT (lead zirconate titanate)	4000	30	
Water	1498	1.50	0.0022

Data from A. B. Wolbarst, *Physics of Radiology*. Appleton and Lange, 1993.

where the attenuation coefficient, μ, is often expressed in dB cm^{-1} rather than cm^{-1}, as with x-rays. Thus:

$$\mu\left(\mathrm{dB\ cm}^{-1}\right) = -\left(\frac{1}{x}\right) 10 \log\left(\frac{I(x)}{I_0}\right) = 4.343\mu\left(\mathrm{cm}^{-1}\right) \qquad (4.7)$$

The attenuation coefficient is characteristic of the material (Table 4.1) and is approximately proportional to frequency for most tissues. At 1 MHz, the attenuation coefficient for soft tissue is about 1 dB cm^{-1}; for air and bone, at the same frequency, it is much higher: 45 dB cm^{-1} and 8.7 dB cm^{-1}, respectively. Increasing the ultrasound frequency increases spatial resolution but decreases penetration. This trade-off between resolution and attenuation, and therefore range, is the fundamental design limitation in ultrasonic imaging. The basic rule is to use the highest frequency that reaches the required depth to display the anatomical structures of interest.

In order not to confuse this continuous attenuation with the attenuation occurring at the reflection of a surface, which is used to characterize the brightness of the image at that location, the former can be circumvented by using *time gain compensation* (TGC). This amplifies the echo signal as a function of time of travel, so as to compensate for continuous attenuation along the line of travel. There are limits to such compensation, since amplifying small echoes results in noisy signals.

Using the echoes to find the depths of tissue boundaries is the basis of *A (amplitude)-mode* ultrasound. A-mode ultrasound has been used, for example, in detecting eye tumors, liver cirrhosis and myocardial infarction.

B (brightness)-mode ultrasound is more common, and is used to produce a two-dimensional tomographic or slice image of anatomical structure by sweeping the beam repeatedly back and forth through the patient's body. Each sweep is used to form a single vertical line of the B-mode image comprising a series of bright dots. The brightness of the dots is determined by the intensity of the reflected echoes, after correcting for attenuation along the path by time gain compensation. The sweeping is achieved either mechanically, using a rocking or rotating transducer, or electronically by using an array of piezoelectric elements, rather than a single crystal, and delaying the voltage pulse to each element of the array relative to its neighbor (Fig. 4.3). Activity 4.1 shows an animated simulation of beam-steering. After all the echoes have been produced along a particular beam direction, the beam direction is changed electronically by introducing time delays to the piezoelectric elements of the transducer, and a second line of data is acquired. By sweeping the beam, further lines, typically 128 to 256 per image, can be used to build up a sector-shaped image (Fig. 4.4). The time

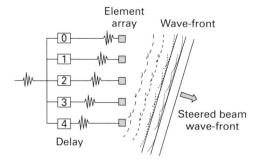

Figure 4.3   Schematic of a swept array as used in B-mode scanning.

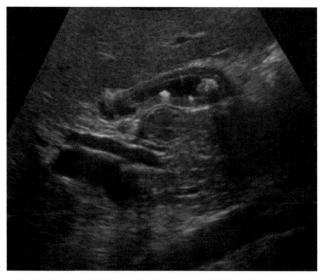

Figure 4.4   A B-mode image of a gall bladder, showing the presence of polyps.

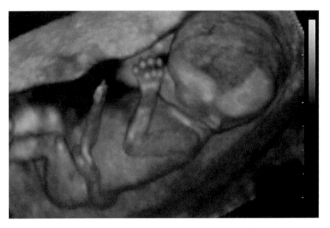

Figure 4.5   Rendered three-dimensional image of a 12-week old fetus.

required to acquire the echoes along a single line is of the order of 100 μs, so that a single image can be acquired in tens of milliseconds, and continuous sweeping of the beam allows the image to be updated in real time.

Worked example

A 5 MHz transducer has 128 elements and is required to give a 12 cm image depth. What time is taken to collect a single image?

At a speed of $1540 \, \mathrm{m \, s^{-1}}$ the returning echo from 12 cm depth takes 156 μs. A single image takes 128×156 μs, i.e. 20 ms.

Three-dimensional ultrasound images can be obtained by adding additional rows of crystal elements to permit sweeping in a direction perpendicular to the plane of the B-mode scan. If a small number of rows is added, typically 3–10, only limited sweeping in this direction can be achieved. If a large number of rows is added, comparable to the number of elements in each row, then the geometry of the array is truly two-dimensional and sweeping gives three-dimensional imaging (Fig. 4.5). Applications include the study of fetal and uterine malformations, and the detection of various tumors.

4.1.1   Image quality

The spatial resolution along the direction of propagation of the ultrasound wave is known as the *axial resolution*. It is defined as the closest separation of two surfaces in that direction which results in distinguishable backscattered signals, and is equal to half the spatial pulse length. The shorter the pulse, the better is the axial resolution of the image.

> **Worked example**
>
> What is the axial resolution in soft tissue of a 5 MHz ultrasound transducer that produces pulses 5 cycles long?
>
>   The wavelength of the ultrasound is 0.308 mm (using Equation (4.2)). The spatial pulse length is therefore 1.54 mm; and the axial resolution is 0.77 mm.

Resolution in the plane perpendicular to the direction of propagation is known as the *lateral resolution*. It is determined by diffraction of the ultrasound beam from its initial cross-sectional size. Diffraction causes the beam to diverge by an angle of about $\sin^{-1}(1.2\lambda/w)$, where w is the diameter of the transducer. Diffraction also results in side lobes which remove energy from the main beam and can introduce artifacts into an image. Because a single crystal transducer typically has a diameter of 1–5 cm, the lateral resolution is intrinsically very poor. It can be improved by focusing the beam, for example by manufacturing the face of the crystal itself concave rather than plane.

The signal-to-noise ratio (SNR) of the backscattered signal depends on the intensity and bandwidth of the ultrasound pulse, the degree of transducer damping and the amount of focusing used. If the speckle from small inhomogeneities is included then the signal-to-noise ratio typically drops to around 2.0, which is very low compared with other modalities. Contrast can be improved using ultrasound contrast agents, usually consisting of small gas-filled microspheres or microbubbles with a diameter less than 10 μm injected directly into the blood stream. The microspheres increase the backscattered echo signal from the blood.

Image artifacts can result from a variety of effects. Because bone has a high attenuation coefficient, transmission of ultrasound through bone is minimal; however, reverberations can occur from very strong reflectors, such as bone or air, giving rise to a characteristic series of equidistant bright lines in an image. Acoustic shadowing occurs when either a strong reflector such as a gas/tissue boundary or a highly attenuating structure hides or "shadows" a deeper-lying organ.

4.1.2   Doppler imaging

Blood velocity measurements are essential in calculating cardiac output and diagnosing *stenosis*, narrowing, of the arteries. The Doppler effect can be used to determine blood velocity and interlace this information with B-mode scanning, as a so-called *duplex scan*.

The Doppler effect is familiar in the form of the increased frequency of a moving sound source, such as a train whistle or police siren, as it approaches, and the reduced frequency, as it passes by. The relative change in frequency, $\Delta f/f$, depends on the velocity of the sound emitter, v, relative to the speed of sound in air, v_s. Thus:

$$\frac{\Delta f}{f} = \pm \frac{v}{v_s} \tag{4.8}$$

where the $\pm$ refers to the sound source traveling towards (+) or away from (−) the receiver.

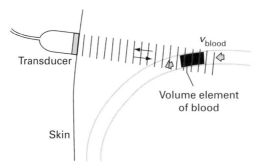

Figure 4.6   Continuous wave (CW) method of measuring blood velocity. (After Wolbarst, 1993, p. 437.)

Red blood cells (RBCs) traveling towards an ultrasound transducer receive pulses at higher frequency because of their velocity, and then they act as moving sources themselves when they scatter the ultrasound in all directions. The backscattered signal is thus Doppler shifted twice, and the overall frequency shift of the echo received at the transducer is given by

$$\Delta f = \frac{2fv(\cos\theta)}{v_s} \tag{4.9}$$

where θ is the angle that the ultrasound beam makes with the direction of blood flow (Fig. 4.6). For $f = 5$ MHz, $\theta = 45°$ and $v = 50$ m s^{-1}, the Doppler shift is 2.26 kHz, which is within the audible range. The received signal can be amplified and mixed with the original signal, and the resulting difference (beat) signal sent to a speaker so that it can be heard. If a spectrum analyzer is used to measure the Doppler shift, then the blood velocity can be obtained, if the direction is known. The angle θ is usually estimated from simultaneously acquired B-mode scans, and the Doppler flow measurements interlaced with the anatomical B-mode images to form duplex images, also known as color Doppler or color flow (CF) images.

The flow information is used to color the appropriate pixels. Common mapping formats are BART (Blue Away, Red Towards, i.e. velocity away from the transducer is colored blue, towards it is colored red), and enhanced or variance flow maps, where saturation and intensity are used to indicate higher velocities and turbulence or acceleration, respectively. A color *look-up table* (LUT), indicating how velocity is mapped into the displayed colors, is usually included beside the image for reference (Fig. 4.7). Activity 4.2 shows ultrasound images of the heart with color Doppler information added to show blood flow.

In continuous wave (CW) Doppler imaging two crystals are used, one as the transmitter and the other as the receiver, both usually embedded in the same transducer. Instead of the pulse–echo principle, the oscillator used to transmit the ultrasound wave is used to "demodulate" the received signal. The mixed signal is filtered, amplified and digitized; and its frequency spectrum is used to obtain the range of blood velocities. CW

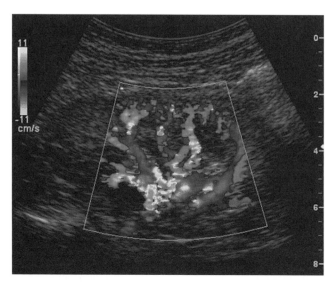

Figure 4.7   Color Doppler duplex image. The color look-up table is related directly to the blood velocity. See also color plate.

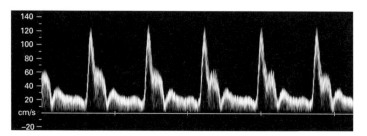

Figure 4.8   Two-dimensional display of spectral Doppler plots as a function of time over several cardiac cycles.

Doppler measurements are usually displayed as a time series of spectral Doppler plots (Fig. 4.8); there is no spatial (i.e. depth) information.

4.1.3   Clinical applications of ultrasound

There are a wide range of applications of ultrasound imaging as a result of its non-invasive, non-ionizing nature, and its ability to form real-time axial and three-dimensional images. The tissues of interest need to reflect sufficient ultrasound energy; this limits the method to soft tissues, fluids and small calcifications preferably close to the surface of the body and unobstructed by bony structures.

Ultrasound is most commonly employed in examinations of the abdomen and pelvis. In obstetrics, fetal head size and fetal length are used as measures of fetal maturity and health, while spinal morphology can be used to detect the presence of abnormalities such as spina bifida. Doppler imaging can be used to measure fetal blood velocity and cardiac function.

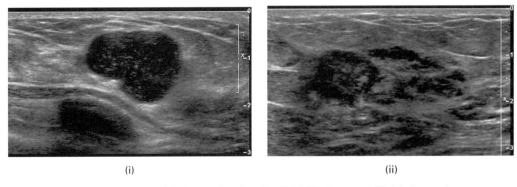

(i) (ii)

Figure 4.9   Ultrasound images of the breast showing (i) a fluid-filled cyst and (ii) lobular carcinoma.

Ultrasound imaging can be used to complement x-ray mammography in the diagnosis of breast cancer (Fig. 4.9). It can help determine whether a lump is a fluid-filled cyst or a solid mass, and is particularly useful in women with dense breast tissue and with young women, because their tissue is relatively opaque to x-rays.

4.2   Magnetic resonance imaging

Magnetic resonance imaging (MRI) is a non-ionizing technique that uses radiofrequency (200 MHz–2 GHz) electromagnetic radiation and large magnetic fields (around 1–2 tesla (T), compared with the Earth's magnetic field of about 0.5×10^{-4} T). The large magnetic fields are produced by superconducting magnets, in which current is passed through coils of superconducting wire whose electrical resistance is virtually zero.

MRI images provide anatomical and physiological details, i.e. structure and function, with full three-dimensional capabilities, excellent soft tissue visualization, and high spatial resolution (~1 mm). Like x-ray CT, it is a tomographic imaging modality. Image reconstruction, while conceptually equivalent to that in CT, is obtained from the raw signals collected in frequency space. With sufficient slice images, the image data is practically three-dimensional and it is possible to reconstruct the data in different two-dimensional planes at will (see Activity 4.3). Scans last several minutes, rather than a few seconds as in x-ray CT, so that patient motion can be a problem. Furthermore, MRI scanners are several times as costly as a CT scanner because of the expensive superconducting magnet required.

4.2.1   Nuclear magnetic resonance

MRI imaging is based on *nuclear magnetic resonance* (NMR). Nuclei are composed of nucleons, either neutrons or protons. Nuclei with unpaired nucleons behave like small magnets, with an associated magnetic moment. The hydrogen nucleus, a single proton, is of particular importance in MRI imaging because of its abundance in biological tissue, and all current MRI scanners use the proton signal.

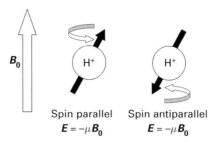

Spin parallel   Spin antiparallel
$E = -\mu B_0$ $E = -\mu B_0$

Figure 4.10 The precession of the nuclear magnetic moments of a hydrogen nucleus about an external magnetic field giving rise to two distinct states, parallel and anti-parallel.

Normally the direction of these magnetic moments is random. However, in an external magnetic field, they line up along the direction of the field, and precess around it (Fig. 4.10) like a gyroscope in a gravitational field. The precessional frequency, known as the Larmor frequency, is proportional to the strength of the external field, B_0. The magnetic moments can either line up in the same direction, parallel, as the magnetic field, which is the lower energy state, or opposite to the field direction, anti-parallel, which is a higher energy state (Fig. 4.10).

This is a small energy difference compared with thermal energies at room temperature, even for large magnetic fields. The protons are continually flipping back and forth between the two states but at any given instant there will be a slight majority aligned parallel to the field, so as to minimize the overall energy. The larger the external field B_0, the greater the difference in energy levels and the larger the excess number aligned parallel to the field. At 1.5 T, for example, for every 2 million protons there is an excess of 9 protons aligned with the field than against it. (For a $2 \times 2 \times 5$ mm voxel of water in a 1.5 T magnetic field, the number of excess protons is about 6×10^{15}.) Higher field MRI scanners produce images with a higher signal-to-noise ratio because it is essentially the number of excess protons which determines the strength of the MRI signal.

In order for the energy difference to be detected it is necessary to apply first a short pulse of electromagnetic radiation. If the energy of this radiation is exactly equal to the energy difference between the two distinct states, it causes some of the parallel spins to jump to the higher energy anti-parallel direction. The frequency of the radiation required to cause these jumps is equal to the Larmor frequency. No other frequency stimulates these transitions, so that this particular frequency is an example of *resonance*. The resonant (Larmor) frequency for hydrogen nuclei in a field of 1–2 T corresponds to *radiofrequencies* (RF). Such jumps would reduce the number of excess protons aligned parallel to the external field, denoted the z direction, and would result in the net magnetization, M_0, spiraling down towards the x–y plane or below it, depending on the strength and duration of the pulse (Fig. 4.11(i)). This is the view from the so-called *laboratory frame* of reference; from the viewpoint of the rotating magnetization vector, the so-called *rotating frame* of reference, visualization is simpler with M_0 smoothly tipping down (Fig. 4.11(ii)), with a tip angle, α, that is a function of the strength and

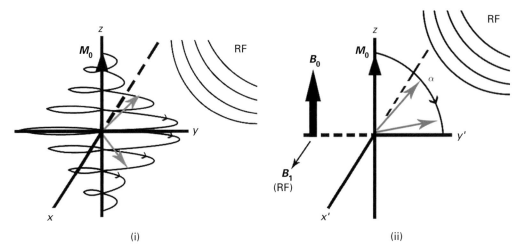

Figure 4.11   The effect of a radiofrequency pulse, at the Larmor frequency, on the net magnetization as seen from (i) the laboratory frame and (ii) the rotating frame of reference.

duration of the RF pulse. The magnetic field of the RF pulse is denoted B_1; it oscillates at the Larmor frequency, and is arranged to be at right angles to the direction of B_0. It is the interaction of B_1, which is much smaller in magnitude than B_0, with M_0 that causes the latter to tip towards the x–y plane.

When the pulse length is such as to produce a tip angle of 90° the pulse is termed a 90° pulse, and the maximum magnetization in the x–y plane is produced. For a pulse twice as long, termed a 180° pulse, the magnetization is tipped to the $-z$ direction and no transverse magnetization is produced.

Once the RF 90° pulse is switched off, the rotating M_0 induces a current in the RF coil that produced the initial pulse, and relaxes slowly back to its original orientation along the z axis. This induced signal is known as the *free induction decay* (FID) signal. The time that it takes to return back to its original (equilibrium) position along the z axis reveals important information about the dynamics of the molecules in the sample.

One of the relaxation processes, known as *longitudinal, T_1, or spin-lattice relaxation*, causes the net magnetization vector to grow back to M_0 in the z direction (T_1 recovery). Physically, this is the result of interactions between the nuclear spins and the lattice, i.e. the surrounding molecules. The process can be described by

$$M_z = M_0\left(1 - e^{-t/T_1}\right) \tag{4.10}$$

with a characteristic time of T_1 (Fig. 4 12(i)), which depends considerably on the tissue type; T_1 is about 100 ms for fat and about 2000 ms for water.

At the same time, the transverse magnetization decays to zero because the individual spins rotate at slightly different frequencies and get out of phase with each other. This

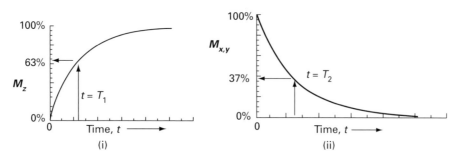

Figure 4.12 (i) Spin-lattice relaxation resulting in M_z increasing to M_0 with a time constant of T_1. (ii) Spin-spin relaxation resulting in $M_{x,y}$ dropping to zero with a time constant of T_2.

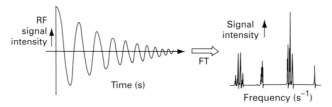

Figure 4.13 The FID signal and its Fourier transform. (After Bushong, 1996, p. 15.)

process is known as *transverse, T_2,* or *spin-spin relaxation,* and results from spins interacting with each other. The process can be described by

$$M_{x,y} = M_0 e^{-t/T_2} \qquad (4.11)$$

where T_2 is the characteristic time (Fig. 4.12(ii)). Although these two processes occur together, T_2 decay almost always occurs more rapidly than the re-growth of longitudinal magnetization; thus, T_2 is always shorter than T_1 for a particular tissue type.

This signal, produced by the decay of transverse magnetization, is called *free induction decay* (FID). It is a decaying harmonic oscillation at the Larmor frequency (Fig. 4.13), since the transverse magnetization is rotating in the laboratory frame; the envelope decays with a time constant of T_2. In practice, de-phasing also occurs due to local variations in magnetic field and non-uniformities within the tissue so that T_2 needs to be replaced by T_2^*, where

$$\frac{1}{T_2^*} = \frac{1}{T_2} + \frac{1}{T_2'} \qquad (4.12)$$

and T_2' characterizes these local variations, and can be 10–100 times shorter than T_2. A so-called *spin echo* technique is often used to record the true T_2 decay rather than the faster T_2^* decay.

To summarize, nuclear spins in the presence of an external magnetic field, $\boldsymbol{B_0}$, align either with or opposed to the magnetic field. The parallel and anti-parallel spins almost cancel each other out, leaving a relatively small number of excess spins aligned parallel with the main magnetic field. If a radiofrequency signal is applied at the Larmor frequency, the individual spins resonate, absorbing the applied energy, and precess in phase. Depending on the magnetic field of the applied pulse and its length, the protons flip towards the x–y plane producing transverse magnetization. The transverse magnetization induces a voltage in an antenna or receiver coil in the x–y plane, often the same coil used to transmit the radiofrequency excitation pulse; this induced signal eventually becomes the MR signal. When the radiofrequency pulse is turned off, the protons de-phase as they try to realign with $\boldsymbol{B_0}$. Two phenomena occur simultaneously. Transverse magnetization decreases (T_2 decay), while longitudinal magnetization increases (T_1 recovery).

Because all the spins are not in identical chemical and magnetic environments, they do not all precess at exactly the same frequency and the FID signal detected is a superposition of all of the individual FID signals. The Fourier transform, FT, of the FID signal gives the information directly in terms of frequencies, the NMR spectrum (Fig. 4.13). Each exponentially decaying sinusoid produces a *Lorentzian* line shape (i.e. of the form $a/(a^2 + (f - f_L)^2)$, where a is the half-width) at the frequency of the sinusoid, its Larmor frequency. Essentially, the positions of the peaks within the Fourier spectrum provide a map of the proton density in the patient, and the fine structure is related to the relaxation times, which are related to the configurations of the protons in the patient.

4.2.2 Magnetic resonance imaging (MRI)

The question remains as to how an MRI image might be obtained from the NMR spectrum, since if the same tissue were in two different positions, the NMR spectrum would still produce only a single peak (Fig. 4.14). Inspection of the spectrum would reveal the presence of protons, but not their location.

If, in addition to the strong static magnetic field produced by a superconducting electromagnet at low temperature, using liquid helium (bp 4.2 K), a linear *magnetic field gradient*, $\boldsymbol{B_x}$, using electromagnetic *gradient coils* to produce small gradients on the order of a few millitesla per meter (mT m^{-1}), were applied, then the total magnetic field would increase across the patient. Since the Larmor frequency is proportional to the

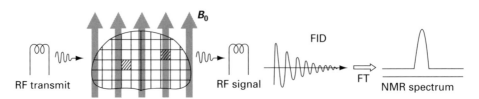

Figure 4.14 The NMR spectrum of a patient with protons at two different positions. (After Bushong, 1996, p. 16.)

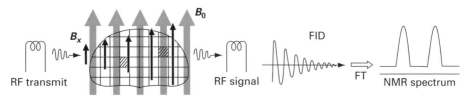

Figure 4.15   The NMR spectrum of two spatially separated clusters of protons when a magnetic field gradient is used. (After Bushong, 1996, p. 16.)

applied magnetic field, it is different for the same tissue located at different positions and the FID signal would be considerably more complicated. For the case of two voxels at two different locations, the Fourier transform of the FID signal would have two peaks at different frequencies, one from each voxel (Fig. 4.15). Thus the two peaks now carry spatial information, and the resulting spectrum can be considered a *projection*, similar to x-ray CT. Unlike B_0, which is always on, the magnetic field gradient is normally only applied transiently during data collection. If multiple projections are obtained around a patient, then an axial image can be reconstructed.

Slice selection is accomplished by using a frequency-selecting RF pulse applied simultaneously with one of the magnetic field gradients. The choice of field gradient, x, y or z, allows us to select the orientation, sagittal, coronal or axial, of the image; if an oblique slice is required, then two gradients are applied, at suitably weighted strengths, simultaneously with the frequency-selecting pulse. From this point on we will consider how an axial image is acquired (i.e. a cross-section perpendicular to the main magnetic field direction). In this case we perform slice selection along the z direction: a gradient in this direction is turned on such that it acts symmetrically about the center of the scanner (the *isocenter*). In this way the resonant frequency is smaller towards the patient's feet, unchanged at the isocenter, and greater towards the head. By simultaneously using a shaped radiofrequency (RF) pulse containing a finite bandwidth, only a section of spins either side of the isocenter is excited into the transverse plane. The slice thickness or position can be varied by using different gradient strengths or RF bandwidths. There is a limit to how thin the slices can be; small values of bandwidth and large magnetic field gradients are technically difficult to generate, and a very thin slice would contain only a few spins and thus have a small signal-to-noise ratio. By changing the center frequency of the frequency-selecting radiofrequency pulse, the slice can be moved to different positions within the patient.

Having selected a slice, the remaining two in-plane dimensions need to be encoded (in this case the "x" and "y" directions) to produce a two-dimensional image. One of the directions is encoded by changes of *frequency* during acquisition. Another gradient is turned on in (say) the x direction. Once again the center of the slice remains unaltered, but to the left of this point the field and therefore the resonant frequency is smaller, and to the right it is larger. Columns of pixels from left to right are therefore discriminated in terms of frequency differences. This is known as *frequency-encoding*.

It can be shown that a gradient applied in the y direction to change frequency in this dimension would not be sufficient to ascribe frequency uniquely to each column and row

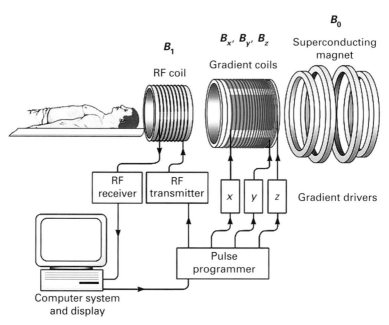

Figure 4.16   Basic components of a MRI scanner.

of pixels. For the last dimension the signal is encoded in terms of *phase*. This is not easy to understand: suffice it to say that a number of gradients are needed to create phase *changes* from row to row prior to acquisition so that the FT is provided with enough information to encode fully the final image. This is known as *phase-encoding*.

Three separate gradient coils are required to encode the three spatial dimensions unambiguously. Multiple projections can be obtained by electronically rotating the magnetic field gradients around the patient. The Fourier transform of the echo signals received produce what are effectively projections of the object along certain directions. These one-dimensional projections can be assembled to give the two-dimensional Fourier transform of the object, which can then be inverse Fourier transformed to give an axial image; this is the direct Fourier reconstruction (DFR) technique (Section 7.8.2), which is almost universally used in MRI reconstruction.

The basic components of a MRI scanner are shown in Figure 4.16. The primary magnet polarizes the protons in the patient. It can either be an electromagnet using superconducting coils, which require cooling to very low temperatures, and which resembles the gantry of a CT scanner; or it can be a permanent magnet constructed of rare-earth alloys, in which case it has a more open structure. The gradient coils produce linear variations on the magnetic field, so that the proton resonant frequencies within the patient are spatially dependent; they are fixed permanently within the primary magnet. The RF coil produces the oscillating magnetic field necessary for creating phase coherence between protons, and receives the FID signal by magnetic induction; it is placed around the body part of the patient to be imaged, with a geometry optimized for that specific part.

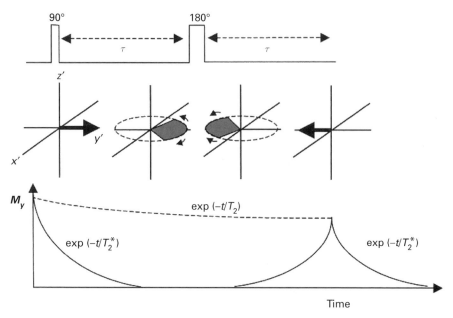

Figure 4.17 The 90° pulse tips the magnetization into the *x–y* plane; after it finishes, de-phasing begins; the 180° pulse flips the individual spins by 180° in the *x–y* plane, so that they start moving into phase again.

4.2.3   Pulse sequences

The spin echo pulse sequence is the mainstay of clinical MRI, because of its simplicity and flexibility in allowing the user to acquire images whose contrast is dominated either by T_1 or by T_2. A 90° RF pulse moves the net magnetization into the transverse plane, and is followed by a 180° RF *re-phasing* pulse. When the 90° pulse is turned off, the phases of the contributing spins begin to change due to local variations and this phase dispersal results in T_2^* decay. However, if a 180° re-phasing pulse is applied before the transverse component dies away, the spins are flipped and then start to move back into focus before beginning to de-phase again (Fig. 4.17). A new echo, called the *spin echo*, evolves as the spins re-phase. A train of 180° pulses causes successive re-phasing by repeatedly changing the direction of the individual rotating spins.

The maximum value of the spin echo following each 180° pulse constitutes a point on the exponential decay describing spin–spin relaxation (Fig. 4.18). Thus, a 90° pulse followed by a carefully timed train of 180° pulses gives an envelope of the T_2 decay in the presence of T_2^* decay, from which T_2 can be measured. The time from the center of the 90° pulse to the center of the spin echo is known as the *echo time*, TE; TE/2 is the time from the center of the 90° pulse to the center of the 180° re-phasing pulse. The pulse sequence is applied multiple times depending on the image size and the required signal-to-noise ratio. The repetition time, TR, is defined as the time from the center of the 90° pulse to the center of the next 90° pulse.

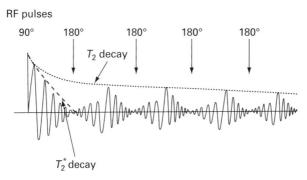

Figure 4.18   A spin echo pulse sequence, comprising a 90° pulse followed by carefully timed 180° pulses produces a series of spin echoes of decreasing amplitudes. Although each individual echo decays as T_2^*, the envelope decays as T_2.

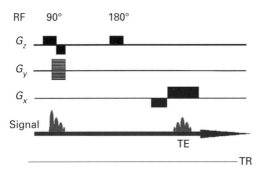

Figure 4.19   Pulse sequence for spin echo imaging.

Figure 4.19 is a spin echo sequence diagram. The bottom line illustrates the evolution of the MR signal (the FID immediately after the 90° pulse and the echo at time TE). Note that the repetition time is also labeled. Gradients are illustrated by rectangular blocks, the area of which represents the amplitude and the sign (i.e. positive or negative) dictated by the position above or below the "time" axis. In this example the phase encoding is in the y direction and the phase encoding gradient (G_y) is drawn as multiple lines to illustrate that the amplitude of this changes each time the sequence is repeated. In contrast, frequency encoding (G_x) is performed all at once at the time of signal detection. A de-phasing lobe (negative half of area) compensates for changes in phase, such that at the time of the echo only a frequency change is exhibited. Lastly, the slice-selection gradient (G_z) has to be applied at the time of both RF pulses so that only the spins within the slice of interest are excited and refocused. It also uses a de-phasing lobe.

The acquisition time for the spin echo sequence is given by the product of the TR of the pulse sequence and the number of phase encoding steps (the number of pixels in the phase direction). If multiple acquisitions were done to improve the signal-to-noise ratio (SNR) then the total acquisition time would be multiplied by this factor. By recording the echo more than once the coherent signal is additive but the incoherent noise cancels out.

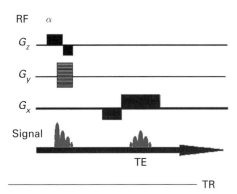

Figure 4.20   Pulse sequence for gradient echo imaging.

In fact, the signal-to-noise ratio improves only as the square root of the number of averages, i.e. taking two acquisitions increases the scan time by a factor of two, but improves the signal-to-noise ratio by only 1.4 (see Activity 4.4). In practice, patient movement and total imaging time limit the number of acquisitions to 6–8.

Multi-slice imaging is achieved by making use of the time between the end of echo collection and the next 90° excitation pulse (TR − TE), referred to as *dead time*. In this period the next slice can be selected and excited; it is possible to acquire 20–30 independent slices during TR. Another consideration is the *cross-talk* (or more correctly "cross-excitation") which occurs between adjacent slices due to imperfect slice profiles. This is accounted for by leaving gaps or interleaving slices, so that even slices are excited first followed by the odd slices.

In order to overcome the relatively long imaging times needed for spin echo imaging, another pulse sequence, known as *gradient echo* (Fig. 4.20), was introduced. In this sequence no 180° pulses are used so that the imaging time is faster. However, the images are influenced by T_2^* rather than T_2, and are therefore prone to susceptibility artifacts. The use of gradient echo imaging is primarily for rapid (short TR) T_1-weighted scans. The use of such short TRs makes it prudent to use partial (non-90°) flip angles. A sequence of pulses, with flip angles usually between 20° and 60°, are used; the particular spin angle can be used to influence the contrast in the final image.

There are very many different pulse sequences, but the majority of them are variants of spin echo or gradient echo imaging. *Inversion recovery* (IR) imaging was introduced as an approach to enhance the T_1-weighted contrast in conventional spin echo imaging. A valuable application of inversion recovery for some clinical applications is the nulling of signal from tissues having a specific T_1 relaxation time such as fat (Fig. 4.21); these sequences are known as *short time inversion recovery* (STIR) sequences. A variant of gradient echo imaging is fast low-angle shot imaging (FLASH), which uses a lower flip angle. Look at the images of the beating heart in Activity 4.5.

Echo planar imaging (EPI) is an extremely fast method of obtaining a magnetic resonance image. To appreciate fully the utility of EPI we must first consider *k*-space, which is an array of numbers whose Fourier transform (Chapter 7) gives the magnetic

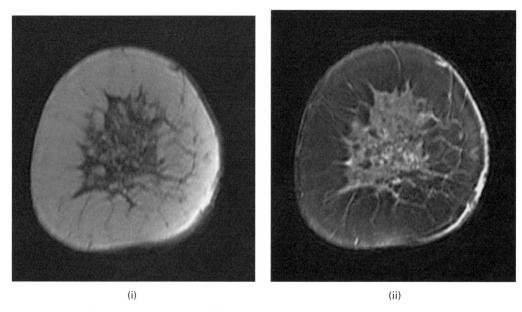

(i)   (ii)

Figure 4.21   Axial breast images (i) pre and (ii) post fat suppression.

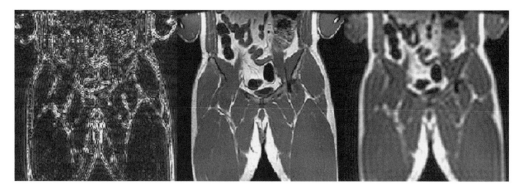

Figure 4.22   Images acquired with full and partial *k*-space (see text).

resonance image. Each row in *k*-space corresponds to the echo data collected with each application of the phase-encoding gradient. The cells in *k*-space *do not* equate one-to-one with the pixels in the image; in fact each cell contains information about every image pixel. Rows near to the center of *k*-space correspond to low-frequency detail obtained from small-amplitude phase-encoding steps; while the edges of k-space correspond to higher-frequency detail obtained using large-amplitude gradient steps. To image an object fully data in the whole of *k*-space must be collected. By acquiring only part of *k*-space (or fewer "lines") the scan is much faster but image quality is compromised.

The central image in Figure 4.22 was acquired with full *k*-space, while for the left-hand image only the outer edges of *k*-space were collected and as a result only the edges or detail are present in the image. Conversely by acquiring only the central portion of k-space (right image) more of the signal is produced but the detail is missing. In normal imaging one line of k-space is collected and the sequence is repeated with an increment of the phase-encoding gradient in order to acquire the next line "up" and so on. In echo planar imaging, the gradients are played out so that all lines of k-space are acquired in one TR (*single-shot technique*). This means that the sequence is extremely fast, typically acquiring a slice every 50 ms. Usually fewer phase-encoding steps are collected compared to a normal sequence (e.g. 64 instead of 256) so the images are not of the same quality. Being so gradient intensive, echo planar imaging is also prone to artifacts. Nevertheless, it is useful for pediatric studies or functional MRI where speed is essential.

4.2.4 T_1- and T_2-weighted images

A magnetic resonance image is a map of the relative strengths of the NMR signals originating from different voxels. It depends on the proton density and on the values of T_1 and T_2, which are a consequence of the neighborhoods of the protons. Various protocols, e.g. spin echo, gradient echo, inversion recovery, etc., using pulse sequences of different lengths and separations, can be used to improve the contrast resolution of the image. Images produced in such a way as to reflect differences primarily in tissue T_1 are said to be "T_1-weighted"; other images might be "T_2-weighted," "proton density weighted," etc.

To achieve T_1-weighting, a spin echo sequence needs to reduce the contributions due to T_2 and spin density; thus both TR and TE should be short (≤ 500–600 ms and ≤ 20 ms, respectively). The short TR ensures that there are maximum differences in the longitudinal recovery between tissues with different T_1 relaxation times; and the short TE ensures that transverse magnetization does not de-phase appreciably and lose these differences.

T_1-weighted images look like CT images and are more focused than other MRI image types. They allow for the overall visualization of structures in the body and can be further enhanced using a contrast medium which renders blood vessels white. In T_1-weighted images of the head, fat tissue appears bright and cerebral spinal fluid (CSF) dark (Fig. 4.23).

In T_2-weighted imaging, TR is long (2000–4000 ms) to reduce T_1 effects, and TE is long (80–150 ms) to produce contrast differences that depend on the T_2 values. In T_2-weighted images, both CSF and areas that have abnormally high water content (those affected by tumor, infection or stroke) appear bright (Fig. 4.24). A problem with T_2-weighted images is that if TE is extended excessively image contrast improves, but the signal-to-noise ratio decreases.

In many MRI imaging situations there is sufficient contrast to distinguish pathological from healthy tissue. When there is not, contrast agents, often based on gadolinium, which is paramagnetic, are used. *Magnetic resonance angiography* (MRA) is fast replacing x-ray angiography as the preferred diagnostic tool for the detection of plaques and blockages (stenoses) in the blood vessels, because it is less invasive and significantly less time consuming. MRI is also developing a tremendous potential not only for showing the structure or anatomy of the body, but also the function or physiology of the body. *Functional MRI* (fMRI) can be used to show the function of the cardiac muscle and even glimpse at the neural activity of the brain itself, for example using pattern

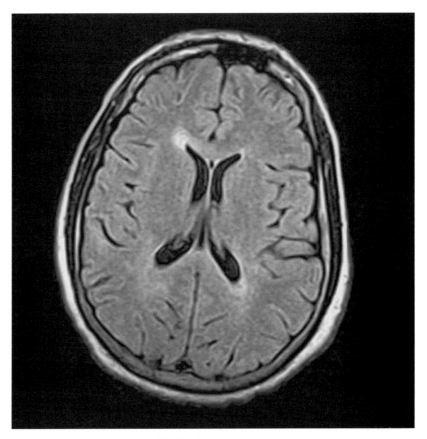

Figure 4.23 T_1-weighted spin echo image of the head.

recognition studies. New applications are being discovered all the time: MRI has been used to show atrophy changes of the brain common in Alzheimer's disease, and it can detect tumors at earlier stages than most other forms of medical imaging.

4.2.5   Image characteristics

The most important parameter affecting the signal-to-noise ratio (SNR) is the strength of the magnetic field, B_0. A larger B_0 results in more spins participating and consequently a larger net magnetization. The improvement in signal-to-noise ratio scales approximately linearly with increases in B_0; thus, other things being equal, a 1.5 T system produces images with a signal-to-noise ratio three times higher than images from a 0.5 T system. However, this is partially offset by increased T_1 times and increased artifacts. Increasing the voxel size, by increasing the field of view, the slice thickness or the coarseness of the matrix, increases the number of protons contributing to each voxel value and hence the signal-to-noise ratio, but at the price of reduced spatial resolution.

Spatial resolution is determined by the number of frequency-encoded projections and phase-encoded projections for a given field of view (FOV). An increase

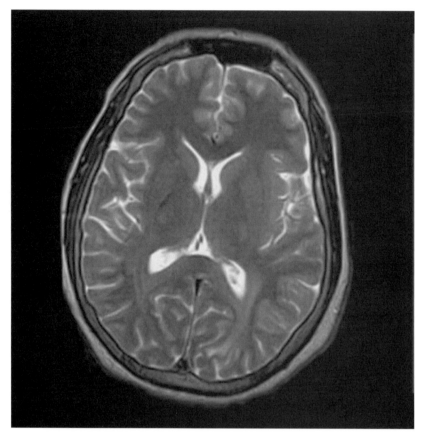

Figure 4.24 T_2-weighted spin echo image of the head.

in spatial resolution along the phase-encoded axis requires an increase in the number of phase-encoded projections, N, each with a different strength of the phase-encoding gradient. This increases the acquisition time. The penalty for increasing spatial resolution along the frequency-encoded axis is that there are fewer protons in the smaller voxels, which decreases the signal-to-noise ratio. In conventional clinical MRI imaging, the overall spatial resolution is similar to that obtained with CT imaging, i.e. 0.5–1.0 mm.

Contrast in MRI images is a complex function of many different factors, including T_1 and T_2 and the proton density of the tissues, the pulse sequence, and flow and diffusion effects. Regardless of the details, however, MRI is capable of delivering outstanding soft tissue contrast and the ability to image flow effects.

Artifacts are usually attributable to instrumentation defects, such as field and gradient non-uniformities and non-linear coil response, or to the patient, such as movement during signal acquisition. Especially problematic with regard to patient-related artifacts are pulse sequences which require long acquisition times, over many heart beats or respiratory cycles. The use of cardiac gating to acquire signals in synchrony with the cardiac

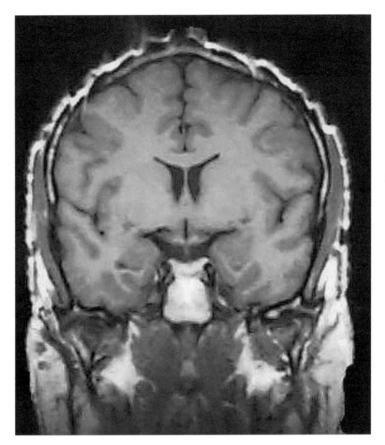

Figure 4.25 T_1-weighted spin echo image showing distortion along the scalp, due to the presence of ferromagnetic material (small metal fragments embedded in the hair or scalp) causing distortion of the local magnetic field.

cycle reduces cardiac-related motion and artifacts due to chest motion. Ringing artifacts are often seen at bright edges, such as at the edge of the brain–fatty scalp boundary in a transverse image of the head. Partial volume effects can result when a voxel contains a mixture of very different tissues. Other artifacts can arise due to the presence of ferromagnetic materials (Fig. 4.25), or due to finite sampling (Section 7.4.2).

Since magnetic resonance imaging does not use ionizing radiation, it is considered safe. There are safety aspects concerned with the high static magnetic field and large field gradients. Due to the adverse effect of large magnetic fields on electrical circuitry, patients with pace-makers or similar devices cannot be examined by magnetic resonance imaging. Those with surgical clips or ferrous metallic implants are also excluded. Although there is little evidence to suggest any problem, pregnant women, especially in the first trimester, are also usually excluded. Peripheral nerve stimulation can occur at field gradients above $60\,\mathrm{T\,s^{-1}}$, which although harmless may be painful. The repetitive use of radiofrequency pulses deposits energy which in turn causes heating in the patient. For fields up to $3.0\,\mathrm{T}$, the heating is proportional to the square of the field but at high fields the body becomes increasingly conductive necessitating the use of increased radiofrequency power. On rare occasions minor patient burns can result. The scans themselves can be quite noisy. The forces acting on the gradient coils due to current passing through them in the presence of the main field causes them to vibrate. These mechanical vibrations are transmitted through to the patient as acoustic noise. As a consequence patients often wear earplugs or head phones while being scanned.

4.3 Picture archiving and communication systems (PACS)

A *picture archiving and communication system* (PACS) is essentially a network system (Fig. 4.26) that allows digital or digitized images from any modality to be retrieved, viewed and analyzed by a relevant expert, or by an appropriate expert system, at different workstations. These images may be held in archives, i.e. be stored "permanently" on DVD, and/or be transmitted to/from remote sites, "teleradiology." The Digital Imaging

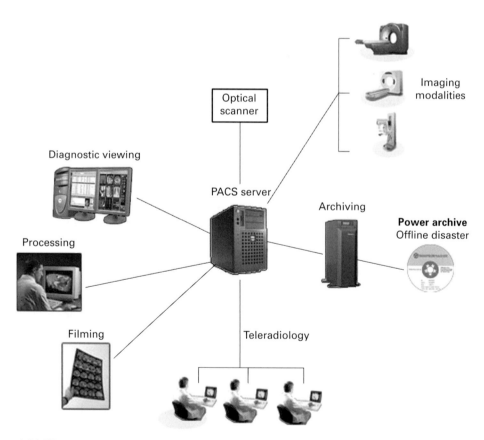

Figure 4.26   A PACS system.

and Communications in Medicine (DICOM) format allows images, and cine-loop images, with associated patient information and reports, including voice notes, to be stored and exchanged readily over the network. PACS systems can be integrated into radiological/hospital information systems (RIS/HIS), with the inclusion of administrative information such as billing and inventory.

Most modalities, including mammography, are now becoming digital. Increasingly, plain-film radiography is being replaced by *computed radiography* or by direct *digital radiography*. The advantages of PACS systems include:

(i) film-less radiology (no darkroom required, no chemical developers to purchase, no bulky storage rooms);
(ii) easy access to images, including those from remote sites;
(iii) easy image processing/enhancement;
(iv) easy registration of images from different modalities;
(v) compression of images for quicker communication.

Major disadvantages are the large capital cost of setting it up and training personnel, and the inevitable difficulties of phasing it in. Nevertheless, it is the obvious way to proceed, and a large number of hospitals have implemented or are implementing PACS systems.

4.3.1   Multimodal registration

Different medical imaging techniques may provide scans with complementary and occasionally conflicting information. The combination of images can often lead to additional clinical information not apparent in the separate images. When images are available from a number of different modalities it becomes possible to combine the information, for example from an anatomical image such as from CT or MRI with a functional image from, say, SPECT, PET or fMRI, as long as the images are properly aligned or *registered* with each other. In a functional image, for example, there is often not sufficient anatomic detail to determine the position of a tumor or other lesion. Figure 4.27 shows a co-registered SPECT–MRI image, where the SPECT image was pasted in "opaque" mode on the top of the black-and-white MRI image, which provided an anatomical template.

The registration can be

• intra-subject registration, i.e. different views of the same subject;
• inter-subject registration, i.e. different subjects (e.g. to assess the variability of structures over different individuals); or
• serial registration, i.e. to monitor changes within an individual over time.

The initial stage involves addressing differences in the acquisition parameters (different pixel/voxel size, different matrix size and different orientations). When registering SPECT images, which are generally 64×64 pixels, with MRI or CT images the SPECT image needs to be expanded to, say, a 512×512 matrix; in order to preserve the quality of images enlarged to this extent, some form of interpolation needs to be used.

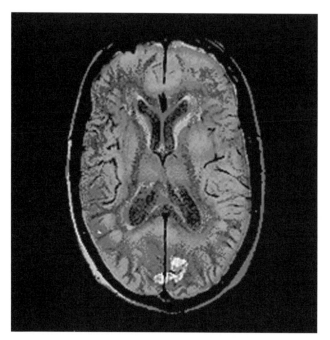

Figure 4.27 Co-registered SPECT–MRI image through the head. (Courtesy of Dr. Karin Knesaurek, Mt. Sinai Medical Center.) See also color plate.

The process of registration is based on a transformation that transforms an image from one modality to the image of the other modality. Each point in one image should map on to the corresponding point in the second image. The process is simplified if external markers can be attached to the patient, but this is often time-consuming and invasive; using internal anatomic markers, e.g. the rib cage, ventricles, bone surfaces, is more frequently used. The registration could be done interactively by a radiologist, assisted by software that gives feedback on the quality of the alignment, but automatic registration is generally preferred. The simplest situation is inter-subject registration where there is no distortion; and then just two rotations and two translations are required for two-dimensional images (Fig. 4.28). If distortion is present in one or both of the images non-rigid registration involving affine transformations (Section 6.3) that include the effect of shear need to be applied.

Medical image registration has also been utilized in radiotherapy, mostly for brain tumors, and by cranio-facial surgeons to prepare for and simulate complex surgical procedures. Radiologists often have difficulty locating and accurately identifying cancer tissue, even with the aid of structural information such as CT and MRI because of the low contrast between the cancer and the surrounding tissues in CT and MRI images. Using SPECT and radioactively labeled monoclonal antibodies it is possible to obtain high-contrast images of the concentration of antibodies in tumors. Registration of both structural and functional images can significantly aid in the early detection of tumors and other diseases, and help in improving the accuracy of diagnosis.

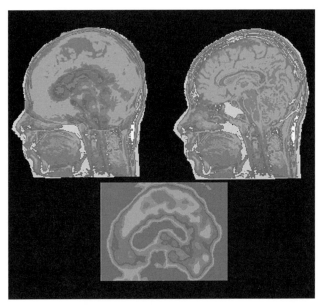

Figure 4.28   MRI (upper right) and SPECT (lower center) head sagittal slices of the same patient and the co-registered (MRI + SPECT) image (upper left). The lesion on the top of the skull is more prominent in the composite image, although it can be visualized in both modalities. See also color plate.

Computer-based activities

Activity 4.1 Beam steering

Double-click **beamsteering.html**, and then click on **Beam steering**. An array transducer comprising seven elements is shown. Element #1 receives a voltage pulse first, and emits an ultrasound pulse; and then each of the other elements receives a voltage pulse, delayed by a fixed amount relative to its neighbor on the left. The resulting ultrasound beam wavefront is almost linear, and travels at an angle which depends on the constant time delay between voltage pulses.

Activity 4.2 Echocardiogram image sequences

Start ezDicom, then **File/Open Dicom** and open the file **US0001**. This is a series of eight images of the heart (i.e. echocardiography) with color Doppler added, showing the action of the heart after exercise, i.e. post-stress. Use the **Video** icon to animate the sequence; different speeds are available, 1 through 5. After viewing the animated sequence, move Video to 0 (still) and use the slider to view the eight images sequentially. Can you see the four chambers of the heart? Can you visualize the direction of the blood flow through the heart, using BART (Blue Away, Red Towards)? Look at **Image/View Image Information** to view the DICOM header with details of the procedure.

What is an advantage of the echocardiogram over other imaging techniques?

Activity 4.3 MRI images of the head

Using ImageJ, open **HeadMRI** to get a stack of 55 MRI images of the human head. From what plane are you viewing these images? Go to **Image/Stacks/Start Animation** to animate the stack. Stop the animation and browse through the stack using the slider under the image.

Use **Image/Stacks/Z Project . . . Max intensity** to see the slices superimposed.

This image data is virtually three-dimensional, although the spacing between stacks is larger than the pixel size. It is possible to reconstruct the data in a different plane. Use the straight line selector in the toolbar to draw a horizontal line (hold down the shift key) in slice number 30, at about the level of the nose. Go to **Stacks/ Reslice**, and choose 2.2 for the input and output Z spacing and 55 for the slice count. The new image appears compressed, and you should scale the x direction by about 20 (you may need to assign more memory in **Edit/Options/Memory**) to see a more accurate view.

Activity 4.4 Noise in MRI images

In order to reduce noise in MRI images, the acquisition is repeated several times, and the resulting frames are averaged. The result is an improved signal-to-noise ratio (SNR). Open the six images **liver_n**, where $n = 1, \ldots, 6$, in ImageJ.

Determine the signal-to-noise ratio in **liver_1** using **Plugins/Ch.5 Plugins/ SNR**, which requires you to select a region of constant grayness in the image (e.g. a rectangle from about (109 186) to (171 303)). Now add the six images: you do this by adding two (**Process/Image Calculator** and get a 32-bit result each time), then adding a third to the result, then a fourth, and so on. Finally divide the final result by six (Process/Math) to obtain the average of the six images. Determine the signal-to-noise ratio of this image. How do you expect it to have changed? Do your results confirm this?

Activity 4.5 The beating heart

Play the movie of the beating heart, **heart.avi**. (Double-clicking the file starts it playing in Windows Media Player.) Also look at the individual frames. Note the aorta in the lower right corner of the image and the clear definition of the heart's four chambers.

Start ezDicom, then **File/Open Dicom** and open the file **MR0001**. This is a series of sixteen images of the heart; use the **Video** icon to animate the sequence. Can you see the four chambers of the heart? Look at **Image/View Image Information** to view the DICOM header with details of the procedure. How does this sequence compare with the avi sequence?

Activity 4.6 Rigid registration using points

Start Scion PC; strangely I have not been able to find a straightforward plugin for ImageJ that registers images with selected fiducial points. Open (**File/Open**) the four images **HeadMRI01**, **HeadMRI 02**, **HeadMRI 03** and **HeadMRI 04**. (If you have trouble reading the images ("unable to open the selected file"), copy them into the Images subdirectory within the Scion Image directory.) Look for corresponding salient anatomical points (landmarks) in the images, e.g. points in the orbits, positions of the ears, identifiable points on the base of the skull. Three landmarks or fiducial points, preferably well-separated, should be identified. They are used to scale, translate and rotate the second, third and fourth images into alignment with the first image, by optimizing the distances between the corresponding points in each image.

Combine the images into a stack (**Stacks/Windows to Stack**) and navigate through the stack using the slider bar. Click **Stacks/Register**, and check "**Select fiducial points on screen**." Now click on the three corresponding fiducial points in the same order for each image of the stack, double-clicking on the third point in each case (which automatically advances to the next image). Be careful with the order of points in image 04! Click on "**Register**." Observe the registered stack to check how well individual images have been registered.

Exercises

4.1 Why is the low megahertz range used in ultrasound imaging?

4.2 Do you expect sound to travel faster in soft tissue or bone? Why?

4.3 How much energy is reflected back when an ultrasound pulse passes from muscle to bone? How much is transmitted? (Use values for Z from Table 4.1.)

4.4 An ultrasound pulse passes through soft tissue and reflects off an interface, producing an echo 0.1 ms later. How deep is the reflecting interface?

4.5 If the delay between successive ultrasound pulses is 0.5 ms, what is the maximum range over which the system can successfully produce images, assuming the speed of the pulses in soft tissue is $1540 \, \mathrm{m\,s^{-1}}$. Note: The echo from one pulse should be received before the transmission of the next.

4.6 The intensity of an ultrasound beam falls by a factor of 100 in passing through a material. Express this drop in decibels.

4.7 Calculate the distance at which the intensity of a 1 MHz ultrasound pulse is reduced by half while traveling through (i) air, (ii) bone and (iii) muscle. (The attenuation coefficients for bone, air and muscle are 45, 8.7 and $1 \, \mathrm{dB\,cm^{-1}\,MHz^{-1}}$, respectively.)

4.8 What is the axial resolution of an ultrasound imaging system that uses 5 MHz pulses which are three wavelengths in length?

4.9 What is the velocity of the blood if a 3 kHz beat signal is heard with a 5 MHz Doppler ultrasound system?

4.10 What is meant by the term "resonance" in magnetic resonance imaging?

4.11 In a magnetic resonance imaging system, the signal is coherent and the noise is random. What is the effect on the signal-to-noise ratio of signal averaging four observations from each voxel?

4.12 What is the purpose of the radiofrequency transmit and receive coils in magnetic resonance imaging?

4.13 What is meant by the free induction decay signal in magnetic resonance imaging?

4.14 You wish to produce an image of hydrogen nuclei in the z–x plane. What directions should the slice-, phase- and frequency-encoding gradients be applied in?

Part II

Fundamental concepts of image processing

5 Fundamentals of digital image processing

Overview

Images can be usefully characterized by their gray-level histograms, from which global qualities, such as brightness, contrast, entropy and signal-to-noise ratio, can be determined. Histograms are simple to calculate, and are the basis for a number of real-time image processing techniques. Display look-up tables allow grayscale transformations to be made, so that the visual appearance of an image is changed without altering the pixel values comprising it. The histogram of an image can be used to determine the parameters for look-up tables which implement various effects.

Learning objectives

After reading this chapter you will be able to:

- describe the basis of the gray-level histogram as a probability density function;
- distinguish between the brightness and the contrast of an image;
- explain the relationship between dynamic range and contrast;
- interpret the concept of entropy applied to an image;
- compute the compression ratio of an image file from the entropy of the image;
- estimate the signal-to-noise ratio (SNR) of an image;
- describe the use of a look-up table (LUT) as a mapping function;
- explain the effects of histogram stretch and histogram equalization, and distinguish between them;
- illustrate the effect of power-law and logarithmic histogram transforms;
- choose an appropriate look-up table to best display a particular image;
- distinguish between global and adaptive processing.

5.1 The gray-level histogram

The *gray-level histogram* is a concise initial characterization of an image, which can be used to assess its overall qualities and determine the appropriate processing steps required to enhance it. The histogram is a plot showing the number of pixels, anywhere

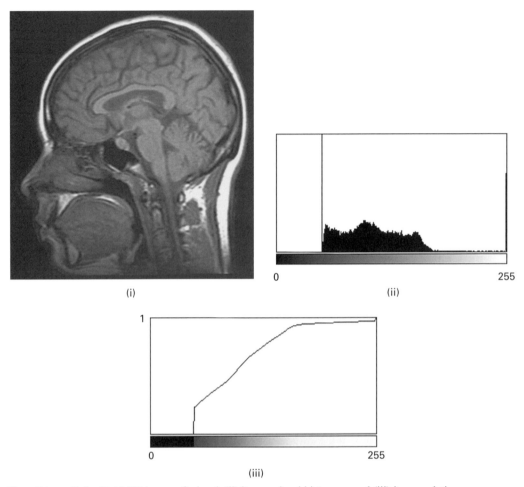

(i)   (ii)

(iii)

Figure 5.1   (i) Sagittal MRI image of a head, (ii) its gray-level histogram and (iii) its cumulative distribution function.

in the image, that displays each of the possible discrete pixel values, a_i. Each pixel value, plotted along the horizontal axis, is represented by a histogram bin whose height represents the number of image pixels with that particular value. A more accurate name for the gray-level histogram is the pixel value histogram, since pixel values and gray levels are not synonymous. We can change the displayed gray levels in an image without changing the pixel values by using a look-up table (LUT).

Figure 5.1(i) is an 8-bit deep MRI image of a head through the sagittal plane, and Figure 5.1(ii) is its gray-level histogram, with pixel values, a_i, from 0 to 255 along the horizontal axis. The bin heights are scaled relative to the largest bin height, which occurs at a pixel value of $\sim$50 for this image and corresponds to the dark gray background surrounding the head. The process of constructing the gray-level histogram involves scanning the image in a raster fashion, for each of the possible pixel values, and filling the corresponding bin as each pixel value is found. The histogram shows the number of pixels that have each pixel value, but it does not record where those pixels are located in the image. Thus, spatial information is discarded. The histogram is unique for a particular image, but different images could have the same histogram. Nevertheless, it does succinctly display some useful properties of the original image.

The sum of all the bin heights in the histogram equals the total number of pixels in the image. A normalized histogram may be obtained by dividing the bin heights by this number, so that the sum of the bin heights equals unity. In statistical terms, the normalized histogram is the *probability density function* (PDF) of the digital image, and indicates the probability, on a scale of 0 to 1, of observing a particular pixel value in the image. The integral of the normalized histogram/PDF is the *distribution function* or *cumulative distribution function,* CDF, of intensity in the image (Fig. 5.1(iii)), and indicates the probability of a pixel having a value equal to or less than a given value. The cumulative distribution function increases monotonically from 0 to 1 because the probability density function values are all positive. The cumulative distribution function value for a particular pixel value is obtained by adding the probability density function values for all the pixel values from zero up to the particular pixel value of interest. The minimum and maximum pixel values within the image can easily be obtained, either from the histogram/probability density function plot or from the cumulative distribution function plot; the median pixel value can be conveniently obtained from the cumulative distribution function plot by finding the pixel value corresponding to a cumulative probability of 0.5.

The gray-level histogram shows whether an image is overall dark or light (Fig. 5.2). The mean pixel value, $\bar{a}$, can be obtained from the histogram by adding the products of pixel value and corresponding bin heights, and dividing by the total number of pixels. A mean pixel value close to half of the maximum possible value, i.e. 127 or 128 for an 8-bit (256 gray levels) image, indicates optimum brightness. A value significantly below or above this indicates that the image is overall dark or bright, respectively, and by how much pixel values need to be changed in order to correct this. Activity 5.1 illustrates these concepts.

5.1.1 Dynamic range and contrast

The range of pixel values, defined as the difference between the maximum ($a_{\max}$) and the minimum ($a_{\min}$) pixel values found in the image, ignoring any obvious outliers, is known as the *dynamic range* of the image. It can be expressed either as the difference in pixel values or (in decibels (dB)) as

$$\text{dynamic range of image} = 20 \log_{10} (a_{\max} - a_{\min}) \tag{5.1}$$

Thus a 12-bit deep CT image, spanning the full range of pixel values (or CT numbers!) available to it (i.e. 4096, from -1000 to $+3095$), has a dynamic range of 72 dB, while a typical 10-bit deep fluoroscopy image spanning its full range (i.e. 1024, from 0 to 1023) has a dynamic range of 60 dB.

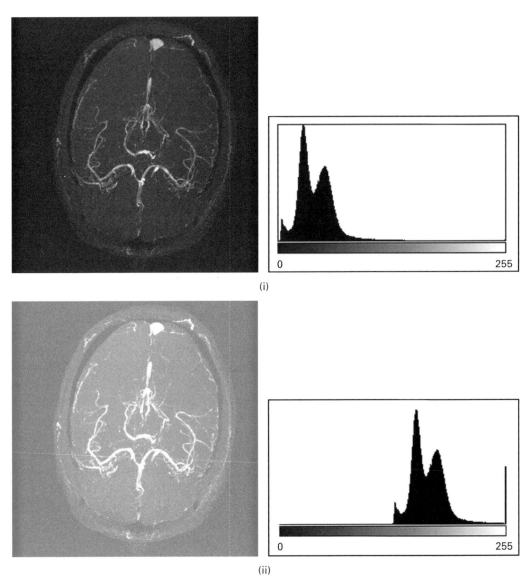

(i)

(ii)

Figure 5.2   (i) An overall dark image with its gray-level histogram, and (ii) an overall bright image with its gray-level histogram.

Ideally, the dynamic range of the radiation from the scene being imaged should be close to the available dynamic range of the detector in the imaging system (2^n for an n-bit system). In this case all the shades of gray in the scene are captured by the detector and represented in the image (Fig. 5.3(i)). If the dynamic range of the radiation from the scene is larger than the dynamic range of the detector, the image histogram has its low and/or high end cut off (Fig. 5.3(ii)). Pixel values underflow or overflow into the values that mark the available limits, and information is irretrievably lost. Even if such underflow or

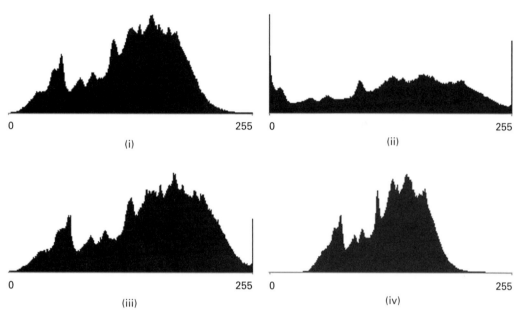

(i)   (ii)

(iii)   (iv)

Figure 5.3   Gray-level histograms which indicate: (i) the full dynamic range of the scene is optimally captured by the detector; (ii) the dynamic range of the scene is larger than the dynamic range of the detector, resulting in overflow at the top end of the histogram and underflow at the bottom end of the histogram; (iii) the dynamic ranges of the scene and the detector are matched, but incorrect exposure has resulted in the recorded pixel values being too large and overflowing at the top end of the histogram; (iv) the dynamic range of the scene is lower than the dynamic range of the detector.

overflow occurs at only one extreme of the histogram (Fig. 5.3(iii)), and the pixel values are subsequently shifted away from that extreme, the information lost cannot be recovered. A more favorable situation is when the dynamic range of the object is smaller than the dynamic range of the detector (Fig. 5.3(iv)). In this case, the dynamic range can be stretched to cover the whole range available (see Activity 5.2), although the number of bins in the original histogram is maintained. The dynamic range of the detector and the display should also be matched. If they are not, for example a camera or scanner digitizing to 7 bits (128 levels) and the image displayed on an 8-bit display (256 levels), the recorded levels are spread out over the available display levels and the image histogram shows 128 levels each separated by an empty level. Thus the histogram often serves as an indicator to ensure the best image quality at the image acquisition stage.

A closely related concept to dynamic range is *contrast*. When the dynamic range of an image covers the available range of the imaging system (2^n for an n-bit system), the image exhibits *high contrast*. Conversely, when the dynamic range is low, i.e. only a small range of closely spaced gray levels are present in the image, the image has *low contrast* and looks dull and washed out. Look at the series of images in Figure 5.4. Which images have the lowest contrast and which have the highest contrast? The relationship

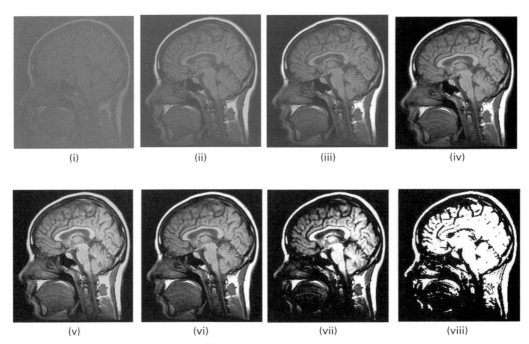

Figure 5.4   A series of images showing different contrasts. (The lowest contrast image is (i), and the highest contrast image is (viii).)

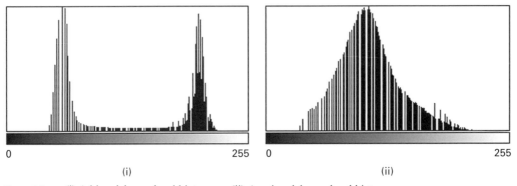

Figure 5.5   (i) A bimodal gray-level histogram. (ii) A unimodal gray-level histogram.

between dynamic range and contrast is explored further in Activity 5.2. Activity 5.3 illustrates the use of macros in ImageJ to record a series of processing operations.

Contrast and dynamic range are not synonymous. While the contrast does depend on the dynamic range, it is also related to the bin heights and to the average separation of pixel values in the image. For example, an image with a *bimodal* histogram (Fig. 5.5(i)), i.e. having two peaks, generally exhibits a higher contrast than an image with a *unimodal* histogram (Fig. 5.5(ii)), i.e. having a single peak.

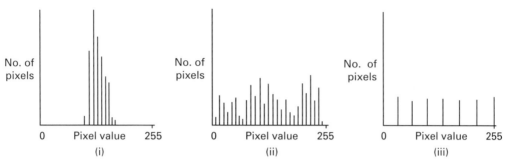

Figure 5.6 Histograms showing (i) low dynamic range and low contrast, (ii) maximum dynamic range and high contrast and (iii) maximum dynamic range and even higher contrast.

The histogram of an image with a low dynamic range, and low contrast as a consequence, is shown in Figure 5.6(i). An image with the maximum dynamic contrast available (256 for an image with 8-bit pixels) is shown in Figure 5.6(ii); it has significantly higher contrast. Although the dynamic range cannot be increased further, the contrast can be increased. Figure 5.6(iii) shows the histogram of such an image; the full dynamic range, combined with an increased separation of pixel values as a result of missing intermediate values, results in an image of higher contrast. Contrast can be increased further by continuing to increase the separation of pixel values, up to the limit where the only pixel values present are 0 and 255; this so-called *binary* image has the maximum possible contrast. However, as the number of pixel values in an image is reduced, *false contouring* or *posterization* becomes increasingly evident. This process of increasing the dynamic range to the maximum available, and then increasing the separation of the pixel values to increase contrast further, produced the series of images in Figure 5.4, culminating in the binary image of Figure 5.4(viii).

5.1.2   Entropy

Entropy is a measure of the amount of disorder or randomness in a system. An organized, highly ordered system has low entropy, whereas a less ordered system has higher entropy. One way of understanding entropy is to consider the spread of states which a system can adopt: a low-entropy system occupies a small number of such states, while a high-entropy system occupies a large number of states.

In the case of an image, these states correspond to the gray levels which the individual pixels can adopt. For example, in an 8-bit pixel there are 256 such states. If all such states are equally occupied, as they are in the case of an image with a uniformly distributed gray-level histogram, the spread of states has the maximum possible value. On the other hand, if the image has only two states occupied, i.e. all the pixels are either black or white, the entropy is low. And if all of the pixels have the same value, the entropy of the image is zero. Note that as the entropy of the image is decreased, so is its information content.

Entropy measures the average global *information content* of the image in bits per pixel. The concept of entropy comes from information theory, where information can be thought of as the reduction of uncertainty. The information content of a single message state in units of information is given by

$$I(E) = \log(1/P(E)) = -\log P(E) \tag{5.2}$$

where $P(E)$ is the prior probability of occurrence of the message. Intuitively, the amount of information carried by a message is inversely related to the probability of its occurrence. Messages with a high probability of occurring carry little information, and conversely, messages that are least expected carry most information. Data and information are different. We all have received long emails (data), many of which contain little information because they tell us what we already know; only when they tell us something unexpected do they carry real information.

If only two events are possible (0 and 1) the base of the logarithm in Equation (5.2) is 2, and the resulting unit of information is the *bit*. if the two events are equally likely $(P_1(E) = P_2(E) = 1/2)$ then $I(E_1) = I(E_2) = -\log_2(1/2) = 1$ bit, i.e. 1 bit of information is conveyed when one of two possible equally likely events occurs. However, if the two possible events are not equally likely (for example, $P_1(E) = 1/4$ and $P_2(E) = 3/4$) then the information conveyed by the less common event $(I(E_1) = -\log_2(1/4) = 2)$ is greater than that conveyed by the more common event $(I(E_2) = -\log_2(3/4) = 0.415)$.

In an image, the pixel values, a_i, occur with probabilities $P(a_i)$, which are given by the bin heights of the normalized histogram; the available pixel values run from 0 to 2^n-1. *First-order statistics* assume that the statistical properties of the pixels do not depend on neighboring pixels. A first-order estimate of the entropy, H, of an image is given by the sum of the information content of each pixel:

$$H = -\sum_{i=0}^{2^n-1} P(a_i)\, I(a_i) = -\sum_{i=0}^{2^n-1} P(a_i) \log_2 P(a_i) \tag{5.3}$$

Differentiating the function in this equation with respect to $P(a_i)$, it can be shown that the maximum possible entropy occurs when all the gray levels occur with the same probability. In an n-bit deep image, if all the (2^n) bins are occupied and with the same probability, i.e. the gray-level histogram is uniformly distributed, the image is said to be *histogram equalized* (Section 5.2.2). In such a case, $P(a_i)$ is constant and equal to $1/2^n$ and the entropy is n bits pixel^{-1}:

$$H = -\sum_{i=0}^{2^n-1} P(a_i)\, \log_2 P(a_i) = -\Sigma(1/2^n)\cdot\log_2(1/2^n) = +\Sigma(1/2^n)\cdot n = n \tag{5.4}$$

Thus, maximum entropy is achieved when all the bins are occupied and with equal probabilities.

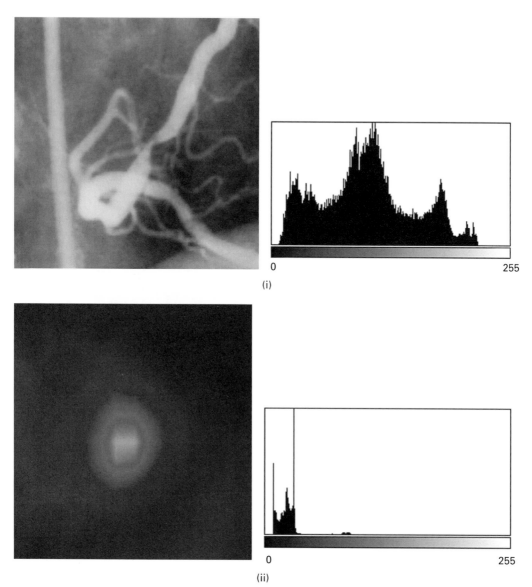

(i)

(ii)

Figure 5.7   Images and their histograms. The corresponding entropies are (i) 7.50 and (ii) 4.95 bits pixel^{-1}.

For an 8-bit deep image, entropy approaching 8 bits pixel^{-1} indicates an information-rich, complex image using all the available pixel values. Such an image tends to have fine details, although first-order entropy only depends on the gray-level histogram, which does not contain information on spatial pattern. Pixel values in the angiogram shown in Fig. 5.7(i) cover a wide dynamic range and the entropy of the image is correspondingly high, although not the maximum achievable value because the histogram does not cover the full range and is not an equalized histogram. Nuclear medicine images tend to have a limited dynamic range and less detail (Fig. 5.7(ii));

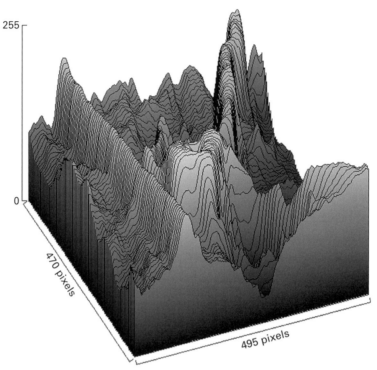

Figure 5.8   A surface plot of the angiogram image shown in Fig. 5.7(i).

their entropy is consequently low. In general, the more occupied bins and the smaller the variation in bin heights the higher the entropy. This can be seen with the images in Activity 5.3.

An image with high entropy has many different pixel values, all occurring at about the same frequency, which is evident from a surface plot, i.e. plotting the pixel values as a function of pixel position (Fig. 5.8). Entropy can characterize the *texture* of regions, whether rough or smooth, within an image because it provides information about the local variability of the pixel values. Texture can be used to distinguish normal from pathological tissue, and has been used with breast tissue to predict malignant versus benign outcomes.

If the histogram shows that some pixel values occur more frequently than others, a more efficient coding system than natural binary coding can be used for the image. Instead of using the same coding length, 8 bits for example, for each pixel value, the pixel values that occur more frequently can be assigned shorter codes, and those that occur less frequently assigned longer codes. The result is that the average code-length can be reduced without loss of information, resulting in *lossless* or *error-free* file compression. This is the basis of variable-length coding systems, such as *Huffman coding*. Entropy is indicative of how much lossless compression can be achieved for a particular image. Images with high entropy cannot be compressed significantly.

Consider an image containing only 4 pixel values (0, 1, 2 and 3), with normalized histogram values of 0.5, 0.25, 0.125 and 0.125, respectively. Sketch the histogram! The average information per symbol, or entropy, is given by

$$H = -(0.5 \ \log_2(0.5) + 0.25 \ \log_2(0.25) + 0.125 \ \log_2 (0.125)$$
$$+ 0.125 \ \log_2 (0.125))$$
$$= -(-0.5 - 0.5 - 0.375 - 0.375) = 1.75$$

This is less than the 2 bits pixel^{-1} that are required using fixed-length binary coding (00, 01, 10 and 11), indicating that the image could be compressed using appropriate coding. If the codes 0, 10, 110 and 111 were used, the average codeword length, L, would be:

$$L = (0.5 \times 1) + (0.25 \times 2) + (0.125 \times 3) + (0.125 \times 3) = 1.75$$

which is equal to the entropy; this is the condition for the best possible code, and this is therefore an *optimal* code.

Using this code results in a *file compression ratio*, C, the ratio of the size of the original file to that of the compressed file, of 2:1.75, i.e. 1.14:1, although there is a small overhead in having to attach the code table to the image. With so few pixel values, the saving in file space due to using a variable-length coding system is not great, but as the number of pixel values increases, so do the potential savings.

The entropy of the image defines the limit of compressibility by variable-length coding. An image with an *equalized* histogram, for example, cannot be compressed in this way.

5.1.3 Signal-to-noise ratio

The signal-to-noise ratio (SNR) of an image can often be estimated from the image itself, in a straightforward way. The signal, or mean intensity, of the image is characterized by the square of the mean pixel value of the entire image, $\bar{a}^2$. Noise is characterized by the variance of pixel values, σ_a^2, but needs to be measured in a region within the image which is expected to have constant gray values and is large enough so that all significant variations are included in the noise measurement. This is required so as not to confuse variations of pixel values due to local information, i.e. features, with variations due to noise. Alternatively, the noise could be measured in a second, completely uniform image acquired under the same conditions as the first image, if such an image is available. In radiography it can be obtained by imaging, for example, a block of acrylic or a uniform water "phantom," or even doing an "air scan" with only air in the beam. In each case the noise in the second image can be calculated, so long as it contains only random statistical fluctuations and no correlated noise, and assumed to be applicable to the first image.

The SNR of an image, in decibels (dB), is:

$$\text{SNR} = 10 \, \log_{10}(\bar{a}^2/\sigma_a^2) = 20 \, \log_{10}(\bar{a}/\sigma_a) \tag{5.5}$$

which is obtained from Equation (2.13), where the signal power is determined from the square of the average pixel value in the entire image and the noise power is determined from the variance within a region of interest (ROI) containing no features. Practice in finding the signal-to-noise ratio of images is given in Activity 5.4.

In many images, the goal is to distinguish a foreground structure from the background, for example a tumor from surrounding normal tissue. In such cases it is the contrast-to-noise ratio, CNR, rather than the signal-to-noise ratio, SNR, which is more useful:

$$\text{CNR} = 20 \, \log_{10}((\bar{a}_{\text{foreground}} - \bar{a}_{\text{background}})/\sigma_a) \tag{5.6}$$

where the signal, or average pixel value for the whole image, is replaced by the contrast, or difference in the average pixel values of the foreground and background. The contrast-to-noise ratio is equal to the difference in signal-to-noise ratios for the foreground and background, respectively, since the noise is similar whether measured using the foreground or background pixels.

5.1.4   Other histogram features

Spatial *moments* are a very simple and powerful way to describe the spatial distribution of values within a distribution provided that there is a sufficiently strong central tendency, i.e. a tendency to cluster around a modal value. They can be applied either to a one-dimensional distribution, such as the gray-level histogram, or to a higher-dimensional distribution, such as the image itself.

Applied to a one-dimensional discrete distribution with N possible values, x_i, the nth moment is defined by

$$m_n(x) = \sum_{i=0}^{N} P(x_i) \cdot x_i^n \tag{5.7a}$$

Central moments are defined relative to the mean, $\bar{x}$; thus the nth central moment is defined by

$$\mu_n(x) = \sum_{i=0}^{N} P(x_i) \cdot (x_i - \bar{x})^n \tag{5.7b}$$

The first moment of the histogram gives the average pixel value,

$$m_1 = \sum_{i=0}^{255} P(a_i) \cdot a_i = \bar{a} \tag{5.8a}$$

and its second central moment gives the variance,

$$\mu_1 = \sum_{i=0}^{255} P(a_i) \cdot (a_i - \overline{a})^2 = \sigma_a^2 \qquad (5.8b)$$

where the summation over $i = 0$ to 255 applies to an 8-bit deep image. The third central moment gives the *skewness* of the distribution. If it is numerically equal to zero, the histogram is symmetric. A negative value for the skewness indicates that the histogram is asymmetric to the left (i.e. its tail extends left of the center or average value); a positive value indicates that it is asymmetric to the right (i.e. its tail extends right of the center or average value). The fourth central moment gives the *kurtosis*, which is a measure of how close it is to a normal or Gaussian shape. A kurtosis of zero indicates it is Gaussian, while a negative/positive value indicates that it is flatter/more peaked than Gaussian.

5.2   Histogram transformations and look-up tables

We have seen that an image is stored as a matrix (array) of pixels, with pixel values in the range 0 to 255 if 8 bits (one byte) are used to store each pixel value. These pixel values determine the brightness of the displayed image via a display look-up table (LUT). The pixel values are addresses in the look-up table and are used to "look up" the brightness information (gray level) for that pixel (Fig. 5.9(i)), which is sent to the monitor and used to "paint" that pixel on the screen. In the identity or *default look-up table* pixel values give the gray level directly, i.e. pixel value 0 gives the 0th gray level (black), pixel value 255 gives the 255th gray level (white), pixel value 127 gives the 127th gray level (mid-gray) and so on (Fig. 5.9(ii)). The look-up table may be represented either graphically as a plot of input pixel value along the x axis against output gray level (running from black up to white) on the y axis, or as a vertical window of gray levels (Fig. 5.9(iii)).

The look-up table maps pixel values to gray values and can be used to display an image differently, by changing the distribution of pixel values into a differing distribution of gray values without changing the stored pixel values. The process can be described with the *mapping function*

$$g = M(a) \qquad (5.9)$$

where a and g are, respectively, the stored pixel values and the displayed gray levels. The form of the mapping function M determines the effect of the operation. Image transformation using a look-up table is an example of a *point operation*, where the output pixel value depends only on its corresponding input value.

The brightness of an image can be changed by either adding a fixed value to all the pixel values to brighten the image, or subtracting a fixed value from all the pixels to darken the image. However, this changes the pixel values in the image file. An alternative way to change the brightness of a displayed image, which preserves the

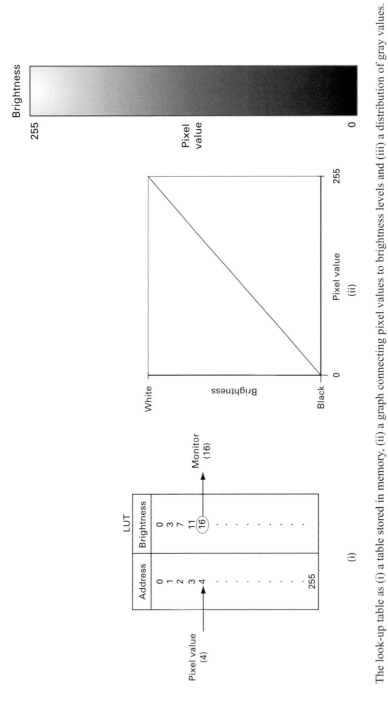

Figure 5.9 The look-up table as (i) a table stored in memory, (ii) a graph connecting pixel values to brightness levels and (iii) a distribution of gray values. (In this case, (ii) and (iii) represent the identity or default look-up table.)

original pixel values, is to use a display look-up table in which pixel values are looked up to give lighter (or darker) grays than those using the default look-up table. This could be achieved by using a look-up table that is parallel to the default look-up table, but above (or below) it.

The contrast of a displayed image can also be changed by using an appropriate look-up table, rather than multiplying or dividing pixel values by a fixed value. The contrast could be increased (or reduced) by using a look-up table with a gradient greater (or less) than the default look-up table. These changes are illustrated in Activity 5.5.

In many vision applications, it is useful to be able to separate out or *segment* the regions of the image corresponding to objects in which we are interested, from the regions of the image that correspond to background. *Thresholding* often provides an easy and convenient way to perform this segmentation on the basis of the different intensities or colors in the foreground and background regions of an image. The input to a thresholding operation is typically a grayscale image and the output is a binary image, comprising black and white pixels only, representing the segmentation. Usually black pixels correspond to background and white pixels correspond to foreground, although this can be reversed. In simple implementations, the segmentation is determined by a single parameter known as the *intensity threshold*. Each pixel in the image is compared with this threshold. If its value is higher than the threshold, the pixel is set to white in the output; if it is less than or equal to the threshold, it is set to black. The use of a step-function look-up table enables us to display the result of the thresholding, without actually changing the stored pixel values.

For more sophisticated applications, multiple thresholds can be specified, so that a *band* of pixel values in an image can be set to white while everything else is set to black, or various bands can be assigned different false colors. Identifying multiple bands is referred to as *density slicing*. For color images, it may be useful to set different thresholds for each color channel. Another common variant is to set to black all those pixels corresponding to background, but leave foreground pixels at their original intensity (as opposed to forcing them to white), so that that information is not lost.

5.2.1 Histogram stretch

An image with a dynamic range lower than the full dynamic range available (2^n) can be displayed with the full dynamic range if its histogram is stretched. The simplest solution would be a linear stretch, without otherwise changing the shape of the histogram (Fig. 5.10(i)). The operation is referred to as *histogram stretch* or *contrast stretch*. It can be implemented by a specific look-up table which leaves the pixel values unchanged but maps them to gray values covering the full range from black to white. This new look-up table maps the minimum pixel value in the image, $a_{\min}$, to black, the maximum pixel value in the image, $a_{\max}$, to white and all intermediate pixel values

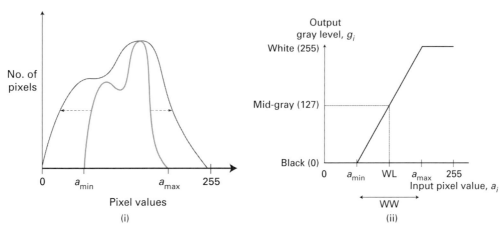

Figure 5.10   (i) The concept of linearly stretching a histogram. (ii) The look-up table required to implement a linear histogram stretch.

linearly to gray values; thus the transform from pixel values, a_i, to gray values, g_i, is given by

$$g_i = \frac{2^n - 1}{a_{max} - a_{min}} \cdot a_i \tag{5.10}$$

The required look-up table is shown in Fig. 5.10(ii). The range of values that is stretched, in this case ($a_{max} - a_{min}$), is known as the *window width* (WW), and the midpoint of the window is known as the *window level* (WL). The look-up table transforms each pixel value to its own gray level value, i.e. it is a one-to-one transform, so that the number of bins in the histogram remains the same. Since they are spread further apart by the histogram stretch, there are intervening empty bins. This can be seen in Fig. 5.11. This form of look-up table is used to implement windowing in computed tomography. A value of window level is chosen from the range {−1000 3095}, together with a value of window width, both depending on the anatomy of interest; the bottom of the window is mapped to black, and the top of the window to white.

For some images the majority of pixels may fall within a narrow range but there may be a few outlier pixels with values near the extremes of black or white. If these outlier pixels are included the window may span almost the full dynamic range possible, and very little stretching is possible. A more robust approach is to choose the window such that a certain percentage, say p%, of the pixel values is ignored. This has the effect of saturating the tails of the histogram of the modified image, by forcing $p/2$% of the pixels into the black bins, and $p/2$% into the white bins. (This can be **Process/Enhance Contrast**, selecting **Normalize** and entering the percentage of saturated pixels, p.)

For an RGB color space digital image, histogram stretching can be accomplished by converting the image to a hue, saturation, intensity (HSI) color space representation of the image and applying the brightness mapping operation to the intensity information alone.

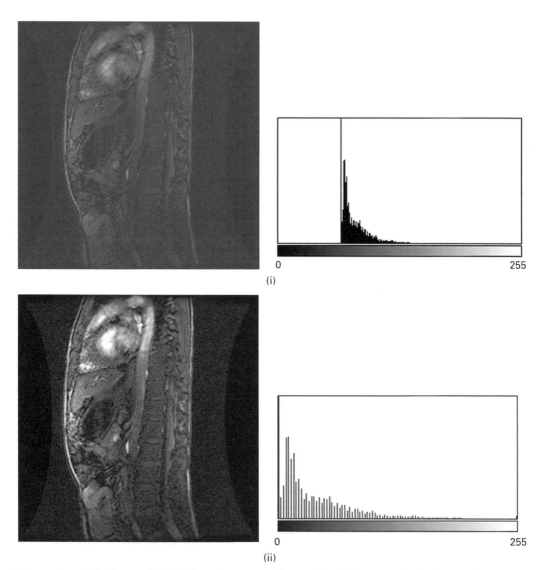

Figure 5.11 (i) An image of limited dynamic range and its gray-level histogram. (ii) The image after a linear histogram stretch, with its gray-level histogram.

In *floating-point* images the pixel values are represented by signed floating-point (FP) numbers, i.e. real numbers rather than integers, in scientific notation with a sign, a number and an exponent. In (single-precision) 32-bit numbers, the first bit is the sign bit, "S," the next eight bits are the exponent bits, "E," and the final 23 bits are the fraction, "F":

S   EEEEEEEE FFFFFFFFFFFFFFFFFFFFFFF
0   1   8 9   31

This allows a huge range of values, useful when the pixel values represent some physical quantity. When converting floating-point pixel values to 8-bit integer pixel values, the range is first *normalized* to 0–255 before conversion to 8-bit integers. This can be done with a mapping function similar to the look-up table for histogram stretch, such as

$$g_i = \text{round}\left(\frac{(2^n - 1) \cdot \text{FP}_i}{(\text{FP}_{\text{max}}) - (\text{FP}_{\text{min}})}\right) \tag{5.11}$$

where *round* indicates quantization on to the 256 available levels. Obviously some information is lost in the normalization process, but the relative intensities of the pixels are preserved. *Double-precision* floating-point numbers assign 64 bits to a number to encompass an even bigger range: one bit for the sign, "S," 11 bits for the exponent, "E," and 52 bits for the fraction, "F."

5.2.2   Histogram equalization

When it is necessary to compare several images, which may have been acquired under differing conditions, on a specific basis, such as for quantitative texture measurement, it is usual to try to standardize their histograms. The most common standardization technique is histogram equalization, where one attempts to change the histogram into a flat, uniform or equalized histogram, in which every pixel value occurs equally frequently. The expectation is that this maximizes the information conveyed in the image and that the transformed image has an enhanced appearance.

Consider an "input" image, A, with a normalized histogram or probability density function (PDF), $p(x)$. A transfer function, $y = T(x)$ (Fig. 5.12), will map its probability

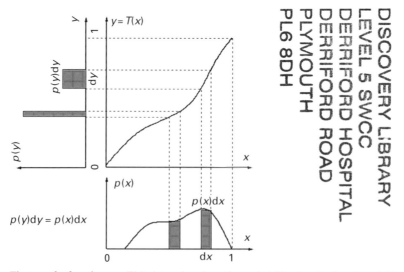

Figure 5.12   The transfer function, $y = T(x)$, determines how the probability density function $p(x)$ is transformed into the probability density function $p(y)$.

density function into an alternative probability density function, $p(y)$, describing the intensity levels of an "output" image, B. Since the number of pixels mapped from x to y is unchanged,

$$p(y)\mathrm{d}y = p(x)\mathrm{d}x \tag{5.12}$$

If we want the "output" image to have a flat, equalized probability density function then $p(y)$ should be constant (and equal to 1/255 for an 8-bit image). Thus

$$\mathrm{d}y = p(x)\mathrm{d}x \tag{5.13a}$$

or

$$\mathrm{d}y/\mathrm{d}x = p(x) \tag{5.13b}$$

The mapping function, $y = T(x)$, for histogram equalization is therefore

$$A(x, y) = \mathrm{CDFB} - 1\{\mathrm{CDFA}(A(x, y))\} \tag{5.14}$$

where

$$T(x) = \int_0^x p(u)\mathrm{d}u, \quad T(0) = 0 \tag{5.15}$$

Intuitively, we can see that

- if $p(x)$ is high, $T(x)$ has a steep slope, $\mathrm{d}y$ will be wide, causing $p(y)$ to be low to keep $p(y)\mathrm{d}y = p(x)\mathrm{d}x$;
- if $p(x)$ is low, $T(x)$ has a shallow slope, $\mathrm{d}y$ will be narrow, causing $p(y)$ to be high.

For discrete gray levels, the gray level of the input image, x, takes one of the discrete values, $x = \{0, 1, 2, \ldots, 255\}$, and the continuous integral transfer function becomes discrete

$$T(x) = \sum_{i=0}^x p_i \tag{5.16}$$

and is the cumulative distribution function (CDF) of the input image. Thus the transfer function, or look-up table, required to achieve histogram equalization is the cumulative distribution function (CDF), suitably scaled to the range $0 < y \leq 255$, which is obtained by integrating the pixel value histogram of the image (Section 5.1). Each image requires its own specific look-up table, obtained from its histogram (Fig. 5.13(i)). It is monotonic and, in general, non-linear, unlike the linear look-up table used in histogram stretching.

In the discrete implementation, the output image will not necessarily be fully equalized. The scaled look-up table may yield values that are not equal to the available

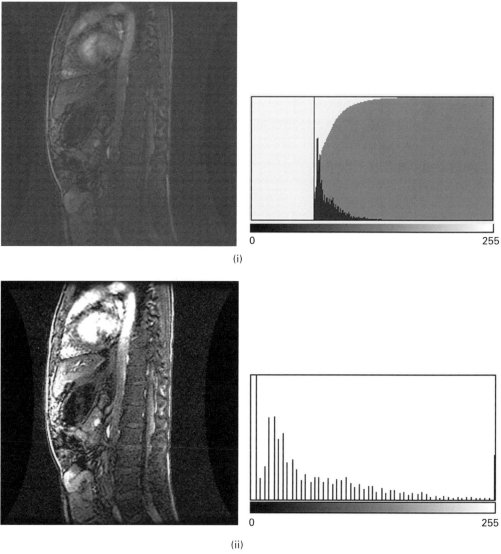

Figure 5.13 (i) An image of limited dynamic range (same as Fig. 5.10(i)) and its gray-level histogram with superimposed cumulative distribution function. (ii) The image after histogram equalization, using the cumulative distribution function of the original image as a look-up table, and its gray-level histogram. Compare the resulting histogram with that of the histogram stretched image of Fig. 5.11(ii).

quantized gray levels, and the values will have to be quantized to the nearest available levels. Indeed transformed values may be quantized to the same level, even though they were different in the original image; this renders the (discrete) histogram equalization technique non-unique and irreversible, and the entropy of the transformed image lower, rather than higher, than the original image. There will generally be gaps (i.e. unused intensity levels) in the histogram of the output image, because pixels of the same gray level in the input histogram cannot be separated to satisfy a completely constant distribution in the output histogram. This results in only an approximately flat histogram (Fig. 5.13(ii)). These effects decrease as the number of pixels and intensity quantization levels in the input image are increased. Despite these drawbacks, histogram equalization remains a popular method for image enhancement.

In Figure 5.14, the histogram (PDF) and cumulative distribution function (CDF) of an "input" image in Figure 5.14(i) is shown in Figure 5.14(ii). The cumulative distribution function is used as the transfer function (or look-up table) to produce an "output" image (Fig. 5.14(iii)). Although the histogram of the "output" image is not completely flat/equalized (Fig. 5.14(iv)), it is considerably flatter than that of the "input" image; and the cumulative distribution function of the histogram of the "output" image is close to a linear ramp (as expected for a flat histogram).

The use of the cumulative distribution function as a look-up table to implement histogram equalization is illustrated in Activity 5.6. An advantage of histogram equalization is that it is fully automatic; i.e., given an image, we can extract its gray-level histogram

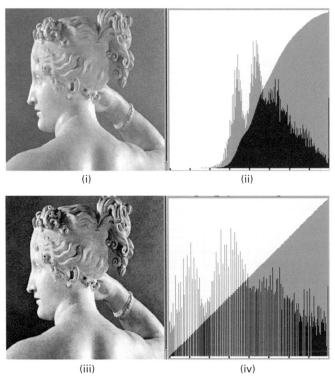

(i) (ii)

(iii) (iv)

Figure 5.14 (i) "Input" image. (ii) Histogram with cumulative distribution function (CDF) overlaid. (iii) Histogram-equalized "output" image, using the scaled cumulative distribution function of the "input" image as the look-up table. (iv) The histogram and cumulative distribution function of image (iii).

and then obtain its cumulative distribution function, which after scaling is used as the look-up table, without the need for specifying any parameters. The computation is simple since it only involves repeated additions of the histogram values.

However, the use of a global transform and the consequent merging of gray levels that had low probabilities of occurrence in the original image can be a significant problem in medical images. Attempts have been made to address this issue by applying histogram equalization on a local basis, so-called *local-area histogram equalization*. The histogram of the pixels within a sliding rectangular window, centered on the current pixel being processed, is applied only to that pixel and the process repeated for every pixel in the image. The method is computationally expensive and can introduce artifacts due to the artificial rectangular shape of the moving window. *Adaptive local-area histogram equalization* has also been used, where the window used for a particular pixel is not constrained to a particular shape or size but can adapt to its environment.

5.2.3   Histogram matching

Sometimes it may be useful to transform an image so that its histogram has a certain shape or matches that of another image. Histogram matching, in general, requires non-linear and non-monotonic look-up tables to map between pixel values in the input and output images.

Suppose we wish to transform an image, A, so that its histogram matches that of image B. This can be achieved in a two-step process. First, the image is transformed so that it has an equalized histogram using its cumulative density function, CDF_A, as the LUT. Now the cumulative distribution function of image B, CDF_B, can be used to histogram-equalize image C. Conversely, the inverse of that cumulative distribution function could be used to transform an image with a flat histogram into an image with the histogram of B; that is what is required for the second stage of the transformation of image A. Thus

$$A'(x,y) = CDF_B^{-1}\{CDFA(A(x,y)\}$$ (5.17)

transforms image A into an image A', having a histogram that matches image B.

This can be used in *photometric calibration*, by transforming an image produced by a digitizer with photometric non-linearity (i.e. its output gray level has a non-linear relationship with input film density) to what it would have been using an ideal, linear digitizer.

5.2.4   Local histogram transformations

The histogram transformations discussed above are global in that they apply a transform or look-up table whose form is based on the gray-level distribution of an entire image.

Although this method can enhance the overall contrast and dynamic range of an image, there are cases in which enhancement of details over small areas is desired. The solution in these cases is to derive a look-up table based upon the gray-level distribution in the local neighborhood of every pixel in the image.

The procedure involves defining a neighborhood around each pixel and, using the histogram characteristics of this neighborhood, deriving a look-up table which maps that pixel into an output intensity level. This is performed for each pixel in the image. Since moving across rows or down columns only adds several new pixels to the local histogram, updating the histogram from the previous calculation is possible.

5.2.5 Other histogram transformations

There are a number of other commonly used gray-level histogram transformations that can be implemented by display look-up tables (Fig. 5.15). The linear or identity line is the default value. A line of negative slope transforms an image into its *complement* or *inverse*, i.e. the equivalent of its photographic negative. This transformation is sometimes made when looking at bones or mammographic images (Fig. 5.16). The logarithmic and square root transformations expand the displayed brightness at the dark end of the scale,

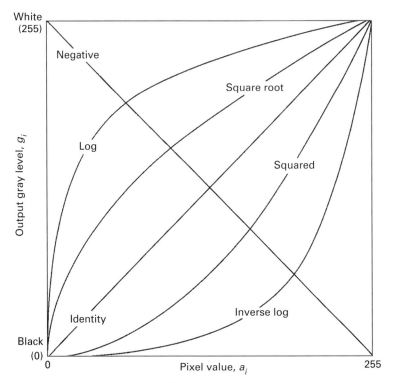

Figure 5.15   Examples of look-up tables used for enhancing images.

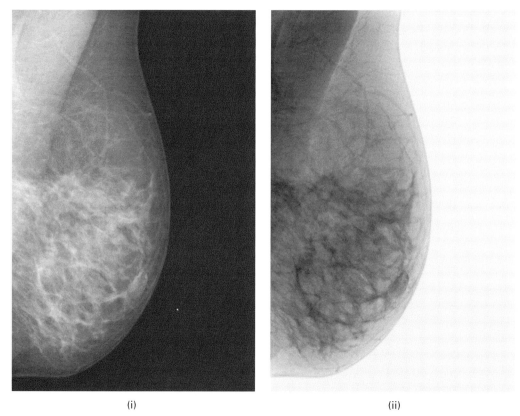

| (i) | (ii) |

Figure 5.16   (i) Original mammographic image and (ii) its complement.

and compress them at the bright end. This type of relationship can be used to convert an image from a camera with a linear response curve to the logarithmic brightness curve of the human visual system. It is also used to compress the dynamic range of images, such as astronomical images. The effects of the log look-up and the inverse log look-up tables is illustrated in Activity 5.7.

Power-law transformations have the general form:

$$\text{output gray level} = \text{factor}^*(\text{input pixel value})^\gamma \tag{5.18}$$

where the exponent is known as the *gamma* of the transformation, e.g. $\gamma = 1/2$ for the square root transformation and $\gamma = 2$ for the square transformation. Pixel values are "raised to the power" of the gamma value, and the output values are scaled to 8 bits (0–255). Faint objects can be made brighter without saturating bright objects by using $\gamma < 1$, or bright objects can be dimmed without losing less bright objects by using $\gamma > 1$. Rather than directly computing the transformation for each pixel in an image, which

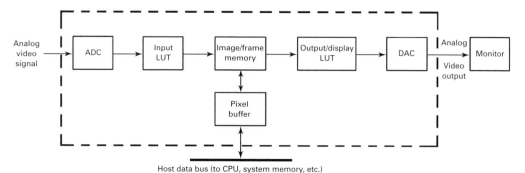

Host data bus (to CPU, system memory, etc.)

Figure 5.17   Schematic of frame-grabber board containing input and output LUTs.

would be very computer intensive, the output values are pre-calculated for the 256 possible input values and stored in a look-up table. Gamma correction can be important when using computer monitors, which generally have a power-law response function with an exponent close to 2. In order to display an image accurately on a monitor with an exponent of 2.5, for example, the image should be pre-processed using a power-law look-up table with a gamma of $(2.5)^{-1} = 0.4$.

In most imaging systems, look-up tables are implemented in hardware on a frame-grabber board (Fig. 5.17). An input look-up table may be located between the analog-to-digital converter (ADC) and the frame or image memory. Its use is generally limited to the situation where the digitization precision is higher than the storage precision, or for compressing a large dynamic range using a non-linear look-up table. The output or display look-up table, located between the image memory and the digital-to-analog converter (DAC), is much more versatile since it does not change the stored pixel values. Figure 5.17 shows how the frame-grabber board interfaces with the host computer, which performs the image processing tasks using its central processor unit (CPU). Display look-up tables can also be used to convert a grayscale image into a *pseudocolor* or false color image, thus enhancing the visibility of particular structures in an image; this is frequently the case with ultrasound images. Three look-up tables are required, one for each of the three digital-to-analog converters used for the primary colors red, green and blue.

Digital medical imaging systems have a suite of transforms, stored in memory as look-up tables, which can be selected by the operator to modify the appearance of a stored image. The image can be displayed using various look-up tables until the operator judges that the features of most interest are best shown. Computed radiography (CR) systems, for example, allow the user to display the image using the linear look-up table applicable to the image plate (IP) detector or to use a sigmoidal display look-up table that mimics the shape of a film characteristic curve. Many imaging systems allow the user to custom-build a look-up table interactively using the mouse. The effect of using different look-up tables to view an image is explored in Activity 5.8.

Computer-based activities

Activity 5.1 Image brightness

Open the image **mri** in ImageJ. Note that it is rather dark. Display its gray-level histogram (**Analyze/Histogram**), and note its mean pixel value. Note that although the vertical scaling of the bin heights is not displayed, any individual bin height can be found by moving the cursor within the histogram; the pixel value is shown as "Value," and the bin height as "Count." Click on the **mri** image, to ensure that it is the current image, and go to **Image/Adjust/... Brightness/Contrast**. Move the **Brightness** slider to lighten the image. Once you are satisfied with the setting, click **Apply**, and then look at the histogram of the lightened image (**Analyze/Histogram**). Note its shape and mean pixel value. How does it compare with the histogram of the original image?

Do the same for the image **dsa stent**, which has been acquired by Digital Subtraction Angiography (DSA) and which shows the pelvis of a patient who has had a kidney transplant and a stent placement. Note that there is significant pixelation.

Activity 5.2 Contrast and dynamic range

Open the image **MRIhead** in ImageJ. Go to **Analyze/Histogram** to see the histogram of pixel values. Note the minimum and maximum pixel values (a_{min} and a_{max}); the difference between them is the dynamic range. Click the menu bar of **MRIhead** again. Move the contrast slider (in **Image/Adjust... Brightness/Contrast**) to the left (for lower contrast) and to the right (for higher contrast), watching the image as you do this. The contrast of the image changes, as does the look-up table in the "B&C" box (but the histogram does not change). Move the slider as far to the right as you think is needed to obtain an image of acceptable contrast, and click **Apply** to see the histogram update in the "B&C" box. Note that the original histogram has been stretched; the "new" image has a higher dynamic range and a better contrast. The pixel values have been spread out, but there are the same number of bins, so that gaps or missing values appear in the histogram. You can see these more clearly if you close the "histogram" window and then re-open it, so that it is updated too. What happens to the histogram as you continue to increase the contrast of the image?

Lower the contrast of the image with the contrast slider, and note that the number of pixel values is reduced so that periodically the pixel values pile up and produce higher spikes.

Activity 5.3 Entropy

Open image **noise** in ImageJ and obtain its gray-level histogram (**Analyze/ Histogram**). Use the entropy plugin (**Plugins/Ch.5 Plugins/Entropy**) to obtain its entropy in bits pixel^{-1}. Repeat using the following images: **histeq**, **16 gray-bands**, **8 gray-bands**, **4 gray-bands** and **2 gray-bands**.

Comment on the entropy values obtained and their relationship to the gray-level histograms referencing Equation (5.3).

Open image **dsa stent**; how does its entropy relate to its gray-level histogram? Adjust the contrast of the image using histogram stretch (**Process/Enhance Contrast** and check "Normalize," with saturated pixels set to 0%) and save the image using a different name: view its histogram and record its entropy. Now histogram-equalize the original **dsa stent** image (**Process/Enhance Contrast** and check "Equalize Histogram") and save this image using another name: view its histogram and record its entropy. Compare the entropies of the three images. Note that the number of bins in each of the three histograms is the same. The bin heights stayed the same as the original with histogram stretch, they just moved further apart; whereas in histogram equalization the bin heights changed and became more equal.

Repeat the exercise with the **broken foot** and **thermography** images.

Look at the surface plots of the three original images (**Analyze/Surface Plot** and check "Draw Wireframe"). Is there a connection between the shape of the surface plots and the entropy of the images?

Activity 5.4 Signal-to-noise ratio

Open the **angiogram** image in ImageJ. View its histogram using the **Live Histogram Plugin** (in **Plugins/Ch.5 Plugins**). Select as large a region as possible with constant gray values, using the polygon selection tool. Find the signal-to-noise ratio, as both a ratio and in decibels (dB), using the **SNR** plugin in **Plugins/Ch.5 Plugins**.

Smooth the image (**Process/Smooth**). How does this affect the shape of the histogram? How do the mean and standard deviation change? Try several iterations of smoothing to see the trend clearly. Now sharpen the original image (**Process/ Sharpen**). How does this affect the shape of the histogram? How do the mean and standard deviation (and dynamic range) change? Again, try several iterations to see the trend clearly. Explain the changes.

Add Gaussian noise (**Process/Noise/Add Specified Noise**) with a standard deviation of 10 to the original **angiogram** image. Compare the updated histogram with the histogram of the original image, in terms of its overall shape, its standard deviation and its dynamic range. Estimate the signal-to-noise ratio of the noisy image. Repeat after adding noise of standard deviation 20 to the original image. How does the signal-to-noise ratio change with added noise?

Activity 5.5 Look-up tables

Open up image **normal mri** in ImageJ, and display its histogram (**Analyze/ Histogram**). Click on the image, and go to **Image/ Adjust/...Brightness/ Contrast**; the histogram of pixel values is shown again, with the identity look-up table overlaid on it. The displayed image changes interactively as the brightness slider is moved, first to the left of center, and then to the right: the image becomes darker, then brighter. Watch what happens to the display look-up table. The darker display is caused by the look-up table moving to the right but remaining parallel to the default look-up table; a pixel value from the image file is looked up on this shifted look-up table to give a smaller (darker) gray-level value. The brighter display image is a consequence of the look-up table shifting to the left but remaining parallel to the default look-up table, causing pixel values to be looked up as higher gray-level values. Pressing the "Reset" button returns the display look-up table to its default values, namely the identity look-up table. (Note that the histogram shown is the histogram of pixel values and does not change, unless the "Apply" button is pressed.)

Click "Reset" to return to the original look-up table. Now move the contrast slider first to the left and then to the right. Note how the displayed image changes, and how the look-up table changes to produce these effects. The gradient or slope of the look-up table changes to modify the displayed contrast; a look-up table with a higher gradient produces a higher contrast displayed image, and vice versa. If these changes are made permanent, by pressing the "Apply" button, the histogram changes: a high-contrast histogram corresponds to one with a large dynamic range.

The contrast can be continuously increased by dragging the slider to the right, which increases the slope of the look-up table, to the extreme when the look-up table approaches a step function with a very steep slope at a particular pixel value. This pixel value is known as the *threshold* and the look-up table implements *thresholding* by displaying all pixels up to and including that value as black, and those above it as white. The resulting image has the maximum possible contrast, comprising just black and white pixels. A look-up table with an increasingly shallow slope produces a displayed image of low contrast; the extreme in this direction is obtained when the look-up table becomes horizontal, resulting in all pixels being displayed as mid-gray and the image having no contrast at all.

Activity 5.6 Histogram equalization

Open the `dsa stent` image in ImageJ and apply the **Live Histogram Plugin**. Make a duplicate of the image, apply histogram equalization (**Process/ Enhance Contrast** and check **Equalize** (the saturated pixels are ignored)) and save the result. What effect does histogram equalization have on the appearance of the image? How has the shape of its histogram changed?

Using the original image, go to **Image/Color/Show LUT** to see the default (identity) LUT. Click "List" to see a text listing, comprising four columns; the first column contains the pixel values 1–155, and the next three columns contain the looked-up values of red, green and blue; because this is a gray-scale LUT each of these three columns is identical. (The LUT can be viewed as a 16×16 array of grayscales with **Image/Color/Edit LUT**.)

Click on `dsa stent` and start the **CDF** plugin (in **Ch. 5 Plugins**). A window opens, containing the histogram and the cumulative density function (CDF) superimposed in gray, as well as a results box containing the pixel values and the cumulative bin counts. The cumulative density function values are written to a file **CDF_LUT.txt** in the form of a LUT recognized by ImageJ. Import this text file into ImageJ, using **File/Import/LUT**. This look-up table immediately applies to the image **dsa stent**, which is now histogram-equalized: you can view the look-up table using **Image/Color/Show LUT**.

The same result can be obtained using ImageJ's built-in histogram equalization (**Process/Enhance Contrast/Histogram Equalization**).

Activity 5.7 Log and inverse log look-up tables

Open **dsa stent** in ImageJ, and check that the display look-up table is the identity look-up table, using **Image/Color/Show LUT**.

Make a duplicate of the stent image. Using **File/Import/LUT...** import the text file **logLUT.txt**. The imported log look-up table is immediately applied to the duplicate image. Note the difference in appearance. Observe the log look-up table using **Image/Color/Show LUT**.

Make another duplicate of the original stent image. Using **File/Import/LUT...** import the text file **invlogLUT.txt**. The imported inverse log look-up table is immediately applied to the duplicate image. This particular image becomes very dark! Observe the inverse log look-up table using **Image/Color/Show LUT**.

A number of transforms can be applied directly to images in ImageJ using **Process/Math** and selecting the appropriate look-up table from the list.

Activity 5.8 Applying different look-up tables

Open up **chest radiograph**, and display its LUT using **Image/Color/Show LUT**. Make a duplicate of the radiograph. Go to **File/Import/LUT** and choose **s-curve LUT.txt**. Note the changed appearance of the image. Display its look-up table, which is sigmoidal in shape like the characteristic curve of film. Thus the original image data may have been collected by computed radiography (CR) and viewed with the identity look-up table; the duplicate is viewed with a sigmoidal look-up table which is one of several available on most computed radiography systems, and shows how the image would appear if captured on film.

Exercises

5.1 Suppose that you had a scene of three objects of different distinct intensities against an extremely bright background. What would the histogram of the corresponding image look like?

5.2 Draw annotated sketches of the histograms of the following types of images:
   (i) a collection of objects of the same gray level placed on a uniform background of another gray level;
   (ii) a collection of relatively dark objects on a relatively bright background, both having a spread of gray levels;

(iii) an under-exposed radiograph;

(iv) an over-exposed radiograph.

5.3 Draw the look-up tables that would display the following:

(i) a band of pixels, between Thr_1 and Thr_2, as white (foreground) and all other pixels as black (background);

(ii) a band of pixels, between Thr_1 and Thr_2, as their "normal" (default) shades of gray, and all other pixels as black (background).

Suggest a possible application for each of these look-up tables.

5.4 Imagine you have an image taken in low light and which, as a result, has low contrast. What are the advantages of using contrast stretching to improve the contrast rather than simply scaling the image by a constant factor (i.e. multiplying all the pixel values by the constant factor)?

5.5 Explain the advantage of using a logarithmic look-up table to view astronomy images.

5.6 Sketch the corresponding cumulative distribution functions, CDFs, for the probability density functions, PDFs, shown in Figure E5.1.

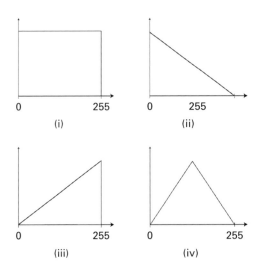

Figure E5.1

5.7 Table E5.1 gives the number of pixels at each of the gray levels in a 4-bit deep (i.e. 16 gray levels) image. Draw the gray-level histogram, perform histogram equalization and draw the resulting histogram. What is the objective of histogram equalization?

Gray level	Number of pixels
0	20
1	40
2	60
3	75
4	80
5	75
6	65
7	55
8	50
9	45
10	40
11	35
12	30
13	25
14	20
15	30

5.8 Suppose that you histogram-equalize a digital image. Explain why histogram-equalizing the result does not lead to any significant change.

5.9 Perform histogram equalization on the image of a cell colony (Fig. E5.2), and describe the resulting image. Can you obtain a better result by using histogram stretch and parameters of your choosing? (In what way do you think the image is better?) When the contrast is improved, it becomes more apparent that the illumination of the field of view was uneven. Can you think of a way to improve this unevenness?

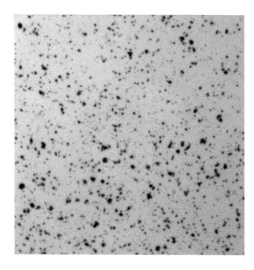

Figure E5.2

5.10 What is the dynamic range of the image shown in Figure E5.3? Use whichever method you consider gives the best improvement in contrast, and comment on the resulting image.

Figure E5.3

6 Image enhancement in the spatial domain

Overview

Image enhancement is the processing of images to improve their appearance to human viewers, in terms of better contrast and visibility of features of interest, or to enhance their performance in subsequent computer-aided analysis and diagnosis. Because the objective of image enhancement is dependent on the application context and is often poorly defined, and the criteria are often subjective, image enhancement techniques tend to be ad hoc. Enhancement techniques include *point operations*, where the output pixel value depends only on its corresponding input value, and *local or neighborhood operations*, where the eventual output pixel value depends on the neighborhood of input pixel values. These latter operations include convolution, which uses appropriate masks or kernels to produce smoothing or sharpening of an image.

Learning objectives

After reading this chapter you will be able to:

- describe the effect on the signal-to-noise ratio (SNR) of averaging noisy images;
- remove uneven background in an image;
- outline applications of image multiplication and division;
- describe the applications of logical and geometric operations;
- explain the process of convolution and the role of the point spread function (PSF) in imaging;
- recognize the benefits of using a variety of masks, including the median and Gaussian masks, for smoothing;
- distinguish between convolution masks used for smoothing and those used for sharpening an image;
- separate two-dimensional masks into one-dimensional masks where possible;
- choose appropriate techniques to sharpen an image, including an image with significant noise;
- compare the use of first and second derivative masks in finding edges.

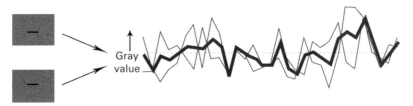

Figure 6.1   Noisy CT images of a water phantom, with a profile from each (solid lines) and the mean of the two profiles (thick solid line).

6.1   Algebraic operations

Algebraic operations produce an output image which is the pixel-by-pixel sum, difference, product or quotient of two or more input images.

6.1.1   Averaging

A noisy image contains random fluctuations above and below the image data. Figure 6.1 shows two x-ray computed tomography (CT) images taken of a *water phantom*, a container of water used as a homogeneous subject for scanning, under identical conditions. Profiles along corresponding lines in the images indicate that the pixel values in each profile fluctuate randomly around the mean gray value, which corresponds to a CT number of zero. The profiles are not identical because the fluctuations are random. However, if the two profiles are averaged, then the resulting profile fluctuates by a lesser amount.

In some imaging systems, it is possible to obtain multiple images of the same object each differing only in the amount of random noise which has been added during the imaging process. For example, we may have M images in which the essential part of the image is unchanged, but each has a random noise pattern superimposed, i.e.

$$D_i(x, y) = S(x, y) + N_i(x, y) \qquad (6.1)$$

where $S(x, y)$ is the unchanged feature that is being imaged, and $N_i(x, y)$ is the additive noise. The latter is either quantum (or statistical) noise arising from the discrete nature of electromagnetic radiation, or it is electronic noise introduced by the imaging system. We saw in Section 2.5.3 that most medical images are quantum limited, i.e. the quantum noise component is dominant, and quantum noise follows Poissonian statistics with a signal-to-noise ratio (SNR) given by the square root of the signal strength. Electronic noise follows Gaussian statistics, resulting in a bell-shaped distribution curve. Both are examples of *uncorrelated* noise. If the M images are averaged, each pixel value in the resulting image is formed by adding M pixels from corresponding positions in each image and dividing the sum by M. During addition the signal values add, but the noise pattern builds up more slowly since the squares of the noise add rather than the noise values themselves. As a consequence, the stationary component of the

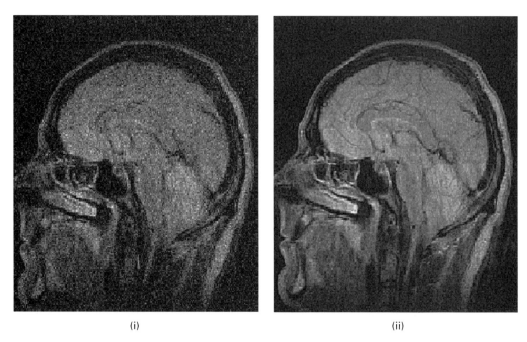

(i)   (ii)

Figure 6.2   MRI images reconstructed from (i) one and (ii) eight measurements.

image remains constant and the noise is reduced by $\sqrt{M}$ to give an increased signal-to-noise ratio (SNR).

Averaging images to increase the signal-to-noise ratio of the resulting image can be implemented in a number of medical imaging systems. It is frequently done in nuclear medicine imaging (Section 3.2), for example, either by adding M sequentially acquired images pixel-by-pixel or by acquiring a final image over a time M times longer than initially planned. Both methods result in an increased dose of radiation to the patient, and therefore should only be used if there is no alternative to acquire an image of diagnostic quality. Averaging can be performed in magnetic resonance imaging (MRI) by reconstructing the image from the average of a number of measurements (Fig. 6.2).

Given the finite range of gray values (say, [0, 255]), it is very important to ensure that the addition step does not result in overflow and subsequent clipping of the pixel values. This can be avoided if the pixel values are added into a temporary matrix which is stored with a greater depth (say, 12 or 16 bits per pixel) prior to division and re-scaling to [0, 255].

6.1.2   Image subtraction

If an image is contaminated by an uneven background shading pattern, caused by uneven illumination of the scene or variations in detector sensitivity, it can be improved by subtracting the background image from it. If the background image cannot be acquired independently, it can often be synthesized by blurring the original image to such an extent

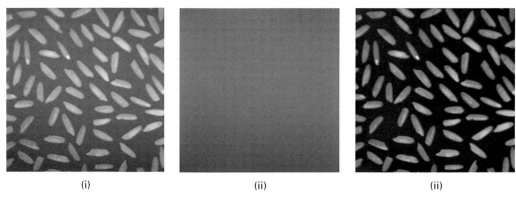

Figure 6.3   (i) An image and (ii) its background, obtained by blurring it with a Gaussian mask. (iii) The result of subtracting the background (ii) from the original image (i) and stretching the contrast.

that the features within it are spread out so much as to be no longer identifiable and only the underlying shading remains (Fig. 6.3). Practice in applying the appropriate blurring to obtain a background is provided in Activity 6.1.

Subtraction can lead to an underflow, i.e. pixel values less than zero. Again, to avoid clipping, a temporary storage matrix with a greater depth (say, 12 or 16 bits per pixel) or the use of *signed floating-point numbers* (i.e. numbers which are non-integral and can be positive or negative) is needed to store the differences prior to re-scaling to [0, 255].

In digital subtraction angiography (DSA), images taken immediately before (the *mask* or pre-contrast image) and just after (the *live* or post-contrast image) an injected bolus of iodinated contrast material reaches the region of interest are subtracted, ideally leaving an image of just the iodinated blood (Fig. 3.23). In practice, it is the logarithm of the images that are subtracted, equivalent to division of the original images.

In practical computer vision, motion analysis requires the storage and manipulation of image sequences rather than single images. Each image in a sequence is often called a *frame*, and the time which elapses between each frame being digitized is called the *frame interval*. The inverse of the frame interval, the number of frames per second, is the *frame rate*. For many applications, such as automatic control, the ideal is to process each frame as it arrives, i.e. in *real time* or *online*. Image subtraction of two images, sequentially acquired from a stationary detector, can be used to detect relative motion of objects if the two images are accurately *registered*, i.e. they record exactly the same region. A problem with this technique is that the gray level changes both where the object *was* in the previous frame and where it *is* in the current frame to give a kind of double view of each object. Both this effect and the residual edges caused if registration is not perfect can be minimized if the difference image is subsequently thresholded.

6.1.3   Multiplication and division

Subtraction of a background image to correct for uneven illumination rests on the assumption that image features are additively superimposed on the scene background. However, in a non-linear system this is not the case, and the intensity associated with a feature is in fact proportional to the background intensity in that part of the image. In such cases, division of the image by a scaled version of its background, rather than subtraction, removes the uneven background. (You can explore this in Activity 6.2.) Division of images is a problem if the divisor image contains a pixel value of zero. This is usually avoided by adding a 1 to the entire pixel values of the background image so that they run from 1 to 256, and then re-scaling after division. The division process also removes artifacts that are caused by variations in the pixel-to-pixel sensitivity of the detector and/ or by distortions in the optical path. The process is often referred to as "flat-fielding," since it seeks to produce a "flat" or uniform background in an image. It is a standard calibration procedure in everything from pocket digital cameras to giant telescopes.

Image division is also used when processing images are collected in different spectral bands; the ratio of the images is an effective way of generating an image at an intermediate spectral band.

Multiplication of images can be used for superposition of texture on to an image, or for masking portions of an image. A potential difficulty with multiplication is that an extreme range of pixel values may be generated. Even with automatic re-scaling a significant loss of precision can result for some values.

6.2 Logical (Boolean) operations

Logical operations also operate on a pixel-by-pixel basis. They often use binarized images as their input. All logical operations can be implemented from a combination of three basic operations, AND, OR and NOT. The effect of each of these is given by a truth table (Fig. 6.4). Bit "1" is associated with "true" (or "ON") and bit "0" with "false" (or "OFF"). The AND operator produces an output that is 1 (true) if both inputs A *and* B

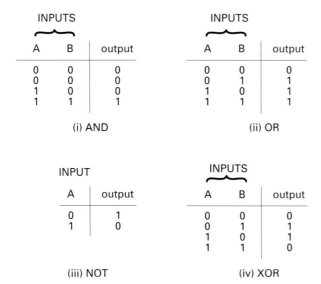

Figure 6.4   Truth tables for (i) AND, (ii) OR, (iii) NOT and (iv) XOR.

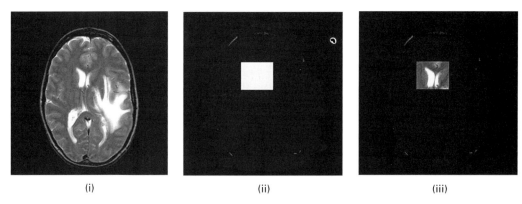

(i)   (ii)   (iii)

Figure 6.5   (i) Original image; (ii) AND mask; (iii) result of ANDing (i) with (ii).

are 1 (true); otherwise it produces a 0 (false). The OR operator produces an output that is 1 (true) if either inputs A *or* B (or both) are 1 (true); otherwise it produces a 0 (false). And the NOT operator produces an output that is *not* equal to the (single) input.

The operator, XOR (exclusive OR), produces an output that is 1 (true) if either inputs A *or* B (but not both) are 1 (true); otherwise it produces a 0 (false).

The most obvious application of AND is to compute the *intersection* of two images, highlighting all ON (1) pixels common to two input images. The OR operation computes the *union* of the images, highlighting all pixels which represent an object either in the first *or* in the second image. And the XOR operation is used to find positions whose pixel values in the two images differ.

The logical operators can be applied to grayscale images, in which case they are applied bit-wise to the corresponding bits from the pixel values of the input images. For example, for two 8-bit pixels **00100100** and **00100001** from images A and B, the XOR operation produces

A   **0 0 1 0 0 1 0 0**
B   **0 0 1 0 0 0 0 1**
XOR   **0 0 0 0 0 1 0 1**

The NOT operation is used for obtaining the *inverse* or *complement* of an image. The AND, OR and XOR operations are used for masking, i.e. selecting sub-images within an image, often referred to as *region of interest* (ROI) processing. You define a region of interest by creating a *binary mask*, which is a binary image that is the same size as the image you want to process. For the AND mask the pixels that define the region of interest are set to white (1111 1111) and all other pixels set to black (0000 0000), and it is logically ANDed with the image. The pixels in the region of interest within the image remain the same, while the pixels outside the region of interest become black (Fig. 6.5). A similar result can be obtained by logically ORing the image with a mask where the pixels defining the region of interest are set to black.

The AND operation can also be used to perform so called *bit-slicing* of an image to give *bit-planes*. To determine the influence of one particular bit on an 8-bit image, the image is ANDed in a bitwise fashion with a constant number, where the relevant bit is set to 1 and

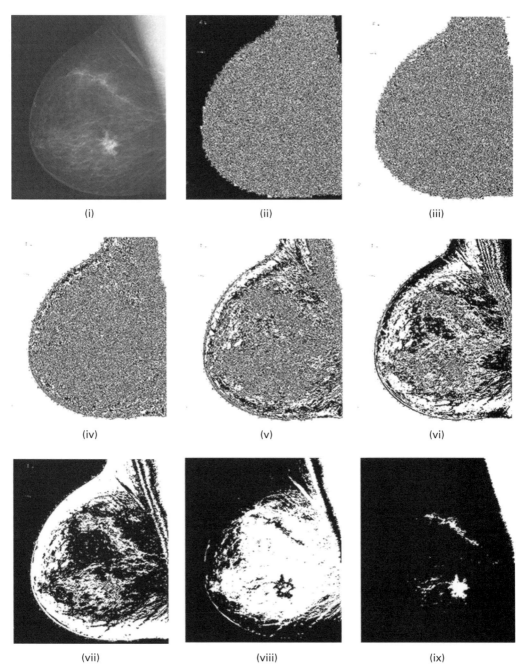

(i) (ii) (iii)

(iv) (v) (vi)

(vii) (viii) (ix)

Figure 6.6   (i) A mammography image and its bit planes: (ii) bit-plane 0, (iii) bit-plane 1, (iv) bit-plane 2, (v) bit-plane 3, (vi) bit-plane 4, (vii) bit-plane 5, (viii) bit-plane 6, (ix) bit-plane 7.

the remaining 7 bits are set to 0. For example, to obtain bit-plane 7 (bp7, corresponding to the most significant bit) the image is ANDed with 128 (10000000 binary); bit-plane 4 (bp4) is obtained by ANDing with 16 (00010000 binary). Figure 6.6 shows a mammography image and its constituent bit-planes. Note that the least significant bit-plane (bp0) is essentially random noise, and the most significant bit-plane (bp7) is actually a threshold of the image at level 127. Activity 6.3 involves finding the bit-planes of an image.

The original image, I, can be obtained from the bit-planes by combining them as a weighted sum, i.e.

$$I = (2^*(2^*(2^*(2^*(2^*(2^*(2^*bp7 + bp6) + bp5) + bp4)$$
$$+ bp3) + bp2) + bp1) + bp0) \quad (6.2)$$

Operations on grayscale images can be problematic. For example, it is not guaranteed that ANDing two high pixel values in a bitwise fashion yields a high output value (for example, 128 AND 127 yields 0). A problem with ORing grayscale images is that the output can fluctuate wildly with a small change in one of the input pixel values. For example, 127 ORed with 128 gives 255, whereas 127 ORed with 126 gives 127. To avoid these problems, it is best to operate on binarized images.

Logical operations are used frequently in *morphological processing* (Chapter 9).

6.3   Geometric operations

It is often necessary to perform elementary geometric operations or transformations on an image such as scaling (zooming), translation, reflection, rotation and shear. Two separate algorithms are required for a geometric operation. First, there is the spatial transformation itself. Then there is an algorithm for gray-level interpolation, since in general integer (x, y) positions in the input image maps to non-integral positions in the output image.

A geometric spatial operation maps pixel values at each pixel location (x, y) in an input image to another location (x', y') in an output image. The basic operations are described by first-order polynomials which take the following form:

$$\begin{bmatrix} x' \\ y' \end{bmatrix} = A \begin{bmatrix} x \\ y \end{bmatrix} + B \quad (6.3)$$

where A is a 2×2 matrix and B is a 2×1 column vector. Translation can be accomplished by specifying values for the matrix B, while scaling, rotation and reflection use the matrix A.

With *homogeneous coordinates*, where the x–y plane is considered to be the $z = 1$ plane of three-dimensional x, y, z space, all the transformations can be done by matrix multiplication. The general (*affine*) transform is

$$\begin{bmatrix} x' \\ y' \\ 1 \end{bmatrix} = \begin{bmatrix} a_{xx} & a_{xy} & b_x \\ a_{yx} & a_{yy} & b_y \\ 0 & 0 & 1 \end{bmatrix} \begin{bmatrix} x \\ y \\ 1 \end{bmatrix} \quad (6.4)$$

It is often used in applications, e.g. remote sensing, where we wish to correct for geometric distortions in the image.

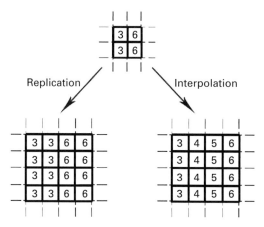

Figure 6.7 Methods of zooming: (i) replication of a single pixel value and (ii) interpolation.

Scaling expands/zooms or compresses/shrinks an image along the coordinate directions. An image (or a RoI within an image) can be zoomed either through pixel replication or interpolation. Figure 6.7 shows how pixel replication simply replaces each original image pixel by a group of pixels of the same value, where the group size is determined by an integral scaling factor. Alternatively, *interpolation* of the values of neighboring pixels in the original image can be performed in order to replace each pixel with an expanded group of pixels. For non-integral scaling factors, (x', y') maps into non-integral locations and gray-level interpolation is necessary. Using homogeneous coordinates, scaling is described as

$$\begin{bmatrix} x' \\ y' \\ 1 \end{bmatrix} = \begin{bmatrix} s_x & 0 & 0 \\ 0 & s_y & 0 \\ 0 & 0 & 1 \end{bmatrix} \begin{bmatrix} x \\ y \\ 1 \end{bmatrix} \tag{6.5}$$

Nearest-neighbor (or *zero-order*) *interpolation* involves assigning the gray value of the nearest integral neighbor. *Bilinear interpolation* uses the weighted average of the four nearest (integral) neighbors, and gives a more pleasing result. The weighting is proportional to the distance or pixel overlap of the nearby projections. Higher-order (polynomial) interpolation or spline-based interpolation can be used, but at a higher computational cost that is often not justified.

Worked example
Suppose we have a (one-dimensional) set of four pixel values, a profile $f(x) = \{100, 150, 75, 125\}$, that we want to scale to eight values, x'. The four values of x are evenly spaced, as are the eight values of x'. We could represent them as in Figure 6.8, where only the first and last points coincide. We need to estimate the values $f(x'_i)$, based on the nearby values of $f(x_i)$.

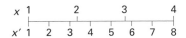

Figure 6.8   Interpolation in one dimension.

One way of doing this is to assign the closer value of $f(x_i)$ to each $f(x'_i)$. Thus, $f(x_1)$ (i.e. 100) would be assigned to $f(x'_2)$, $f(x_2)$ (i.e. 150) would be assigned to both $f(x'_3)$ and $f(x'_4)$, and so on. This is nearest-neighbor interpolation, and would result in $f(x') = \{100, 100, 150, 150, 75, 75, 125, 125\}$. Another way would be to assign intermediate values to $f(x')$, which are a combination of two values of $f(x)$ spanning it, combined as a linear weighted average depending on the two relative distances. For example, $f(x'_2)$ would get a value between $f(x_1)$ (i.e. 100) and $f(x_2)$ (150); and it would be closer to $f(x_1)$ than $f(x_2)$, reflecting its closer proximity. Thus

$$f(x'_2) = (4/7)\cdot100 + (3/7)\cdot150 = 121$$

if values are limited to integers between 0 and 255. Continuing in this way, the new values $f(x')$ would be $\{100, 121, 143, 129, 96, 82, 104, 125\}$. This is linear interpolation.

These methods can be applied to images. Figure 6.9 shows how a 4×4 image would be interpolated to give an 8×8 image. For nearest-neighbor interpolation the new values take on the values of the closest original points. But for bilinear interpolation, interpolation (i.e. linear weighted averaging) is required in two dimensions. First, linear interpolation can be applied along all the rows, and then these values can be interpolated along the resulting columns. (The same method would be used if we were scaling down from a large image to a smaller image.)

Let us calculate the value of the interpolated pixel at position X in Figure 6.10. Using linear interpolation along the rows gives values of 30 and 70 for the middle pixels along the top and bottom rows, respectively. Then interpolating up the middle column would give us a value of 40 for the pixel marked X, taking into account the relative distances.

Now we might expect this to be equivalent to taking a weighted average of the four values at the vertices, weighted according to relative distances to the vertices. The relative distances are $\sqrt{5}$ and $\sqrt{13}$, using Pythagoras' distances, i.e. $\sqrt{x^2 + y^2}$. These are used to weight the bottom and top pixels, respectively. Thus the weighted mean reduces to $(60\sqrt{13} + 140\sqrt{5})/(2\sqrt{13} + 2\sqrt{5})$, which is 45 to the nearest integer. Thus the two-step linear interpolation (or weighted averaging) is not equivalent to a one-step interpolation/weighted averaging, using the Pythagorean distances. Further, if we try a one-step averaging of the four pixel values using the Manhattan or taxicab distances (where we add the distances in the x and y directions, i.e. $(|x| + |y|)$ of 3 and 6, we find an interpolated value of 43 to the nearest integer. We might wonder why we are getting different values, and which one should we use!

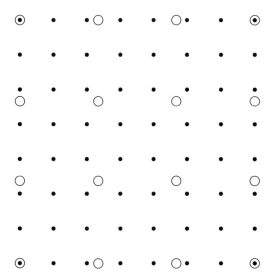

Figure 6.9 Interpolation in two dimensions. The open circles indicate the positions of the original values, and the filled circles indicate the positions of the new values.

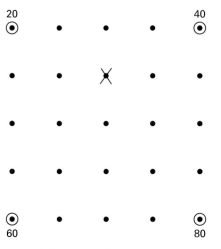

Figure 6.10 Interpolation in two dimensions. We wish to find the pixel value at X, given the four values at the vertex positions.

The key idea of our first method of bilinear interpolation is to perform linear interpolation first in one direction, and then in the other direction. Linear interpolation in the x direction (Fig. 6.11) gives

$$R_1 = \left(\frac{x_2 - x}{x_2 - x_1} \right) Q_{11} + \left(\frac{x - x_1}{x_2 - x_1} \right) Q_{21} \qquad (6.6a)$$

and

$$R_2 = \left(\frac{x_2 - x}{x_2 - x_1}\right) Q_{12} + \left(\frac{x - x_1}{x_2 - x_1}\right) Q_{22} \tag{6.6b}$$

and interpolation in the y direction gives

$$P = \left(\frac{y_2 - y}{y_2 - y_1}\right) R_1 + \left(\frac{y - y_1}{y_2 - y_1}\right) R_2 \tag{6.6c}$$

Substituting from Equations (6.6a) and (6.6b) into Equation (6.6c) gives

$$P = \left(\frac{y_2 - y}{y_2 - y_1}\right) \left[\left(\frac{x_2 - x}{x_2 - x_1}\right) Q_{11} + \left(\frac{x - x_1}{x_2 - x_1}\right) Q_{21}\right]$$

$$+ \left(\frac{y - y_1}{y_2 - y_1}\right) \left[\left(\frac{x_2 - x}{x_2 - x_1}\right) Q_{12} + \left(\frac{x - x_1}{x_2 - x_1}\right) Q_{22}\right]$$

If we choose a coordinate system in which the four points where the pixel values are known are $(0, 0)$, $(0, 1)$, $(1, 0)$, and $(1, 1)$, then the interpolation formula simplifies to

$$P = (1 - x)(1 - y) Q_{11} + x(1 - y) Q_{21} + (1 - x)y Q_{12} + xy Q_{22} \tag{6.7}$$

Contrary to what the name suggests, this interpolant is *not* linear. It is the product of two linear interpolants, and is of the form $b_1 + b_2 x + b_3 y + b_4 xy$. The interpolant is linear along lines parallel to either the x or the y direction, but along any other direction it is quadratic. The result of this bilinear interpolation is independent of the

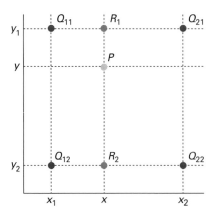

Figure 6.11   The red pixel values are given, and we want to know the value at P, which we get by linearly interpolating along the rows to get values at R_1 and R_2 and then linearly interpolating down the column. See also color plate.

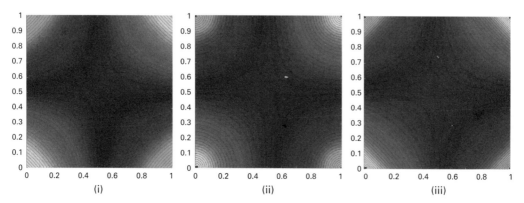

Figure 6.12 Contours of equal distance from four vertices using (i) two-stage linear interpolation, (ii) Euclidean distance and (iii) Manhattan distance. See also color plate.

order of interpolation. If the interpolation is performed first in the x direction and then in the y direction, the result would be the same. The loci of points at various distances from the four vertices are shown as contours in Figure 6.12(i); the contours are hyperbolic.

If we measure distance using Pythagoras' theorem in a Euclidean world, the loci of equal distances from a point are circles; although as we travel further away from the vertices they become hyberbolic (Fig. 6.12(ii)). If we use the Manhattan distance, the loci of equal distances from a point are diamonds; but they become hyberbolic as we travel further away from the vertices (Fig. 6.12(iii)). So, while distance in a one-dimensional world, which results in the weights needed for linear interpolation, is very specific, in two dimensions distance can be defined in various ways giving rise to different weights for two-dimensional interpolation and different contours for equidistance. Caveat emptor ... let the buyer (or user) beware!

Shrinking an image, commonly known as *sub-sampling*, is performed by replacement of a group of pixels either by a pixel from within this group or by interpolating between pixel values in a local neighborhood. Figure 6.13 illustrates these two methods of sub-sampling. In the first, one pixel value within a local neighborhood is chosen to be representative of its surroundings. The second method interpolates between pixel values within a neighborhood by taking a statistical sample (such as the mean) of the values. For non-integral sub-sampling, either nearest-neighbor or bilinear interpolation is used.

Translation by a distance (b_x, b_y) is given by

$$\begin{bmatrix} x' \\ y' \\ 1 \end{bmatrix} = \begin{bmatrix} 1 & 0 & b_x \\ 0 & 1 & b_y \\ 0 & 0 & 1 \end{bmatrix} \begin{bmatrix} x \\ y \\ 1 \end{bmatrix} \tag{6.8}$$

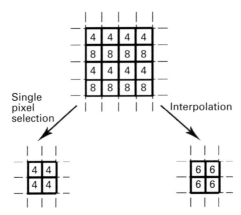

Figure 6.13   Methods of sub-sampling: (i) replacement with upper left pixel and (ii) interpolation using the mean value.

The rotation operator maps the position (x, y) of a pixel in an input image on to a position (x', y') in an output image by rotating it through an angle θ about the origin. The spatial transformation is given by

$$\begin{bmatrix} x' \\ y' \\ 1 \end{bmatrix} = \begin{bmatrix} \cos\theta & -\sin\theta & 0 \\ \sin\theta & \cos\theta & 0 \\ 0 & 0 & 1 \end{bmatrix} \begin{bmatrix} x \\ y \\ 1 \end{bmatrix} \tag{6.9}$$

Rotation about an arbitrary point can be obtained by combining translation with rotation.

The general affine transformation (Equation (6.4)) is defined by six independent parameters: two parameters to align the origins, two parameters for the scaling of the two axes, and two parameters describing the change in angle of each axis. Thus, it is possible to define this transformation completely by specifying the new output image locations of any three input image coordinate pairs.

For most image processing applications, the spatial transform is not amenable to analytic expressions. Instead measurements of at least three corresponding points (*control* or *fiducial points*) in two images are taken and a least squares method is used to find the best fitting transform (see Activity 4.5). In the case of distortion in an imaging system an undistorted image and its distorted counterpart can be used to find the best transform, and the inverse of this transform used to correct subsequent distorted images. Another widely used application is the registering of images acquired from different imaging modalities.

6.3.1   The log-polar transformation

The log-polar transformation is a simple operation that changes the coordinate system of an image from Cartesian to log-polar (Fig. 6.14). It emulates how images appear on the back of the human retina. (The brain then transforms the images back to the Cartesian-like way we perceive them.) The log-polar transformation is a conformal mapping (i.e. it preserves

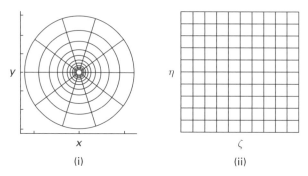

Figure 6.14   Log-polar transformation from (i) points on the Cartesian plane (x, y) to (ii) points in the log-polar plane (ζ, η).

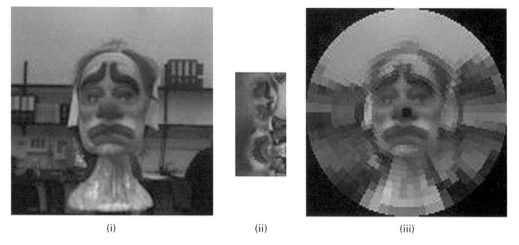

      (i)   (ii)   (iii)

Figure 6.15   (i) A 256×256 image; (ii) its 64×32 log-polar transformation; (iii) retinal representation. See also color plate.

angles and orientations) from the points on the Cartesian plane (x, y) to points in the log-polar plane (ζ, η):

$$\varsigma = \sqrt{x^2 + y^2} \tag{6.10a}$$

$$\eta = \tan^{-1}(y/x) \tag{6.10b}$$

The log-polar transformation converts an image to a form that is rotation and scale invariant, which can be very helpful for object detection, pattern recognition and image registration. Another advantage of log-polar image sampling is data reduction; resolution in the center of the image (i.e. at the fovea of the retina) is high, but at the periphery it is low. For example, 256×256 Cartesian images transform to 128×64 log-polar images achieving an eight times increase in efficiency in both storage and speed (Fig. 6.15). This is useful for tracking in artificial vision systems; objects occupying the central high-resolution part of the visual field become dominant over coarsely sampled background elements in the image periphery. This embeds an implicit focus of attention in the center of the visual field where the target is expected to be most of the time.

6.4   Convolution-based operations

Discrete (digital) convolution in the spatial domain is a fundamental process in image processing, and is used either to smooth or sharpen an image. It comprises a "sum-of-products" and a "shift" operation. The basic concept is that a *mask* or *kernel*, essentially a small image or matrix of $k \times k$ elements, is rotated through $180°$ and moved in a raster pattern across an input image of $M \times M$ pixels; k is usually an odd integer, much smaller than the linear size of the image. Each pixel of the output image is the weighted sum of the input pixels within a region defined by the mask, with the elements of the mask defining the weights. If the input image is F (of size $M \times M$) and the convolution mask is H (size $k \times k$), the output image G is given by

$$G = F \ast H \tag{6.11}$$

Each pixel in the output image is given by

$$g(i,j) = \sum_{m=-a}^{a} \sum_{n=-a}^{a} f(m,n)h(i-m, \; j-n) \tag{6.12}$$

where $a = (k-1)/2$.

The mathematics can seem daunting, but the process is illustrated in Figure 6.16. The mask is rotated through $180°$ and placed on top of the input image, starting at the top left position. The mask elements are multiplied by the corresponding pixel values in the image below, and the products are summed and suitably normalized to form a weighted response which is then the value of the output pixel at the position corresponding to the center of the mask. With most masks k is chosen to be odd, so that the center of the mask is readily apparent. The mask is then moved one position to the right, the sum of products re-calculated and normalized to give the next pixel value in the output image. This process is repeated as the mask is moved across the input image in a raster scan.

In practice, the "sum-of-products" formulation often leads to overflow. Normalization, by dividing by the sum of the elements in the mask, produces a weighted response that remains within the original range of pixel values in the input image. The resulting output image pixels often have non-integral values, so that working with floating-point numbers is necessary in order to avoid "round-off" errors.

The initial rotation of the mask by $180°$ is not apparent if the mask is circularly symmetric, as it is for many common masks used in smoothing and sharpening. However, this is not always the case, e.g. the masks used in locating horizontal and vertical

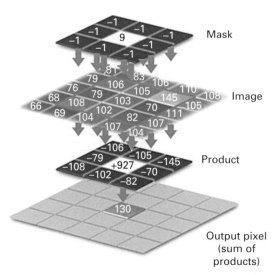

Figure 6.16 Digital convolution: the mask is placed over the source image, mask elements are multiplied by pixel values, and the results added to form an output pixel.

edges in an image. This prior rotation is what distinguishes convolution from correlation: *cross-correlation* involves two images (usually of rather similar sizes) where the sum-of-products, replacement and scanning operations take place without the initial 180° rotation. The resulting *cross-correlation function* is used primarily for locating the features of one image that appear in another, and can be used for aligning or registering images.

Pixels around the borders of the input image lack a full set of neighbors. For convolution with a 3 × 3 mask this involves pixels in a border one pixel wide around the input image, whereas for convolution with a 5 × 5 mask, the border is two pixels wide, and so on. This is not a significant problem if k is much smaller than M. It can be mitigated by extending image A by padding it out with zeroes or by repeating its border pixels, or considering that the input image wraps around in both the horizontal and vertical directions (*cyclic convolution*). However, none of these methods is perfect and a more prudent approach is to ensure that the input image contains no important information within a border of $(k-1)/2$ from its edges.

The computational complexity for convolution of an image of $M \times M$ pixels with a mask of size $k \times k$ is of the order of k^2 per pixel, based on the number of multiply-and-adds (MADDs). This becomes a significant problem for large masks, such that ernative approach to convolution using computation within the spatial frequency domain (Chapter 7) is advantageous.

A *linear* imaging system obeys linear superpositioning, i.e. it produces an output image from a composite input image that is a linear superposition of what it would produce for the component parts. If it is also *shift-invariant*, it produces an output whose features are independent of the position in the input image, i.e. if a feature in the input image is shifted, the corresponding feature in the output image is shifted by the same amount, but not otherwise changed. Many imaging systems exhibit, at least

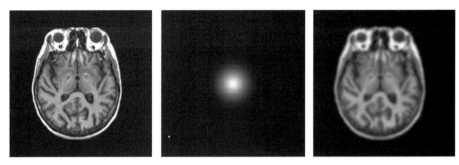

Figure 6.17 Convolution of a sharp MRI image of a human brain (left) with a Gaussian PSF function (center) to give a blurred image (right).

approximately, both these properties and are known as *linear, shift-invariant* (*LSI*) systems. Note that this implies a zero output for a zero input, and a magnification of unity.

If an impulse point of light $\delta(x, y)$ passes through an imaging system the image produced is called the point spread function (PSF), $h(x, y)$. Any discrete image is composed of individual points or pixels. If the system is a linear, shift-invariant (LSI) system, linearity allows the application of an operator to each impulse separately and the addition of the responses; shift invariance allows the use of one response for all the other impulses if the appropriate shifts are made. Thus, if the response to a point image (i.e. the point spread function) is known, the response to any image can be computed. The output image, $g(x, y)$, resulting from an input, $f(x, y)$, is a sum-of-products, described by the convolution of the input with the point spread function (Fig. 6.17), that is

$$g(x, y) = f(x, y) * h(x, y) \qquad (6.13)$$

and the point spread function is described by a convolution mask that completely characterizes the imaging system, and describes its blurring properties due to, for example, imperfect optics, sensors, recorders and displays. Convolution with different-sized point spread functions can be seen in Activity 6.4.

The technique of undoing the effect of these degradations in quality caused by the imaging system would be an inverse process, known as *deconvolution*.

6.4.1   Smoothing masks

The simplest smoothing operation is that of neighborhood averaging, i.e. each pixel in the output image is formed from the average of the pixel values in a neighborhood surrounding the pixel in the input image at that position. The mask that implements this is a $k \times k$ mask, with all coefficients equal to unity (Figs. 6.18(i) and (ii)) and a constant pre-multiplier of $1/k^2$; it is called an averaging or box mask. The averaging process reduces the abrupt variations in local pixel values, smoothing the input image by reducing its noise. A reduced smoothing effect can be obtained by using a weighted-average mask (Fig. 6.18(iii)).

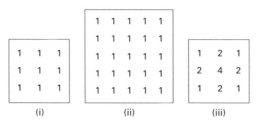

Figure 6.18 Convolution masks: (i) 3×3 averaging mask; (ii) 5×5 averaging mask; (iii) 3×3 weighted-average mask.

Smoothing an image reduces its signal-to-noise ratio and changes its gray-level histogram (Activity 6.5).

One use of such a mask is to smooth out the false contours that occur in images acquired with an insufficient number of gray levels. Another use is to blur out features smaller than the mask. This would be useful as a pre-cursor to *segmentation*, where an image is divided into areas of interest. The rule of thumb is that the size of the mask, k, should be greater than or equal to $2w + 1$ if features of diameter w are to be blurred out; k should be lower or equal to $2w - 1$ if such features are to be retained, while reducing the overall noise.

The masks in Figure 6.18 are examples of *separable* masks. Each two-dimensional mask can be separated into two one-dimensional masks, which can be used successively on an image to produce the same effect but with less computation. For example the two-dimensional mask in Figure 6.17 (i) could be replaced by a one-dimensional horizontal mask, [1 1 1], and its transpose, a one-dimensional vertical

mask, $\begin{bmatrix} 1 \\ 1 \\ 1 \end{bmatrix}$, since convolving these two masks gives the original two-dimensional mask.

Two-dimensional convolution can then be replaced by two one-dimensional convolution operations, the second operating on the result of the first. The order is not important since convolution with linear shift-invariant operators is commutative. This reduces the number of multiplications from k^2 to $2k$ per pixel. The convolution mask can be written as a matrix h and, if it is separable, h can be written as

$$[h] = [h_{col}][h_{row}]^{T} \tag{6.14}$$

where "T" indicates the transpose of a matrix, with rows being substituted for columns.

Averaging masks are subject to a particular effect known as *ringing* as a result of their *brick wall* profile with its discontinuities; we will discuss this drawback in terms of spatial frequencies in Chapter 7. An imaging system that is not well focused can be modeled by a point spread function shaped like a "pill box," that is an averaging mask which is circularly symmetric. The effect on a test pattern is shown in Figure 6.19. Not only is the defocused image smoothed and its edges blurred, but dark radial bands turn to light, and vice versa. This is clearly an unwanted property of masks with sharp discontinuities.

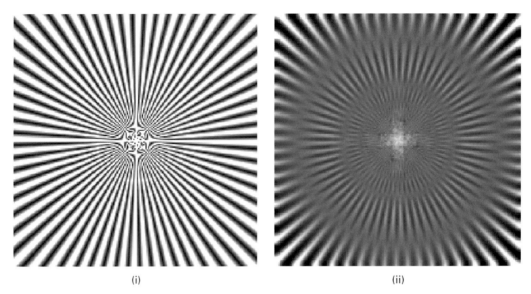

(i)   (ii)

Figure 6.19   Test pattern convolved with a circularly symmetric averaging mask to model defocusing: (i) test pattern, (ii) defocused image.

Gaussian masks have a bell-shaped profile, with a high value element in the center and symmetrical tapering to either side. They produce a response somewhat similar to the weighted average mask, but with even less *ringing* because of the gradual tapering of their profile. The mask elements are given by

$$h(i,j) = A\exp\left[(-1/2)(d/\sigma)^2\right] \qquad (6.15)$$

where A is a scaling factor, d is the distance of a pixel from the center of the mask ($d = \sqrt{(x^2 + y^2)}$) and σ determines the width of the mask (Fig. 6.20). The rule of thumb is to set $\sigma = (2w + 1)/2$, where w is the size of the feature to be blurred out. Gaussian masks are separable, so that they can be implemented by using a one-dimensional horizontal Gaussian, followed by a one-dimensional vertical Gaussian. The Gaussian is in fact the *only* completely circularly symmetric operator which can be decomposed in such a way.

The *Central Limit Theorem* in statistics shows that all distribution shapes tend to a Gaussian when they are combined. The underlying process is convolution. Thus when two averaging masks are convolved the result is triangular, corresponding to the linearly weighted average mask; as more masks are convolved together, the resulting shape approaches a Gaussian. Many imaging systems can be modeled using a Gaussian mask to represent their point spread function (PSF).

The Gaussian mask can be built approximately from one-dimensional binomial masks (Fig. 6.21), whose elements are the coefficients of the binomial expansion $(1 + x)^n$, i.e. the discrete binomial distribution given by Pascal's triangle. The odd-sized masks are of more interest. When a horizontal (e.g. b_2) and a vertical binomial mask (e.g. its transpose,

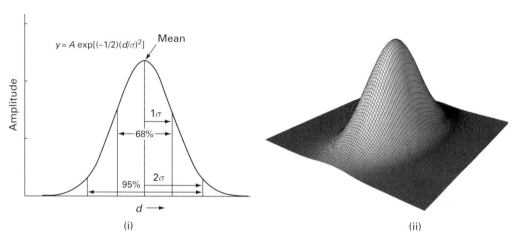

Figure 6.20   (i) Gaussian profile (one-dimensional) and (ii) wireframe image of a two-dimensional Gaussian.

b_1	1/2 (1 1)
b_2	1/4 (1 2 1)
b_3	1/8 (1 3 3 1)
b_4	1/16 (1 4 6 4 1)
b_5	1/32 (1 5 10 10 5 1)
b_6	1/64 (1 6 15 20 15 6 1)
b_7	1/128 (1 7 21 35 35 21 7 1)
b_8	1/256 (1 8 28 56 70 56 28 8 1)

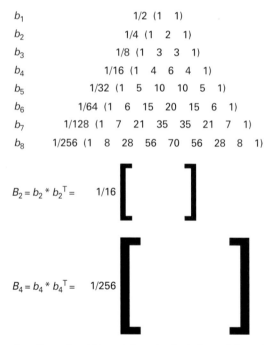

$B_2 = b_2 * b_2^T =$ 1/16

$B_4 = b_4 * b_4^T =$ 1/256

Figure 6.21   One-dimensional binomial masks, b_1 to b_8, and Gaussian masks, B_2 and B_4.

b_2^T) are convolved, they form a two-dimensional mask (in this case, B_2). As the number of terms becomes bigger, the binomial distribution better approximates a Gaussian. The mask B_4, for example, is already a good approximation and can be used as an integer-based Gaussian mask.

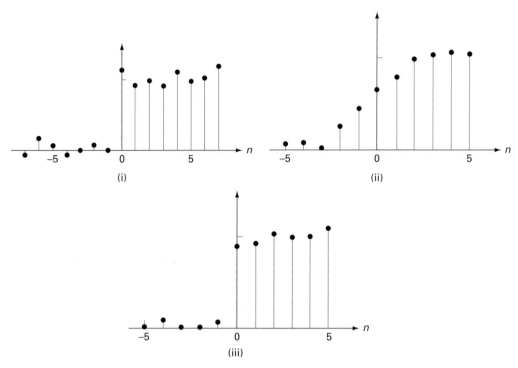

Figure 6.22   Effect of a one-dimensional five-element mask on an edge (i) using (ii) an averaging mask and (iii) a median mask.

A major disadvantage of the averaging mask is that it blurs edges in an image. An edge in an image is a sharp transition between gray levels. Figure 6.22(i) shows a one-dimensional profile perpendicular to an edge: the variation in pixel values on either side of the edge indicates the presence of random noise. The result of convolving the edge profile with a (one-dimensional) averaging mask, five elements long, is shown in Figure 6.22(ii). The mask moves along the profile, and a running average is calculated over five pixels and used to replace the center pixel at each position. When the mask samples only low or high pixel values to either side of the edge, averaging reduces the random noise. However, when the mask includes both low and high values it produces averages that are neither low nor high and the profile of the output image becomes a ramp from low to high values rather than a sharp edge. The longer the mask, the longer the ramp, and the more blurred the edge becomes. A weighted average has a similar, though less severe, effect.

An alternative mask, which smoothes noise but does not blur edges, is the *median mask*. It is a *non-linear* mask, which returns the median or middle value of the pixels within it. It is an example of a *rank-order* (or *order-statistic*) *mask*, other examples being the "*maximum*" and "*minimum*" masks which return the largest and smallest pixel values, respectively, from the neighborhood. The median mask smoothes an image, since it returns a value in the middle of a range of values thereby reducing local fluctuations. It selects one of the existing pixel values, namely the median, rather than calculating the mean or average; no round-off errors are involved if we want to work exclusively with

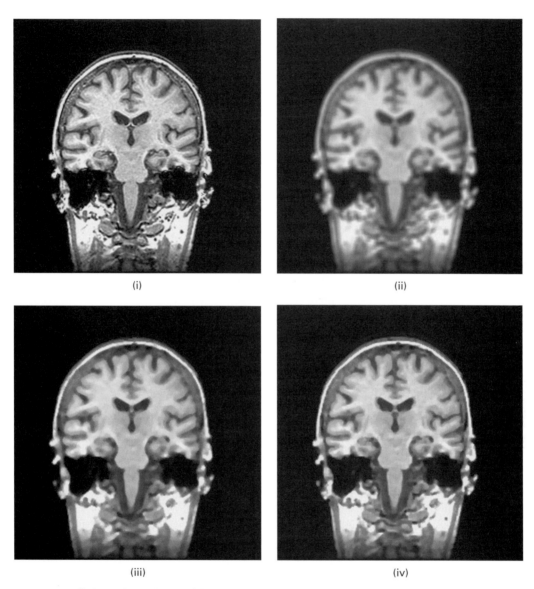

(i)   (ii)

(iii)   (iv)

Figure 6.23   (i) Coronal MRI image of the head. After convolution with (ii) 5 × 5 averaging mask, (iii) 5 × 5 square median mask and (iv) diamond-shaped 5 × 5 median mask.

integer pixel values. Consider the operation of a one-dimensional median mask on the noisy edge profile of Figure 6.22(i). As the median mask moves into the edge, it contains some low and some high pixel values. However, depending on which predominates, the median is always either a low value or a high value, and never an intermediate value. Thus, the edge remains sharp (Fig. 6.22(iii)) and is not degraded into a ramp; the one-dimensional median filter is *edge-preserving*. It should be noted that the square two-dimensional median mask is a non-separable mask. Since edges play an important part in our perception of images, their preservation in processing can be an important asset.

Figure 6.23(i) shows a 256 × 256 MRI image, a coronal section of a head. The effect of averaging with a 5 × 5 mask is shown in Figure 6.23(ii): the image is noticeably smoother, but its edges are blurred. A square 5 × 5 median mask convolved with the original produced the image of Figure 6.23(iii), which has been smoothed but has significantly less blurring of horizontal and vertical edges. Finally, Figure 6.23(iv) shows the effect of a median mask with a diamond shape and a height and width of 5 pixels. The image has been smoothed, but this time all the edges, including those in a diagonal direction, remain essentially free from blurring.

Median masks are particularly good at removing *impulse* or *salt-and-pepper noise* from an image. This type of noise involves isolated pixels being either turned on (white, hence *salt*) or off (black, or *pepper*), as a result of data drop-out often caused by errors in data transmission. Figure 6.24(i) shows a profile though an image where two pixels have suffered from impulse noise. The result of convolving the profile with a (one-dimensional) averaging mask, five elements long, is shown in Figure 6.24(ii): the impulse noise is reduced in intensity but is blurred out over more pixels. With a median mask, the majority of the pixels covered by the mask as it moves through the image profile are of low intensity so that the resulting pixels are not affected by the impulse pixels. Thus in two-dimensional images, isolated clusters of salt or pepper pixels with areas less than half that of the mask are removed (Fig. 6.24 (iii)). The median mask is not as good at smoothing other types of noise as the averaging mask (Activity 6.6); since its output values are always constrained to values already present, it cannot produce new values that might be better matched to produce smoothing.

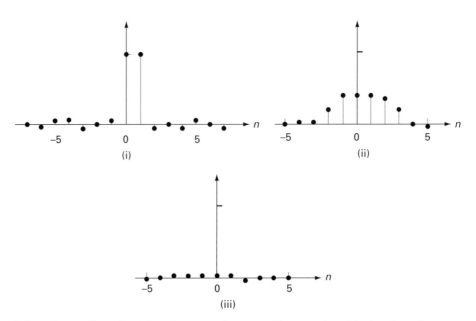

Figure 6.24   Effect of a one-dimensional five-element mask on a profile contaminated by impulse noise (i) using (ii) an averaging mask and (iii) a median mask.

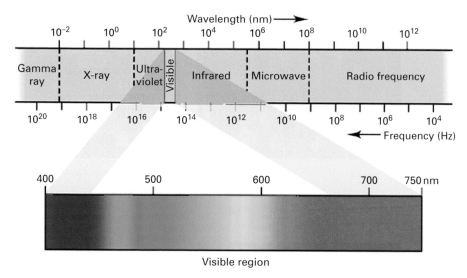

Wavelength (nm) ⟶

Plate 1 The electromagnetic spectrum arranged according to the energy of the photons, or the frequency of the waves.

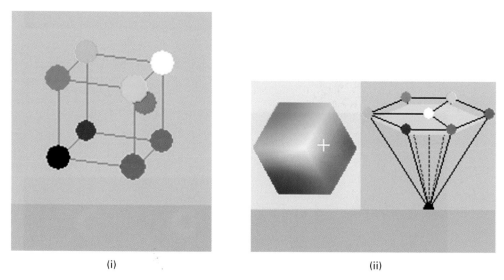

(i)   (ii)

Plate 2 (i) A color (bottom) and its position in RGB space, shown by the gray ball at red = 240, green = 160, blue = 140 and (ii) the same color (bottom) and its position in HSV space, with hue = 0.02, saturation = 0.40 and value = 0.93; in the hexagonal cone, the hue is the angle from the red axis, the distance to the center is the saturation, and the position up the vertical axis is the value.

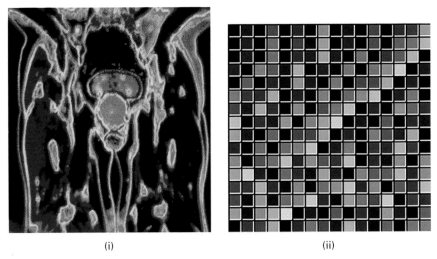

(i)   (ii)

Plate 3   (i) An indexed color image and (ii) its color palette, comprising 256 colors with indices running from 0 at top left to 255 at bottom right.

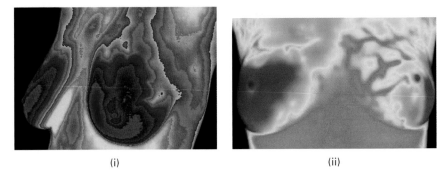

(i)   (ii)

Plate 4   Breast thermograms of (i) normal breasts and (ii) breasts showing a suspicious difference in temperatures.

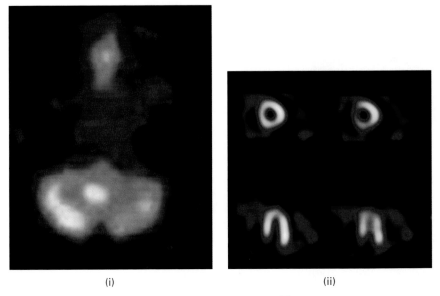

(i)   (ii)

Plate 5   SPECT images showing (i) a brain tumor (in white), using ^{99m}Tc-GH (glucoheptinate), and (ii) thinning of the cardiac wall (reduced intensity), using ^{99m}Tc-sestamibi.

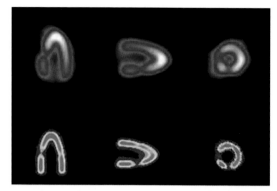

Plate 6   A realistic heart phantom imaged along three axes by SPECT with ^{99m}Tc (top row) and PET with 18F-fluorodeoxyglucose (bottom row).

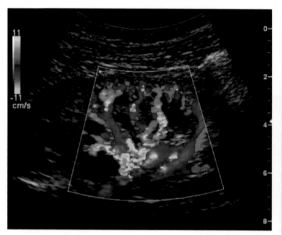

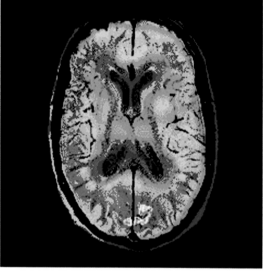

Plate 7   Color Doppler duplex image. The color look-up table is related directly to the blood velocity.

Plate 8   Co-registered SPECT–MRI image through the head. (Courtesy of Dr. Karin Knesaurek, Mt. Sinai Medical Center.)

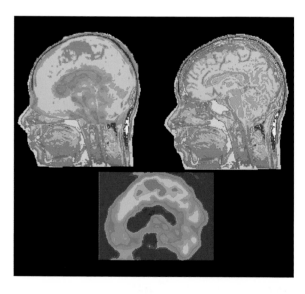

Plate 9   MRI (upper right) and SPECT (lower center) head sagittal slices of the same patient and the co-registered (MRI + SPECT) image (upper left). The lesion on the top of the skull is more prominent in the composite image, although it can be visualized in both modalities.

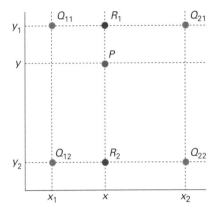

Plate 10   The red pixel values are given, and we want to know the value at P, which we get by linearly interpolating along the rows to get values at R_1 and R_2 and then linearly interpolating down the column.

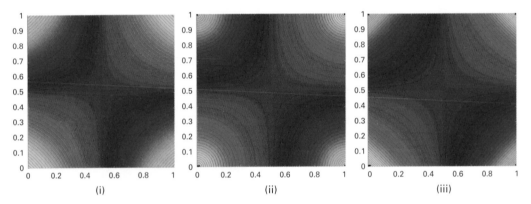

(i)   (ii)   (iii)

Plate 11   Contours of equal distance from four vertices using (i) two-stage linear interpolation, (ii) Euclidean distance and (iii) Manhattan distance.

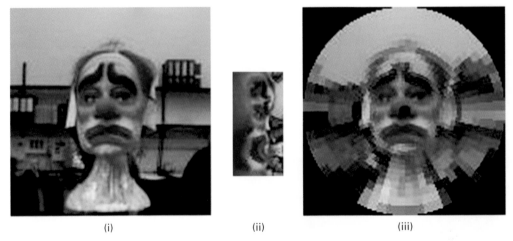

(i)   (ii)   (iii)

Plate 12   (i) A 256×256 image, (ii) its 64×32 log-polar transformation, (iii) retinal representation.

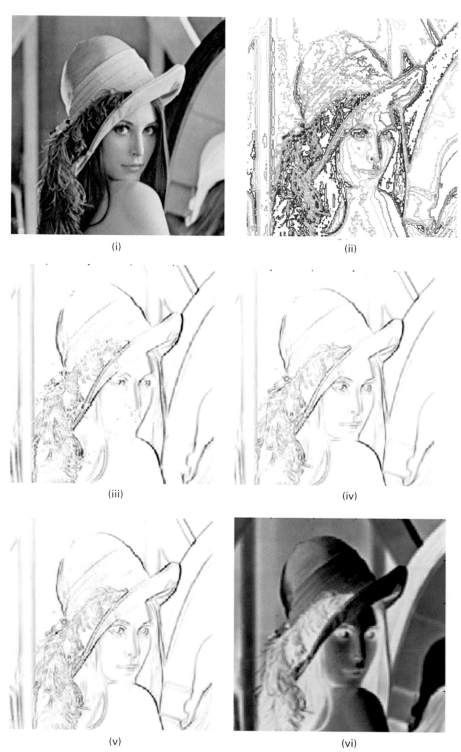

(i)

(ii)

(iii)

(iv)

(v)

(vi)

Plate 13 (i) Original (noiseless) 256×256 image and (ii) its contours. Results of gradient edge detection using (iii) Roberts, (iv) Prewitt, (v) Sobel, and (vi) Frei–Chen operators.

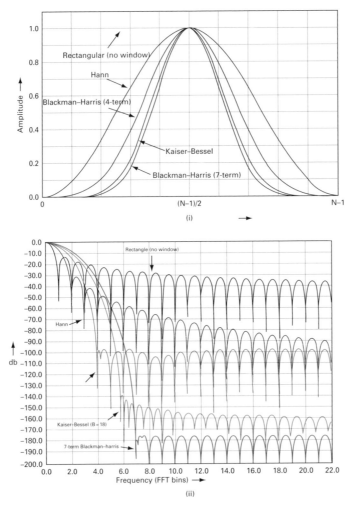

(i)

(ii)

Plate 14 (i) Profiles of several commonly used window functions and (ii) their Fourier transforms.

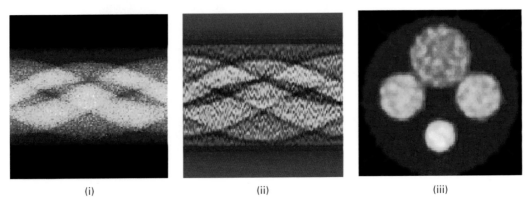

(i)   (ii)   (iii)

Plate 15 The direct Fourier reconstruction method used for two-dimensional image reconstruction from projections.

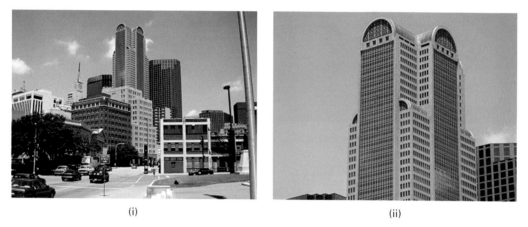

(i)   (ii)

Plate 16   (i) An image taken with a wide-angle lens showing barrel distortion and (ii) an image taken with a telephoto lens showing slight pincushion distortion.

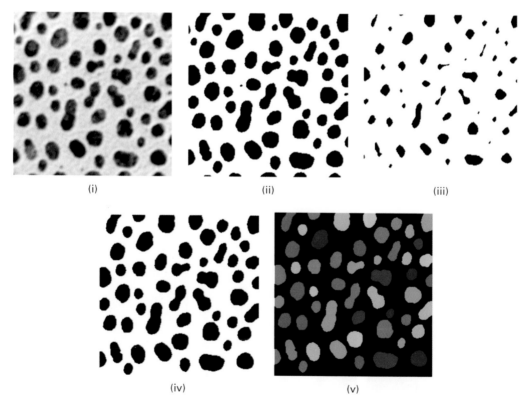

(i)   (ii)   (iii)

(iv)   (v)

Plate 17   (i) Original image; (ii) after thresholding; (iii) after 4 erosions; (iv) after 12 conditional dilations (the small objects have been removed); (v) after labeling and displaying each object in a different color.

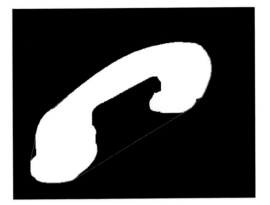

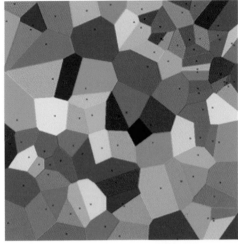

Plate 18 A feature enclosed by its convex hull (shown in red).

Plate 19 The Voronoi diagram of a set of points, showing the polygons of influence.

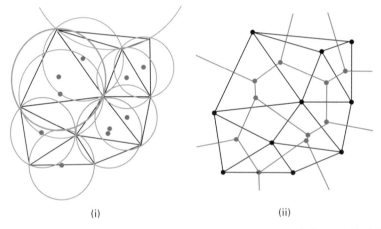

(i)   (ii)

Plate 20 (i) A set of points (in red) with their Delaunay triangulation and circumscribed circles.
(ii) Connecting the centers of the circumscribed points produces the Voronoi diagram (in red).

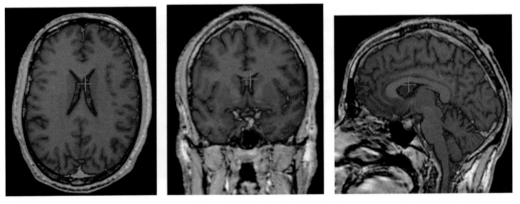

Plate 21 A characteristic shading has been added to the brain following segmentation. The three images show (from left to right) axial, coronal and saggital planes. A common point is marked in each image.

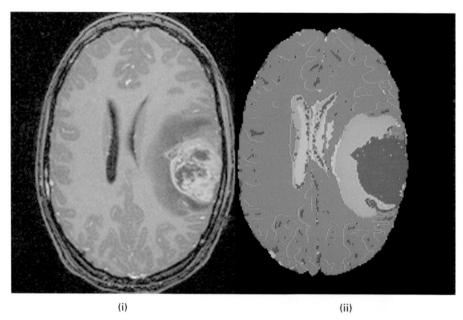

(i) (ii)

Plate 22 (i) Axial slice of MRI brain image and (ii) automatic segmentation into five classes, including a tumor. The segmentation was done in three dimensions. (Courtesy: Prof. Guido Gerig, Department of Computer Science, University of North Carolina at Chapel Hill).

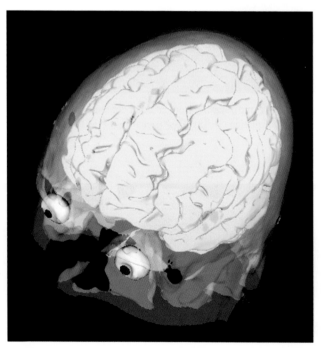

Plate 23 Segmentation of a three-dimensional MRI image by region growing. The white and gray matter regions were combined before three-dimensional rendering (Chapter 12).

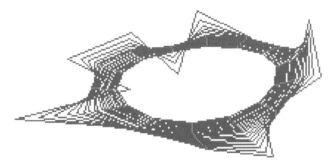

Plate 24   Twenty iterations of a snake (red), starting from an outer contour, moving under an internal elastic function. The trajectories of the control points are shown in green.

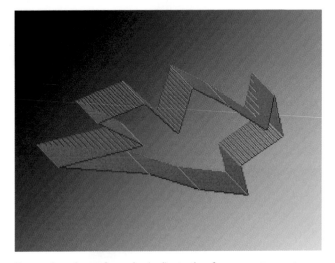

Plate 25   Twenty iterations of a snake (red), starting from an outer contour, moving under an external energy function given by Equation (10.13). The trajectories of the control points are shown in green.

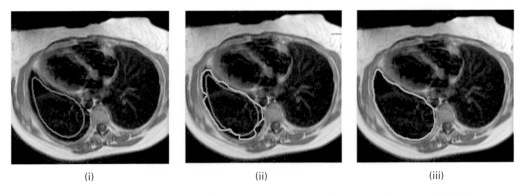

| (i) | (ii) | (iii) |

Plate 26   (i) Initial contour; (ii) intermediate contour in yellow (initial contour in green); (iii) final contour.

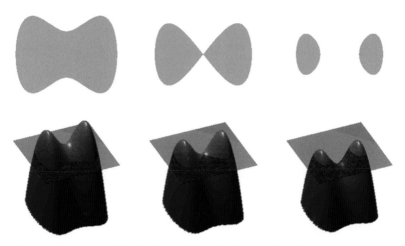

Plate 27   Contours (top row) and their relationship to the level set function, φ.

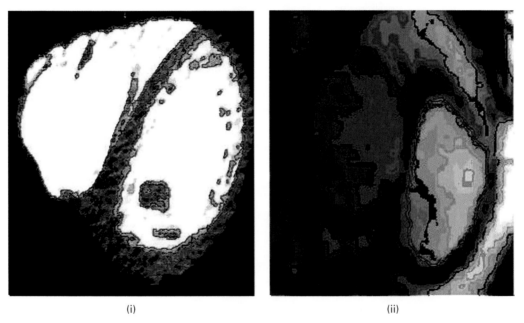

(i)   (ii)

Plate 28   Segmentation of (i) CT and (ii) MRI images of the heart using level sets. Each of these images is part of a time series. The snake is shown in red in (i) and in green in (ii). (Courtesy: Dr. Rene Vidal, Biomedical Engineering, Johns Hopkins University.)

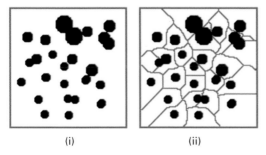

(i)   (ii)

Plate 29   (i) Binary image with overlapping features and (ii) watershed lines (in red) overlaid on the original image.

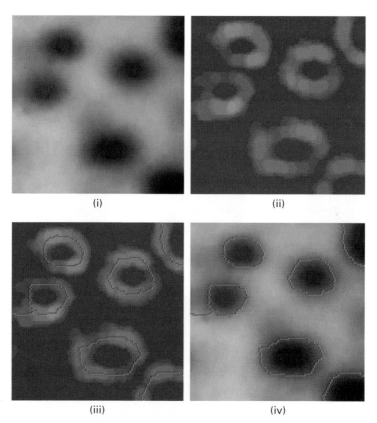

Plate 30 (i) Original image. (ii) gradient image and (iii) Watershed lines overlaid on the gradient image. (iv) Watershed lines overlaid on the original image.

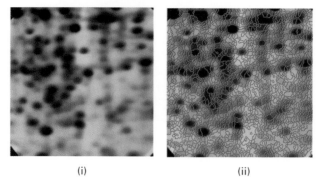

Plate 31 (i) Image of electrophoresis gel. (ii) Watershed transform of the gradient image.

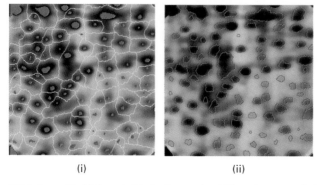

Plate 32 (i) Markers of the blobs and of the background and (ii) marker-controlled watershed of the gradient image.

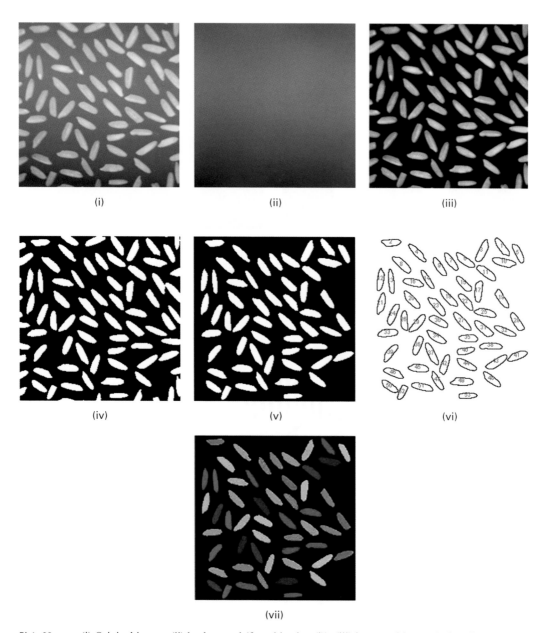

(i)   (ii)   (iii)

(iv)   (v)   (vi)

(vii)

Plate 33   (i) Original image; (ii) background (from blurring (i)); (iii) improved image (= (i) − (ii)); (iv) segmented image (Otsu threshold of (iii)); (v) partial objects removed from (iv); (vi) labeled components image; (vii) color-coded labeled components image.

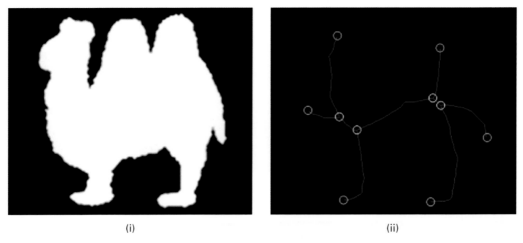

(i)   (ii)

Plate 34   (i) Image and (ii) its skeleton (red), with its branch points (white) and end points (green) circled.

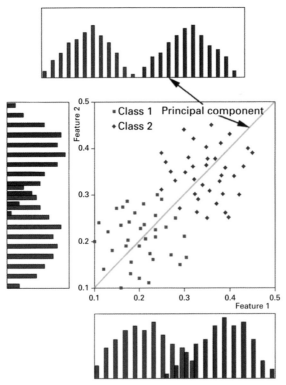

Plate 35   The data set is optimally separated (as shown by the histograms) along a line, the first principal component direction, which is a linear combination of the original features. (After Russ 2002).

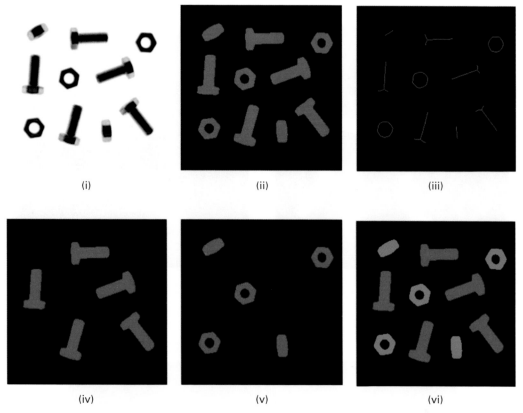

Plate 36 (i) Original image; (ii) after thresholding; (ii) after subsequent skeletonization; (iv) after conditionally dilating the branch pixels from (iii); (v) after logically combining (ii) and (iv); (v) color coding the nuts and bolts.

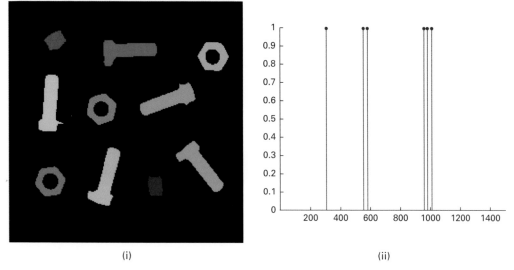

Plate 37 (i) Segmented, labeled image (using Fig. 11.5(i)); (ii) one-dimensional feature space showing the areas of the features; (iii) the features "painted" with their measured areas; (iv) after thresholding image (iii) at a value of 800.

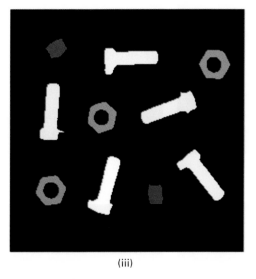 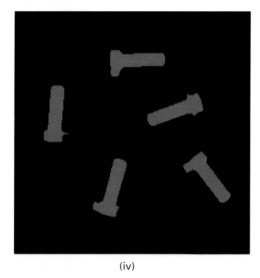

(iii)   (iv)

Plate 37   (Cont.)

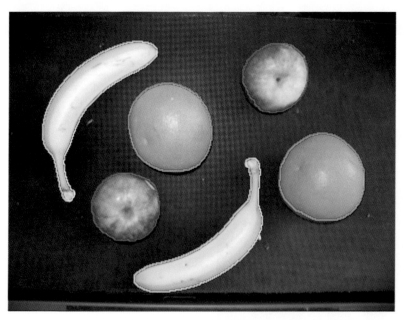

Plate 38   Objects have been classified into three classes of fruit, and outlines superimposed on the
original image.

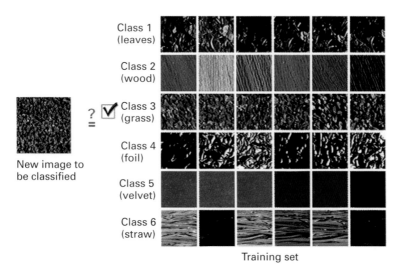

Class 1 (leaves)
Class 2 (wood)
Class 3 (grass)
Class 4 (foil)
Class 5 (velvet)
Class 6 (straw)

New image to be classified

? ☑

Training set

Plate 39   The image at left has to be classified into one of the classes defined by the training set images. A good classifier will assign it to class 3.

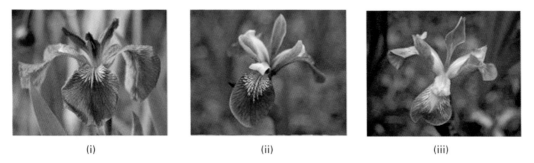

(i)   (ii)   (iii)

Plate 40   (i) *Iris setosa*, (ii) *Iris versicolor* and (iii) *Iris virginica*.

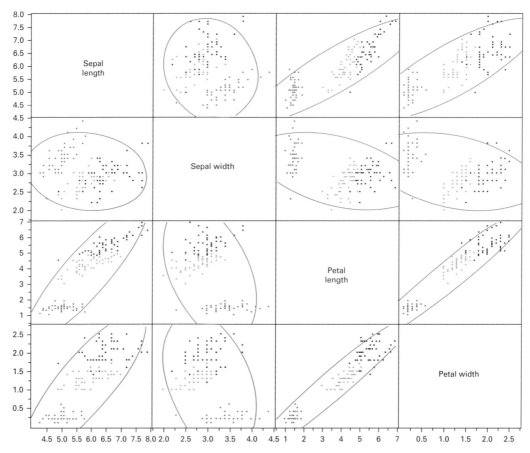

Plate 41　　Scatter plot matrix of Fisher's iris data. (The features from *Iris setosa* are plotted in red, those from *Iris versicolor* are plotted in green, and those from *Iris virginica* are plotted in blue; the elliptical contours enclose 95% of the features in each plot.)

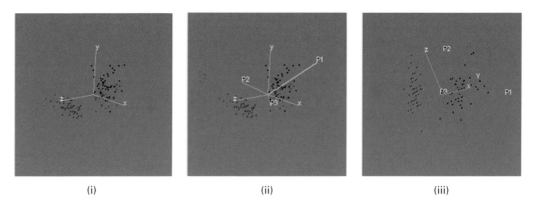

(i)　　　　　　　　　　　　　(ii)　　　　　　　　　　　　　(iii)

Plate 42　　Spinning plots: (i) *x*, *y* and *z* are petal length, sepal length and sepal width, respectively; (ii) the principal components, P_1, P_2 and P_3, are shown overlaid; (iii) a projection in the plane of P_1 and P_2. (The features from *Iris setosa* are plotted in red, those from *Iris versicolor* are plotted in green, and those from *Iris virginica* are plotted in blue.)

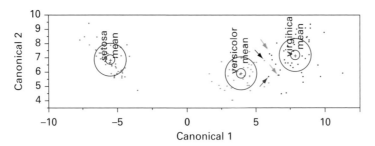

Plate 43   Canonical plot for the Fisher data. The three features that are misclassified (see Table 11.3) using this classifier are marked with colored arrows; the black arrow shows an additional feature that is misclassified if cross-validation is used. (The small colored circles are 95% confidence limits for the positions of the means; and the larger colored circles contain 50% of the features for that class.)

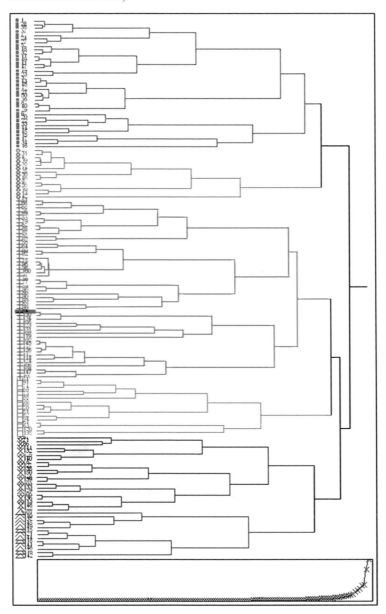

Plate 44   Dendrogram and scree plot obtained by hierarchical of the canonical data from the Fisher iris database. The number of classes can be chosen by drawing a vertical line down the dendrogram at a particular position. The scree plot helps determine this position: as shown it is placed to identify six clusters (shown colorized), although the scree plot suggests just three clusters.

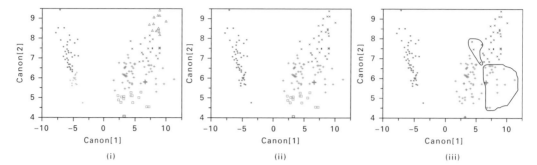

Plate 45   Scatter plots of Fisher's canonicals with data colorized according to the number of clusters chosen in the dendrogram obtained by hierarchical clustering: (i) 6 clusters, (ii) 4 clusters and (iii) 3 clusters.

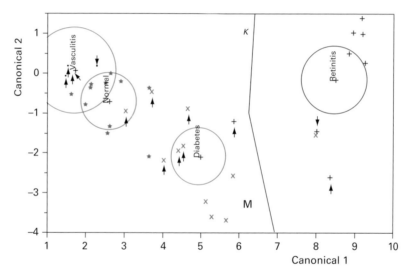

Plate 46   Canonical plot of data from retinal vessels. Data from the ground truth conditions are indicated by separate symbols (• vasculitis; * normal; × diabetes; + retinitis). The directions of the features, M and K, are shown in the canonical space by the labeled rays. The size of each circle corresponds to a 95% confidence limit for the mean (marked with +) of that group; groups with significantly different values of tortuosity have non-intersecting circles. The small arrows indicate misclassified data points.

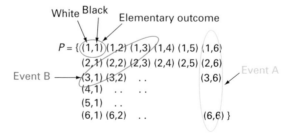

Plate 47   Throwing two dice.

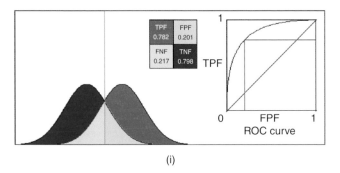

(i)

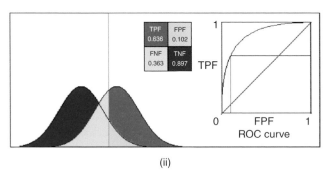

(ii)

Plate 48   Overlapping distributions. Decision threshold at (i) intercept of distributions and (ii) higher value than (i). The corresponding points on the ROC plot are shown.

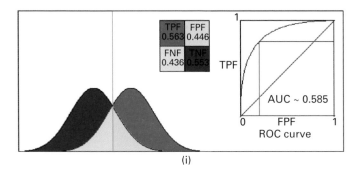

(i)

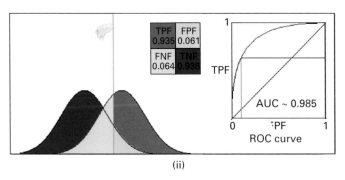

(ii)

Plate 49   Distributions with (i) a large and (ii) a small overlap. The corresponding values of AUC are shown with the ROC plots. (The AUC value for the distributions shown in Figure B.14 is 0.859.)

6.4.2   Sharpening and edge-detecting masks

Sharpening is used to produce a crisper image with sharper edges in order to highlight fine detail. One way of sharpening an image is by *unsharp masking*. The original image is blurred, i.e. unsharpened, and a fraction of it is subtracted from the original. The resulting image, $g(x, y)$, is given by

$$g(x, y) = f(x, y) - cf_S(x, y) \qquad (6.16)$$

where $f_S(x, y)$, the smoothed image, is obtained using an averaging mask and c is a constant. In terms of masks, the unsharp masking operation, UM, is given by

$$\text{UM} = \begin{vmatrix} 0 & 0 & 0 \\ 0 & 1 & 0 \\ 0 & 0 & 0 \end{vmatrix} - \left(\frac{c}{9}\right) \begin{vmatrix} 1 & 1 & 1 \\ 1 & 1 & 1 \\ 1 & 1 & 1 \end{vmatrix} \qquad (6.17)$$

The value of the constant can be varied to give different degrees of sharpening; in the case of $c = 0.9$ the resulting mask would be

$$\text{UM}' = \left(\frac{1}{10}\right) \begin{vmatrix} -1 & -1 & -1 \\ -1 & 9 & -1 \\ -1 & -1 & -1 \end{vmatrix} \qquad (6.18)$$

where the elements add to unity, preserving the average intensity of the original image in the processed image. However this does *not* guarantee that the pixels in the resulting image remain in the range 0 to 255, so that re-scaling is necessary. A sharpening mask typically has a large positive element in the center, surrounded by small negative elements, whereas there are no negative elements in a smoothing mask.

Unsharp masking is illustrated in Figure 6.25. The original image in Figure 6.25(i) was smoothed by Gaussian blurring (Fig. 6.25(ii)). When the two images are subtracted, a sharper image results (Fig. 6.25(iii)).

Figure 6.26 illustrates schematically the consequences of unsharp masking on a one-dimensional profile.

Sharpening is the reverse operation to smoothing. Since smoothing is achieved by averaging, which is essentially integration, intuition suggests that sharpening should be achieved by subtraction or differentiation. Consider a horizontal line of pixels within the image on the left in Figure 6.27. If repeated subtractions of neighboring pixels along each line were executed, the resultant image would be that shown on the right. The only significantly non-zero pixels result from subtractions across the edges, where low values are subtracted from high values, or vice versa. In areas of constant gray levels, whether low or high, the processed pixels are all low, i.e. close to black. The only exception to this would be if there was significant noise in the initial image; in which case subtraction would accentuate its importance.

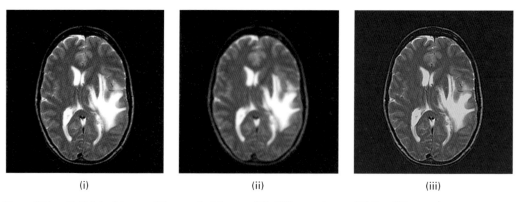

(i)   (ii)   (iii)

Figure 6.25   (i) Original image; (ii) smoothed image; (iii) difference image (2*(i) – (ii)).

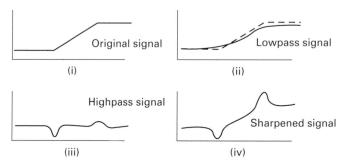

Figure 6.26   (i) Original profile; (ii) profile after smoothing; (iii) smoothed profile subtracted from original profile; (iv) smoothed profile subtracted from twice the original profile.

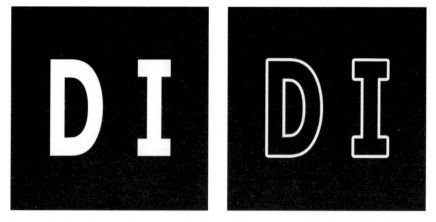

Figure 6.27   Repeated subtractions performed on the pixels of the image on the left result in the image on the right.

Differentiation is essentially subtraction of two values and division by the step separating them; if the step is unity, the division is redundant. It could be argued that since a digital image is not a continuous function of the spatial variables, it is not differentiable. However, since the original analog image was continuous and therefore differentiable, and since subtracting the pixels of the digitized image is an approximation of the derivative of the analog image, it is therefore legitimate.

A first derivative of an image $f(x, y)$ in the x direction is

$$\frac{\partial f}{\partial x} = f(x + 1, y) - f(x, y) \tag{6.19a}$$

and in the y direction it is

$$\frac{\partial f}{\partial y} = f(x, y + 1) - f(x, y) \tag{6.19b}$$

The first derivative in two dimensions, ∇f, or grad f, could be taken as the sum of the magnitudes of the one-dimensional derivatives so that

$$\nabla f \approx f(x + 1, y) + f(x, y + 1) - 2f(x, y) \tag{6.20}$$

which could be implemented by using the two masks

$$\begin{bmatrix} -1 & 1 \\ 0 & 0 \end{bmatrix} \quad \text{and} \quad \begin{bmatrix} -1 & 0 \\ 1 & 0 \end{bmatrix}$$

and adding the two resulting images. A more symmetrical pair of masks can be obtained by rotating these masks by 45°, i.e.

$$\begin{bmatrix} -1 & 0 \\ 0 & 1 \end{bmatrix} \quad \text{and} \quad \begin{bmatrix} 0 & -1 \\ 1 & 0 \end{bmatrix}$$

These are known as the *Robert's cross-gradient operators*. They could be combined to give

$$\begin{bmatrix} -1 & -1 \\ 1 & 1 \end{bmatrix}$$

This is a very simple algorithm to compute, but the small mask makes it sensitive to noise and it produces very weak responses to genuine edges unless they are very sharp.

Masks of even size are awkward to implement because they do not have a well-defined central term. Instead, the differencing could be implemented by 3×3 masks such as

$$\frac{\partial}{\partial x} = \begin{bmatrix} -1 & 0 & 1 \\ -1 & 0 & 1 \\ -1 & 0 & 1 \end{bmatrix} \quad \text{and} \quad \frac{\partial}{\partial y} = \begin{bmatrix} -1 & -1 & -1 \\ 0 & 0 & 0 \\ 1 & 1 & 1 \end{bmatrix} \tag{6.21}$$

which are called the *Prewitt operators*. These compute the derivatives in the x and y directions, respectively, which are then combined to give the total derivative of the image. Each is essentially an edge detector for the horizontal and vertical directions, with both results adding to give all the edges. Each operator is separable, into a derivative and an averaging operator, so that the computation can be implemented with greater efficiency by performing consecutive passes with one-dimensional convolution masks. It is prudent to incorporate some smoothing into the process, since differentiation is so susceptible to noise.
Each of the *Sobel operators*

$$G_x = \begin{bmatrix} -1 & 0 & 1 \\ -2 & 0 & 2 \\ -1 & 0 & 1 \end{bmatrix} \quad \text{and} \quad G_y = \begin{bmatrix} -1 & -2 & -1 \\ 0 & 0 & 0 \\ 1 & 2 & 1 \end{bmatrix} \tag{6.22}$$

takes the derivative in one direction, horizontal or vertical, while smoothing by weighted averaging in the orthogonal direction. The Sobel operators are better at suppressing noise than the Prewitt operators. The terms in all these masks add to zero, indicating that they would give a response of zero in an area of constant gray values as expected from a derivative operator. Note that sharpening increases the signal-to-noise ratio of an image and changes its gray-level histogram (Activity 6.7).

The resulting x and y component edge images from convolution with the Sobel operators (or the Prewitt operators) should be combined, pixel by pixel, as the square root of the sum of the squares of the pixel values $\left(\text{i.e. } \sqrt{(P_x^2 + P_y^2)}, \text{ where } P_x \text{ and } P_y \text{ are the corresponding}\right.$ pixel values in the x and y component edge images) to give a "magnitude-of-the-edges" image, although for computational efficiency sometimes the magnitudes of the two images are simply added. The easiest way to identify those pixels corresponding to an edge is to threshold the gradient image, assuming that all pixels having a local gradient above a certain threshold must represent an edge. Natural edges in images often lead to lines in the output image that are several pixels wide due to the smoothing effect of the Sobel operator. Some *thinning* (Section 9.2.4) may be desirable to counter this effect.

Output values from the Sobel (or Prewitt) operators can easily overflow the maximum allowed pixel value if integer pixel values are used; this problem can be avoided by using an image type that supports pixel values with a larger range.

The direction of an edge, α, is the angle subtended by the edge and the horizontal axis. It can be determined from the x and y component edge images, and a Sobel "phase-of-the-edges" image constructed using $\tan^{-1}(P_y/P_x)$. Activity 6.8 shows how these steps can be implemented.

Some form of thresholding of the "magnitude-of-the-edges" image is generally used to eliminate spurious responses to noise, although this often results in breaks in the contours. To remedy this, *edge linking* is needed to assemble the edge pixels into meaningful boundaries. A simple approach would be to compare the magnitude *and* phase of potential edge points, and link them if their differences were less than particular threshold values, which could be varied interactively.

The *Kirsch (edge) operator* comprises eight convolution masks based on first derivatives, each responding optimally to an edge in a particular direction of the compass

$$
\begin{bmatrix} 1 & 1 & 1 \\ 0 & 0 & 0 \\ -1 & -1 & -1 \end{bmatrix} \quad \begin{bmatrix} 1 & 1 & 0 \\ 1 & 0 & -1 \\ 0 & -1 & -1 \end{bmatrix} \quad \begin{bmatrix} 1 & 0 & -1 \\ 1 & 0 & -1 \\ 1 & 0 & -1 \end{bmatrix} \quad \begin{bmatrix} 0 & -1 & -1 \\ 1 & 0 & -1 \\ 1 & 1 & 0 \end{bmatrix}
$$

$$
\mid N \qquad\qquad \searrow NW \qquad\qquad - W \qquad\qquad \diagup SW
$$

$$
\begin{bmatrix} -1 & -1 & -1 \\ 0 & 0 & 0 \\ 1 & 1 & 1 \end{bmatrix} \quad \begin{bmatrix} -1 & -1 & 0 \\ -1 & 0 & 1 \\ 0 & 1 & 1 \end{bmatrix} \quad \begin{bmatrix} -1 & 0 & 1 \\ -1 & 0 & 1 \\ -1 & 0 & 1 \end{bmatrix} \quad \begin{bmatrix} 0 & 1 & 1 \\ -1 & 0 & 1 \\ -1 & -1 & 0 \end{bmatrix}
$$

$$
\mid S \qquad\qquad \searrow SE \qquad\qquad - E \qquad\qquad \diagup NE
$$

Figure 6.28   Masks making up the Kirsch edge detector.

$$
G_1 = \frac{1}{2\sqrt{2}}\begin{bmatrix} 1 & \sqrt{2} & 1 \\ 0 & 0 & 0 \\ -1 & -\sqrt{2} & -1 \end{bmatrix} \quad G_2 = \frac{1}{2\sqrt{2}}\begin{bmatrix} 1 & 0 & 1 \\ \sqrt{2} & 0 & \sqrt{2} \\ 1 & 0 & 1 \end{bmatrix} \quad G_3 = \frac{1}{2\sqrt{2}}\begin{bmatrix} 0 & -1 & \sqrt{2} \\ 1 & 0 & -1 \\ -\sqrt{2} & 1 & 0 \end{bmatrix}
$$

$$
G_4 = \frac{1}{2\sqrt{2}}\begin{bmatrix} \sqrt{2} & -1 & 1 \\ -1 & 0 & 1 \\ 0 & 1 & -\sqrt{2} \end{bmatrix} \quad G_5 = \frac{1}{2}\begin{bmatrix} 0 & 1 & 0 \\ -1 & 0 & -1 \\ 0 & 1 & 0 \end{bmatrix} \quad G_6 = \frac{1}{2}\begin{bmatrix} -1 & 0 & 1 \\ 0 & 0 & 0 \\ 1 & 0 & -1 \end{bmatrix}
$$

$$
G_7 = \frac{1}{6}\begin{bmatrix} -1 & -2 & 1 \\ -2 & 4 & -2 \\ 1 & -2 & 1 \end{bmatrix} \quad G_8 = \frac{1}{6}\begin{bmatrix} -2 & 1 & -2 \\ 1 & 4 & 1 \\ -2 & 1 & -2 \end{bmatrix} \quad G_9 = \frac{1}{3}\begin{bmatrix} 1 & 1 & 1 \\ 1 & 1 & 1 \\ 1 & 1 & 1 \end{bmatrix}
$$

Figure 6.29   Masks making up the Frei–Chen edge detector.

(Fig. 6.28). The resulting edge image is taken from the maximum pixel values of the eight convolved intermediate images.

The *Frei–Chen (edge) detector* is another first-order operator. Edge detection using the Frei–Chen masks is implemented by mapping the intensity vector using a linear transformation and then detecting edges based on the angle between the intensity vector and its projection on to the edge subspace. The 3×3 image area is represented by a weighted sum of nine Frei–Chen masks, which comprise all of the basis vectors. The image is convolved with each of the nine masks (Fig. 6.29), and then an inner product of the convolution results of each mask is performed. The first four masks are used for edges, the next four for lines, and the last mask is used to compute averages. For edge detection, the appropriate masks are chosen and the image is projected on to it.

The *Canny* operator was designed to be an optimal edge detector. It works in a multi-stage process. The first step is to filter out any noise in the original image before trying to locate and detect any edges. The input image is smoothed by convolution with a Gaussian mask; the larger the width of the Gaussian mask, the lower is the detector's sensitivity to noise. The localization error in the detected edges also increases slightly as the Gaussian width is increased. The next step is to find the strength and direction of the edges, using, for example, the Prewitt operators. Edges give rise to ridges in the gradient magnitude image. The algorithm then tracks along the top of these ridges and sets to zero (i.e. suppresses) all pixels that are not actually on the ridge top so as to give a thin line in the output, a process known as *non-maximal suppression*. Finally, hysteresis is used as a method of preventing the edge contour breaking up due to fluctuations around a single threshold. Instead, two thresholds, T_1 and T_2 with $T_1 > T_2$, are used. Tracking begins at all points on a ridge higher than T_1, and continues in both directions until the height of the ridge falls below T_2. This hysteresis helps to ensure that noisy edges are not broken up into multiple edge fragments. Usually, the upper tracking threshold can be set quite high, and the lower threshold quite low for good results. Setting the lower threshold too high causes noisy edges to break up; setting the upper threshold too low increases the number of spurious and undesirable edge fragments appearing in the output.

Most of the edge detectors work well with noiseless images (Fig. 6.30), although the Prewitt and Sobel operators are superior to the Roberts operator. The more complicated Frei–Chen operator produces the best results. Edge detection operators perform less well on noisy images. The Frei–Chen edge operator is the most successful at enhancing edges within noisy images, and the Laplacian of a Gaussian is fairly successful. The Sobel operator is a little better than the Prewitt operator, which in turn is better than the Roberts operator.

Detecting edges is an essential step in object detection or recognition systems. Edge-detection algorithms are used, for example, to delineate better the edges of coronary arteries in x-ray angiograms. Narrowing of the coronary arteries, which supply blood to the cardiac muscle, results in a compromised supply and possible damage to the muscle. The severity of the resulting condition, coronary heart disease, can be evaluated by comparing the cross-sectional areas in the regions of *stenoses* (narrowings) with the cross-sectional areas in normal regions of the artery. More accurate determinations can be made if the vessel edges are clearly delineated prior to measurement.

6.4.3   Second-derivative masks

The objective of edge-detecting algorithms is to locate regions where the grayscale intensity is changing rapidly. This corresponds to a gradient or first derivative, larger than some threshold value. An alternative would be to look for a zero crossing of the second derivative, since this corresponds to a local maximum of the gradient (Fig. 6.31). The second derivative is the difference between two first derivatives, taken at a small distance apart, so that the second derivatives in the x and y directions could be written as

$$\frac{\partial^2 f}{\partial^2 x} = f(x+1, y) - 2f(x, y) + f(x-1, y) \tag{6.23a}$$

$$\frac{\partial^2 f}{\partial^2 y} = f(x, y+1) - 2f(x, y) + f(x, y-1) \tag{6.23b}$$

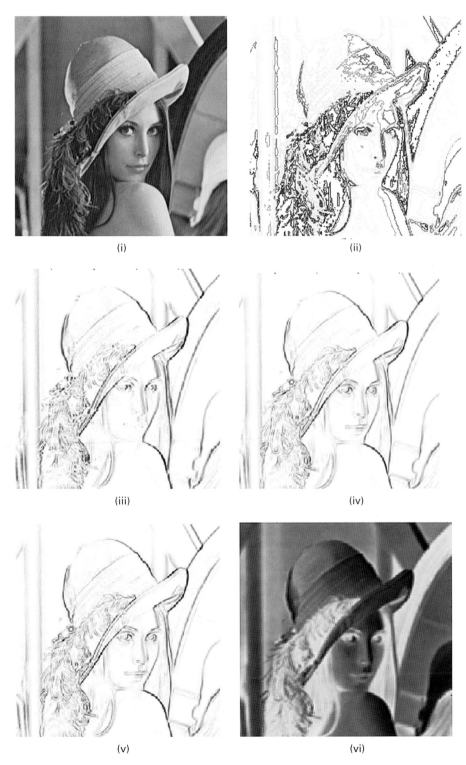

Figure 6.30 (i) Original (noiseless) 256×256 image and (ii) its contours. Results of gradient edge detection using (iii) Roberts, (iv) Prewitt, (v) Sobel, and (vi) Frei–Chen operators. See also color plate.

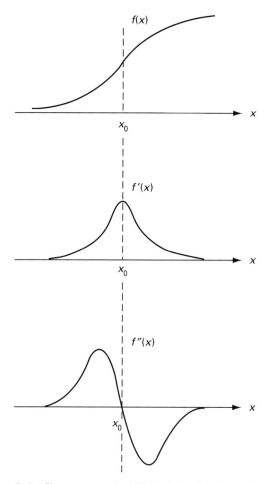

Figure 6.31   (i) Profile across an edge, (ii) its first derivative and (iii) its second derivative.

Combining these two, and writing them as a mask, gives

$$\nabla^2 f = \begin{bmatrix} 0 & 1 & 0 \\ 1 & -4 & 1 \\ 0 & 1 & 0 \end{bmatrix} \qquad\qquad (6.24a)$$

This mask, or its complement, is known as the *Laplacian* mask. Such a formulation is isotropic for rotations of 90°. For rotations isotropic about 45° it would be

$$\nabla^2 f = \begin{bmatrix} 1 & 1 & 1 \\ 1 & -8 & 1 \\ 1 & 1 & 1 \end{bmatrix} \qquad\qquad (6.24b)$$

or its complement. Note this is identical in form to the unsharp mask of Equation (6.17), but without the normalizing factor.

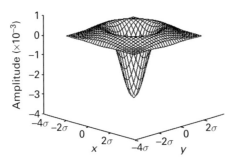

Figure 6.32   The two-dimensional Laplacian of a Gaussian (LoG) function. The x and y axes are marked in standard deviations.

The Laplacian operation is seldom used in practice because it produces double edges and, as a second derivative, it is unacceptably sensitive to noise. However, its location of edges using its *zero-crossing* property is useful if it is combined with some smoothing to minimize its sensitivity to noise. This can be done by convolving it with a Gaussian mask to give the *Laplacian of a Gaussian*, the LoG operator, which is sometimes referred to as the *Mexican hat* operator because of its shape. The two-dimensional Laplacian of a Gaussian function centered on zero and with Gaussian standard deviation, σ, has the following form:

$$\text{LoG} = -\left(\frac{r^2 - \sigma^2}{\sigma^4}\right)\exp\left(r^2/2\sigma^2\right) \tag{6.25}$$

where $r^2 = x^2 + y^2$, and σ determines the degree of smoothing; its form is shown in Figure 6.32. Hence, σ can be set to remove unwanted detail, or noise, as desired. All edges detected by the zero crossing detector are in the form of closed curves, except where the curve goes off the edge of the image (Activity 6.9).

A discrete mask that approximates the Laplacian of a Gaussian function (for a Gaussian width of 1.4) is shown in Figure 6.33. Note that as the Gaussian is made increasingly narrow, the Laplacian of a Gaussian mask becomes the same as the simple Laplacian mask. This is because smoothing with a very narrow Gaussian ($\sigma < 0.5$ pixels) on a discrete grid has no effect.

Gradient (first-derivative) operation is an effective detector for sharp edges where the pixel gray levels change over space very rapidly. But when the gray levels change slowly from dark to bright, the gradient operation will produce a very wide edge. It is helpful in this case to consider using the (second-derivative) Laplace operation. The second-order derivative of the wide edge will have a zero crossing in the middle of edge. Figure 6.34 shows the result of edge detection using the Laplacian of a Gaussian (LoG) operator, which is superior to the first-derivative operators.

The Laplacian and the Laplacian of a Gaussian operator are the basis of *zero crossing detection*. The simplest scheme is simply to threshold the Laplacian of a Gaussian output at zero, to produce a binary image where the boundaries between foreground and

0	1	1	2	2	2	1	1	0
1	2	4	5	5	5	4	2	1
1	4	5	3	0	3	5	4	1
2	5	3	-12	-24	-12	3	5	2
2	5	0	-24	-40	-24	0	5	2
2	5	3	-12	-24	-12	3	5	2
1	4	5	3	0	3	5	4	1
1	2	4	5	5	5	4	2	1
0	1	1	2	2	2	1	1	0

Figure 6.33   Discrete approximation to Laplacian of a Gaussian function with a Gaussian width of 1.4.

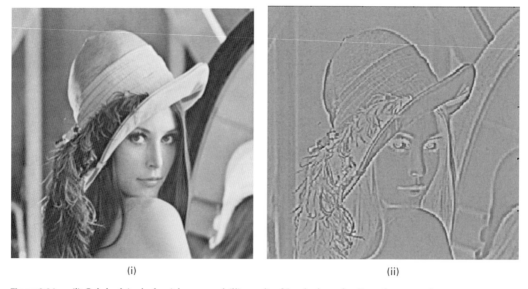

(i)   (ii)

Figure 6.34   (i) Original (noiseless) image and (ii) result of Laplacian of a Gaussian operation.

background regions represent the locations of zero crossing points. A better technique is to consider points on both sides of the threshold boundary, and choose the one with the lower absolute magnitude of the Laplacian, which is hopefully closer to the zero crossing.

It is possible to approximate the Laplacian of a Gaussian mask with a mask that is merely the difference of two differently sized Gaussians, known as a *Difference of Gaussians* (DoG) mask (Fig. 6.35). This corresponds to the subtraction of one smoothed

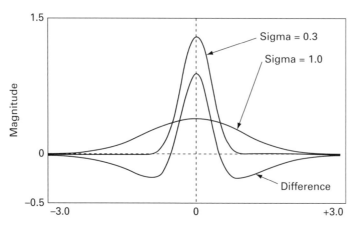

Figure 6.35 The Difference of Gaussians operator in one dimension. Two Gaussian curves with different standard deviations, and their difference.

version of an image from another having a different degree of smoothness, and is a generalization of the unsharp masking technique. It has been suggested that Difference of Gaussians masks are similar to the way that the human visual system locates boundaries.

Computer-based activities

Activity 6.1 Background subtraction

Open the **rice** image in ImageJ and observe its gray-level histogram. The image contains an uneven background, which is darker at the bottom and left-hand side of the image. Blur duplicates of the image using **Process/Filters/Gaussian Blur** and choosing different amounts of blurring (using the **Radius** value). Increase the amount of blurring until the rice grains themselves cannot be seen, but do not continue with too much blur otherwise the background itself gets averaged across the image. Save the optimally blurred image as **background.tif**; subtract it from the original image (using **Process/Image Calculator ... Subtract**), and observe the histogram of the new image. The uneven background has been removed, and the histogram shows a narrow spread of pixel values on a uniform, light background. The image can be seen more clearly if its contrast is stretched (**Process/Enhance Contrast ... Normalize**).

Try the same procedure for uneven background removal on the images **uneven** and **sonnet**.

Activity 6.2 Division of images

Divide the **rice** image by its **background**, as found in Activity 6.1, using **Process/Image Calculator ... Divide**, with a **32-bit result**. Compare the resulting image (after histogram stretch) with the image obtained in Activity 6.1 using subtraction. Which worked better, subtraction or division, at removing the uneven background?

Remove the uneven backgrounds in **uneven** and **sonnet** by division with their respective background images, and compare the results to the use of subtraction in removing uneven backgrounds.

Activity 6.3 Bit-planes

Open **mandrill** in ImageJ, and obtain bit-plane 7 by logically ANDing (**Process/Math/AND ...**) the image with binary 10000000. Enhance the contrast of the result. Now look at the other bit-planes. Which planes contain the most image information, and which contain the finer details and noise?

Can you see how this procedure could be applied to image compression, by retaining the bit-planes with the most information and compressing those with less information?

Activity 6.4 Convolution

Open up **testpattern** and the Gaussian PSF images, **gauss2**, **gauss4** and **gauss8**, in ImageJ. Verify that these latter three images are Gaussian using **Analyze/Surface Plot ...** with **Draw Wireframe** checked. Convolve **testpattern** with each Gaussian PSF in turn using **Process/Filters/Convolve** and choosing the corresponding text file. Note the increased degradation as the width of the Gaussian PSF increases.

Repeat with **testpattern2**.

Activity 6.5 Averaging/smoothing

Open **testpattern** in ImageJ, and observe the effects of (i) 3×3 averaging, (ii) 5×5 averaging and (iii) 3×3 weighted averaging (using the masks **3 x 3 average.txt, 5 x 5 average.txt** and **3 x 3 weighted average. txt**) on (a) the histogram (using the **live histogram** plugin) and (b) the SNR (remember to choose a region of constant gray value before using the **SNR** plugin). Which produces the most smoothing (and blurring of edges), and which the least?

Import the 3×3 weighted average mask as a text image (using **File/Import/Text Image**), scale it to a reasonable size using **Image/Scale** (without interpolation), and display its surface plot with the wire frame drawn (using **Analyze/Surface Plots**: check **Draw Wireframe, Shade, Draw Axis**). Is this what you expect?

Activity 6.6 Noise removal

Open up **noisyS&Pskull**, which is a radiograph of a skull contaminated by salt-and-pepper noise. Use the **live histogram** plugin to display its gray-level histogram: note the large spikes at 0 and 255. Apply a 5×5 average mask using **Process/ Filters ... Mean** with a radius of 2. Note how the histogram changes. Compare the result with that of using a 5×5 median mask (**Process/ Filters ... Median** with a radius of 2 on the original noisy image. Which is more successful at removing this kind of noise? How do the histograms of the resulting images differ? (Hint: Look at the "valley" in each histogram.)

Repeat using **noisyGskull**, which is contaminated with Gaussian noise. Observe the shape of the gray-level histogram of the original image, and how it changes with each mask. Which mask is more successful at removing Gaussian noise? Do you notice much difference in the histograms of the two resulting images?

Activity 6.7 Sharpening

Open **angiogram** in ImageJ and observe the effects of sharpening on (a) its histogram (using the **live histogram** plugin) and (b) its signal-to-noise ratio (remember to choose a region of constant gray value before using the **SNR** plugin). To sharpen use (i) **Process/Filters/Convolve...** and the mask **sharpen.txt** (check its contents) and (ii) **Process/Find Edges**, which implements the Sobel masks.

Repeat with the chest radiograph image, **asthma**.

Activity 6.8 Finding edges using the Sobel operators

Open **brainpathology**, and convert it to a 32-bit image (**Image/Type/32-bit**) to avoid overflow in the subsequent operations. Use **Process/Filters/Convolve...** to convolve it in turn with the two Sobel masks (**Gx.txt** and **Gy.txt**) to get the horizontal and vertical edge images. Go to **Plugins/Macros/Install** and open **ApplyFunctiontoImage.txt**. This makes available several functions when **Plugins/Macros** is next used. Find the square root of the sum of the squares of these two edge images using the (**Sqr**) and Square Root (**Sqrt**) functions within **Plugins/Macros** and the **Add** from **Process/Image Calculator**. The final result can be changed to 8-bit and contrast-stretched, using **Process/Enhance Contrast/Normalize**. It is the Sobel "magnitude-of-the-images" image, showing all the edges in the original image. The result is similar to the result obtained directly from **Process/Find Edges**.

Divide the 32-bit Sobel vertical edge by the Sobel horizontal edge image, using **Process/Image Calculator**. Use the **Atan** function under **Plugins/Macros** to take the inverse tan of this image, which gives the Sobel "phase-of-the-edges" image. This image is useful in linking any broken edges in the "magnitude-of-the-edges" image.

Activity 6.9 The Laplacian of a Gaussian operator

The effect of the Laplacian of a Gaussian operation is to highlight edges in an image. Open **smooth** in ImageJ, and change it into a 32-bit image (**Image/Type/32-bit**) since the Laplacian of a Gaussian operator produces negative pixel values. Convolve it with the Laplacian of a Gaussian mask (using **Process/Filters/Convolve...** and using **LoG.txt**) to see the edges of the image. Verify that the pixel values include negative values, by running the mouse over the image. The contrast of this image can be improved (**Process/Enhance Contrast** and check **Normalize**) with, for example, 10% saturated pixels.

Exercises

6.1 Tracking moving objects is an important problem in computer vision. When the camera is not moving, the problem is often solvable if we know the background, i.e. what the scene looks like when no moving objects are present. Once the background is known, we can find moving objects by finding regions of the current image that are different from the background image. (In practice, this approach is not entirely successful since the background itself usually changes over time due to lighting, camera motion, or other factors. Sophisticated algorithms exist for dealing with these problems. However, we ignore those complexities for this exercise.)

Consider the sequence of images **mall<n>.tif**, where $\langle n \rangle = 1, 2, 3, \ldots, 19$. The images are of the same scene. However, none is a background image since every image contains people in motion. Using all the images together, determine the best background image, using all of the images, and then remove the background (i.e. the stationary scene) from the 19 given images.

6.2 Show, using truth tables, that A XOR B is equivalent to (A OR B) AND (NOT(A) OR NOT(B)).

6.3 Show that ANDing an image with a value N is equivalent to thresholding the image at that value.

6.4 Enlarge the profile 1 4 7 4 3 6 to lengths of (i) 9, (ii) 11 and (iii) 15 pixels, using (a) nearest-neighbor and (b) linear interpolation.

6.5 Enlarge the image

$$
\begin{array}{cccc}
8 & 8 & 13 & 9 \\
1 & 13 & 1 & 15 \\
5 & 4 & 7 & 7 \\
5 & 10 & 3 & 7
\end{array}
$$

to sizes (i) 7×7, (ii) 8×8 and (iii) 10×10, by hand, using (a) nearest-neighbor and (b) bilinear interpolation.

6.6 Suppose an image is scaled upwards in size by a factor k, and the result is then scaled downwards in size by the same factor. Is the final result exactly the same as the original image? If not, why not? What if the image is reduced in size first, and the result enlarged?

6.7 Suppose an image is rotated and then the result rotated back by the same amount (using either (i) nearest-neighbor or (ii) bilinear interpolation). Is the resulting image exactly the same as the original? If not, why not?

6.8 What is the result of convolving the following (symmetric) one-dimensional masks? (In each case you should slide one (M1) past the other (M2), doing a sum-of-products, replacing the center term (pixel) of M2, and then shifting M1 by a single term (pixel).)

(i) $[\,1\,1\,1\,] * [\,1\,1\,1\,]$;

(ii) $[\,1\,1\,1\,] * \begin{bmatrix} 1 \\ 1 \\ 1 \end{bmatrix}$;

(iii) $[\,1\,2\,1\,] * \begin{bmatrix} 1 \\ 2 \\ 1 \end{bmatrix}$;

(iv) $[\,1\,1\,1\,] * \begin{bmatrix} -1 \\ 0 \\ 1 \end{bmatrix}$;

(v) $[-1\,0\,1] * \begin{bmatrix} 1 \\ 1 \\ 1 \end{bmatrix}$;

(vi) $[-1\,0\,1] * \begin{bmatrix} 1 \\ 2 \\ 1 \end{bmatrix}$;

(vii) $[1\,2\,1] * \begin{bmatrix} -1 \\ 0 \\ 1 \end{bmatrix}$.

(Note: the results of (iv) and (v) give the Prewitt operators, and the results of (vi) and (vii) give the Sobel operators.)

6.9 Applying a 3×3 averaging mask twice does not produce the same result as applying a 5×5 averaging mask once. To what is it equivalent?

6.10 Is the 3×3 median mask separable (i.e. can it be implemented by a 3×1 mask followed by a 1×3 mask)? Explain your answer.

6.11 Can unsharp masking be used to reverse the effect of blurring? Choose an image and apply an unsharp mask after a 3×3 averaging mask. Describe the result.

6.12 An averaging mask is applied to an image to reduce noise, and then a Laplacian mask is applied to the result to enhance small details. Would the result be the same if the order of these operations were reversed? Explain.

6.13 What 3×3 mask performs unsharp masking in a single pass through an image?

6.14 What effect does increasing the Gaussian kernel size within the Canny operator have on the magnitudes of the gradient maxima at edges? What change does this imply has to be made to the tracker thresholds when the kernel size is increased?

6.15 Under what situations might you choose to use the Canny operator rather than the Roberts cross-gradient or Sobel operators? In what situations would you not choose it?

7   Image enhancement in the frequency domain

Overview

A number of mathematical transformations can be applied to images to obtain information that is not readily available in the raw image. The *Fourier transform* is the most popular although other transforms, such as *wavelets* and the *Gabor transform*, are being increasingly used. The Fourier transform converts the spatial domain representation of an image into an alternative representation in the Fourier domain, in terms of spatial frequencies. Convolution of the input data with the point spread function of an imaging system results in the formation of an image. The convolution operation in the spatial domain is equivalent to multiplication in the Fourier domain, which is a more efficient method of performing smoothing or sharpening of an image.

Learning objectives

After reading this chapter you will be able to:

- describe how periodic waveforms consist of a linear superposition of sinusoids;
- explain how the Fourier transform is derived from the Fourier series;
- illustrate the concept of the discrete Fourier transform in two dimensions, with its dependence on sample and hold;
- describe the phenomenon of aliasing and apply appropriate procedures to eliminate it;
- outline the properties of the Fourier transform;
- use cross-correlation to perform template matching;
- obtain the spatial resolution of an imaging system both from its point spread function (PSF) and from its modulation transfer function (MTF), and show that they are equivalent;
- use frequency domain filters to smooth or sharpen an image while avoiding ringing artifacts;
- explain the need for filters in filtered backprojection and summarize the filtered backprojection algorithm;
- outline the properties of the Radon transform;
- describe the process of direct Fourier reconstruction.

7.1   The Fourier domain

Although the convolution process provides a model for the formation of an image from input signals by a (linear shift-invariant) imaging system, there exists an alternative and equivalent way of modeling the process in terms of the *spatial frequency* content of the image. Spatial frequency is a measure of how frequently gray values change over distance. High spatial frequencies are characterized by small repeat distances; the gray value changes from dark to bright to dark over small distances, such as occurs for fine details like edges or noise in an image. Low spatial frequencies are characterized by large repeat distances; the gray value changes little with distance, such as occurs for large objects or background in an image.

Just as a sinusoid that varies with time has a frequency (in hertz), which is inversely proportional to the repeat time, the period T (in seconds), so a sinusoid that varies with distance has a *spatial frequency*, which is inversely proportional to the repeat distance, the wavelength λ (in, say, centimeters). The spatial frequency (or wave number), k, is related to the wavelength of the sinusoid, which is the spatial equivalent to the period, by

$$k = \frac{1}{\lambda} \tag{7.1}$$

and has units of cm^{-1} for wavelengths measured in centimeters. In two-dimensional images, the spatial frequency k is related to its components, denoted u and v, corresponding to repeat distances in the x and y directions, respectively, by

$$k = \sqrt{(u^2 + v^2)} \tag{7.2}$$

Figure 7.1 shows sinusoidal patterns of intensity; those that repeat over a short distance have a high spatial frequency (Fig. 7.1(i)), while those that repeat over a long distance have a lower spatial frequency (Fig. 7.1(ii)).

Continuous, periodic waveforms can always be expressed as a series of appropriately weighted sums of sinusoids (sines and cosines), which are integral multiples of a fundamental frequency; the series is known as the Fourier series (Appendix A). Sinusoids are the *basis functions*, comprising a single frequency, from which a more complex, periodic waveform, $f(x)$, can be constructed. They are particularly useful because they are mutually independent or *orthonormal*.

$$f(x) = \frac{1}{2}a_0 + \sum_{n=1}^{\infty} a_n \cos(nx) + \sum_{n=1}^{\infty} b_n \sin(nx) \tag{7.3}$$

The zero-frequency term, $\frac{1}{2}a_0$, if present, constitutes a constant or zero-frequency term, often referred to as the d.c. term borrowing a notation from electrical engineering. The *fundamental frequency* or *first harmonic*, the term with harmonic number n equal to 1, describes the rate at which the whole pattern repeats itself. *Higher harmonics*

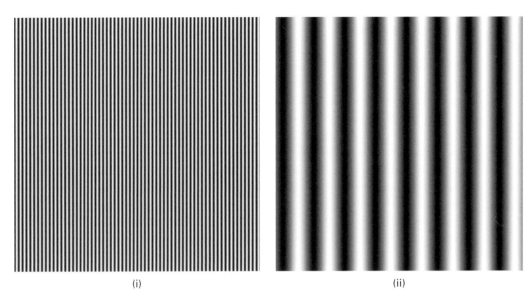

Figure 7.1   Sinusoidal shapes which repeat along the x axis: (i) high spatial frequency and (ii) low spatial frequency.

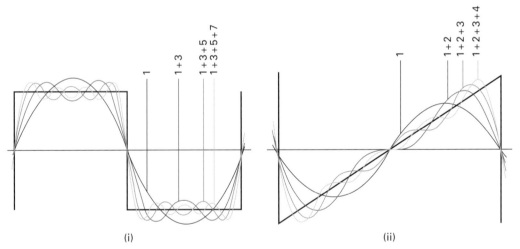

Figure 7.2   Harmonic analysis of (i) square wave and (ii) sawtooth wave. Each comprises a fundamental, i.e. a sinusoid of the same repeat distance (labeled 1) and higher harmonics (labeled 2, 3, 4).

are denoted by higher values of n, e.g. the second harmonic by $n = 2$, the third harmonic by $n = 3$, etc.

Figure 7.2 shows two examples of periodic one-dimensional profiles, and indicates how they can be constructed from sinusoids. Note that sharp edges require high spatial frequencies. The process of decomposing a periodic function into its constituent sine or cosine waves is called *Fourier analysis*. The reverse process, that of combining a series of sines or cosines to give a more complicated function, is known as *Fourier synthesis*.

The notation can be simplified using complex exponential functions

$$f(x) = \sum_{n=-\infty}^{n=\infty} C_n \exp(j \cdot 2\pi nx/L) \tag{7.4}$$

where the Fourier coefficients, C_n, are complex numbers with a magnitude and phase, which can be displayed as the *Fourier spectrum* (see Activity 7.1).

Since a sine wave comprises just a single sinusoidal term, its Fourier spectrum comprises just a single magnitude term (Fig. 7.3(i)). A sawtooth wave comprises a sum of harmonics, with the magnitude of their coefficients decreasing as $1/n$, that is 1, 1/2, 1/3, 1/4,... The phases alternate between 90° and −90°, determining whether the term is a sine or a cosine (Fig. 7.3(ii)). A square wave is composed of odd harmonics only, with Fourier coefficients that go as $1/n$ (Fig. 7.3(iii)). The high-frequency terms contribute to the sharp edges of the square wave. It is not possible to build up a sharp edge or discontinuity exactly; even with an infinite number of terms there are always some residual oscillations, known as *ringing*.

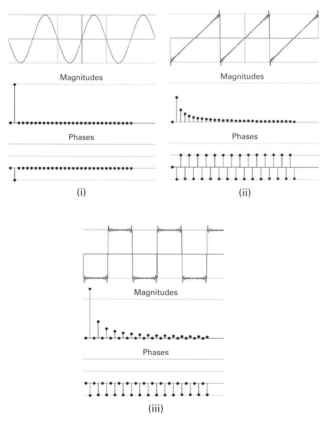

Figure 7.3 The waveform and Fourier spectra (magnitude and phase) of (i) a sine wave, (ii) a sawtooth wave and (iii) a square wave.

7.2   The Fourier transform

When a waveform is not periodic, its repeat distance is effectively infinite. The waveform can still be synthesized from sinusoids, but a continuous range of frequencies is required rather than only integral multiples of a fundamental frequency. This continuous mix of frequencies is known as the *Fourier transform* (FT). The Fourier transform is a complex quantity, with real and imaginary parts; it is often more helpful intuitively to combine these parts into an amplitude and a phase (Appendix A). The *amplitude spectrum* shows the relative amounts of different frequencies in the original waveform, while the *phase spectrum* shows their relative positions. Thus, the Fourier transform converts the original *spatial domain* representation of a waveform or profile, in terms of grayscale intensities, into an alternative *frequency domain* representation, in terms of spatial frequencies.

Figure 7.4 illustrates a number of one-dimensional profiles with their corresponding Fourier amplitude spectra. The rectangular pulse or *rect* function (Fig. 7.4(i)) transforms into a sinc (that is, $\sin \theta/\theta$) shape known as the *sampling function*. Note that it is a continuous function, indicating that all frequencies, not just the harmonics, are present. There are side lobes, separated by zero crossings at $\pm 1/a$, $\pm 2/a$,... and so on. The envelope of the Fourier spectra falls as $1/n$, just like the Fourier series of a periodic rectangular pulse train.

For all pulse shapes, the width of the pulse in the spatial domain (Δx) is inversely proportional to the width of its transform in the frequency domain (Δk); the relationship is

$$\Delta x \, \Delta k \geq 2\pi \tag{7.5}$$

A Gaussian pulse achieves the minimum product due to its smooth shape in both domains; the Fourier transform of a Gaussian pulse is another Gaussian (Fig. 7.4(ii)).

A *delta* or *impulse function*, $\delta(x)$, has zero value except at position $x = 0$, and encloses an area of unity (Fig. 7.4(iii)). Its Fourier spectrum has constant amplitude and phase and extends from $u = -\infty$ to $+\infty$.

Higher-dimensional signals can be treated by a straightforward generalization of the one-dimensional Fourier transform. The Fourier transform of a two-dimensional image, for example, can be displayed as two separate (two-dimensional) images, a *magnitude* (or *amplitude*) *image* and a *phase image*. The spatial frequency, k, increases radially from zero (d.c.) at the center of the images. The frequencies at the horizontal and vertical edges correspond to the highest frequencies or smallest resolvable lengths, namely two pixels, in the spatial domain signal (Fig. 7.5). Some software displays both the magnitude and the phase images, while other software displays only the square of the complex Fourier transform, the *power* (or *power spectral density,* PSD) *image*. Since the high-frequency components of an image are frequently very small, the power image is frequently displayed using a logarithmic look-up table.

Figure 7.6(i) shows two (spatial domain) images, a horizontal sinusoid and a vertical sinusoid, and their Fourier transform (power spectral density) images. Each transform image contains a spot at the center of the image, the zero-frequency term, which contains

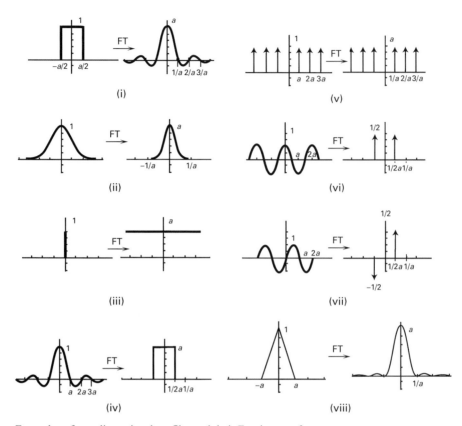

Figure 7.4   Examples of one-dimensional profiles and their Fourier transforms.

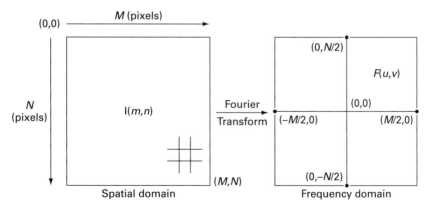

Figure 7.5   Relationship of parameters in the spatial and spatial frequency domains.

information on the average brightness of the spatial domain image, and two spots symmetrically placed about the center. One of these spots is redundant (which one?) and is present because of the symmetry of the Fourier transform operation. The distance of the spots from the center indicates the frequency of the original sinusoid, and the

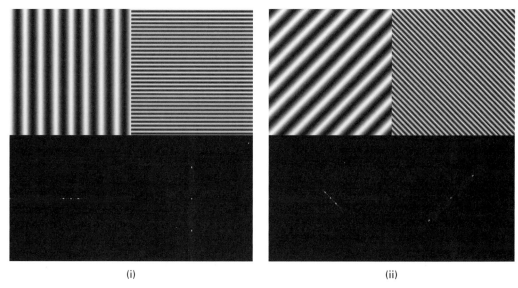

	(i)		(ii)

Figure 7.6   (i) Two sinusoidal images and their Fourier transform (power) images. (ii) The two sinusoidal images of (i) are rotated, causing their Fourier transform images to rotate.

brightness of the spots indicates the intensity of the sinusoid. The sinusoid on the top left of Figure 7.6(i) is of low frequency and runs in the horizontal direction; the spots in its Fourier transform image are on the horizontal (u) axis and close to the central zero-frequency spot. The sinusoid on the top right of Figure 7.6(i) is of higher frequency and runs in the vertical direction; its Fourier transform spots lie on the vertical axis, further from the central, zero-frequency spot. If the original images are rotated, their Fourier transforms are rotated by the same angles (Fig. 7.6(ii)).

Figure 7.7 shows two images, each of which comprises a mixture of a horizontal and a vertical sinusoid. Each component contributes spots to the Fourier transform image, depending on their frequencies and relative strengths. You can experiment with similar images and their Fourier transforms by working through Activity 7.2.

Figure 7.8 shows several images on the left with their corresponding (power) Fourier transforms on the right. The rectangular/square objects (Figs. 7.8(i), (iii), (v), (vii)) result in images with a sinc nature (Figs. 7.8(ii), (iv), (vi), (viii)), whose widths are inversely proportional to the lengths of the objects in that direction. Thus, the smaller the object, the greater the energy content at higher spatial frequencies. Rotating an object (Fig. 7.8(vii)) causes its Fourier transform image to rotate by the same amount (Fig. 7.8(viii)). A circular object (Fig. 7.8(ix)) results in a circularly symmetric Fourier image (Fig. 7.8(x)).

Most images are more complicated than sinusoids, blocks and circles and comprise a mixture of many spatial frequencies. However, their Fourier transform images can still be understood in terms of the basic concepts. The strong periodic pattern in the image of the bricks (Fig. 7.9), especially in the vertical direction, results in prominent spots along the vertical axis of the Fourier transform image. In the Fourier transform image of the

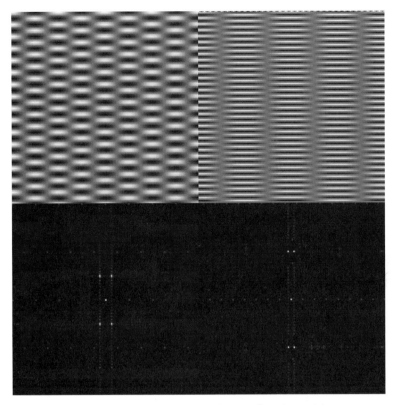

Figure 7.7   Two mixed sinusoidal images and their Fourier transform (power) images.

building blocks (Fig. 7.9), bright lines indicating a collection of frequencies appear perpendicular to the strong edges of the spatial image.

The letters in Figure 7.10 have quite different Fourier transforms, especially at the lower frequencies. Bright lines in the Fourier transform images appear in directions perpendicular to edges in the spatial domain. Note that parallel edges do not introduce any new features since translation in a spatial image has no effect on the Fourier transform. If the letter has circular segments, then so does its Fourier transform.

The concentric ring structure in the Fourier transform of the pellets in Figure 7.11 is due to each individual pellet. The information about the whereabouts of each pellet is contained mostly in the Fourier phase image. The coffee beans (Fig. 7.11) have less symmetry and are more variably colored so they do not show a strong ring structure.

Most images have less repetitive structure and therefore less prominent spots in their Fourier transform (Fig. 7.12). In the Fourier transform image of the young woman, the line from top left to bottom right is due to the edge between her hat and her hair. The Fourier transform of the mandrill image shows more high-frequency power, due to the fine hair. The Fourier transform of the chest radiograph show a broad range of spatial frequencies, with significant vertical and horizontal features, as might be expected from the horizontal ribs and vertical vertebral column in the radiograph.

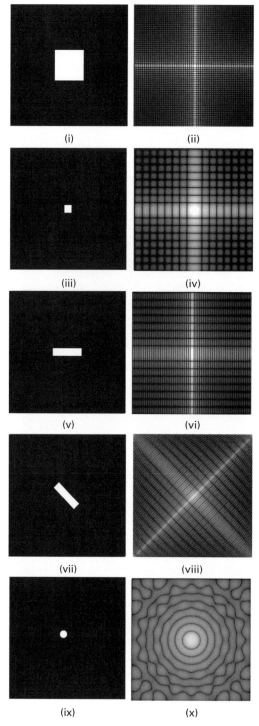

Figure 7.8 All images are 256 × 256 pixels. (i) Image with a white square of size 64 × 64. (ii) Fourier transform of the image in (i). (iii) Image with a white square of size 16 × 16. (iv) Fourier transform of the image in (iii). (v) Image with a white rectangle of size 64 × 16. (vi) Fourier transform of the image in (v). (vii) Image (v) rotated 45° clockwise. (viii) Fourier transform of the image in (vii). (ix) Image with circle of diameter 16 pixels. (x) Fourier transform of the image in (ix).

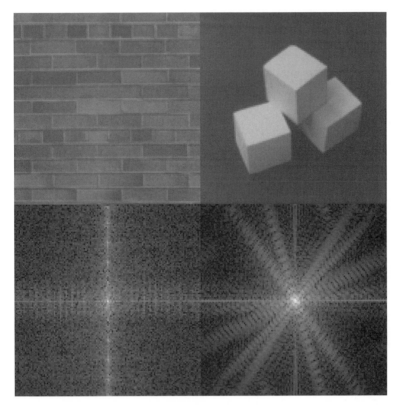

Figure 7.9   Bricks and building blocks (top), and their Fourier transform (power) images (bottom).

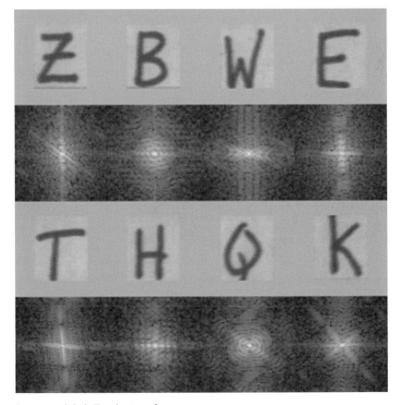

Figure 7.10   Letters and their Fourier transforms.

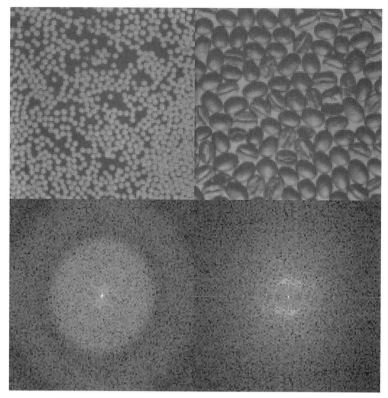

Figure 7.11   Pellets and coffee beans (top), and their Fourier transform (power) images (bottom).

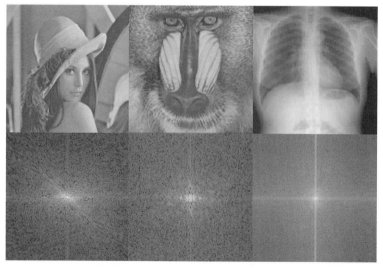

Figure 7.12   Young woman, mandrill and chest radiograph (top), and their Fourier transform (power) images (bottom).

7.3 Properties of the Fourier transform

The Fourier transform has a number of interesting properties, some of which we have discussed already. They can be summarized as follows.

(i) *Separability*   The two-dimensional discrete Fourier transform (DFT) of a matrix (i.e. an image comprising pixel values) can be implemented as two consecutive one-dimensional discrete Fourier transforms, one operating on the rows and the other on the columns. We first calculate the (one-dimensional) discrete Fourier transform of all the rows, and then calculate the (one-dimensional) discrete Fourier transform of all the columns of the result (Fig. 7.13). Since a product is independent of the order, we could equally well calculate the two-dimensional discrete Fourier transform by calculating the (one-dimensional) discrete Fourier transform of all the columns first, and then calculating the (one-dimensional) discrete Fourier transform of all the rows of the result.

(ii) *Linearity* or *linear superposition*   If the Fourier transforms of two signals $f(x, y)$ and $g(x, y)$ are $F(u, v)$ and $G(u, v)$, respectively, then

$$F(af(x, y) + bg(x, y)) = aF(u, v) + bG(u, v) \tag{7.6}$$

(iii) *Translation* or *shifting*   The discrete Fourier transform of a shifted function is unaltered except for a linearly varying phase factor. Translating the original image by (x_0, y_0) does not change the magnitude spectrum of the discrete Fourier transform, just its phase spectrum.

(iv) *Periodicity* and *symmetry*   The discrete Fourier transform and inverse discrete Fourier transform are periodic with period N, and if $f(x, y)$ is real, the Fourier magnitude image has two-fold symmetry.

(v) *Rotation*   If an image is rotated, then its Fourier transform rotates an equal amount.

(vi) *Scaling*   This property is best summarized by "a contraction in one domain produces corresponding expansion in the other domain." Thus a wide Gaussian image transforms to a narrow Gaussian in the frequency domain, and vice versa.

(vii) *Convolution*   Convolution in the spatial domain corresponds to multiplication in the frequency domain, and vice versa. This is represented by Equations (7.7a) and (7.7b):

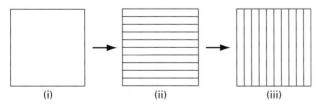

(i)   (ii)   (iii)

Figure 7.13   Calculating a two-dimensional discrete Fourier transform (DFT). (i) Original image. (ii) Discrete Fourier transform of each row of (i). (iii) Discrete Fourier transform of each column of (ii).

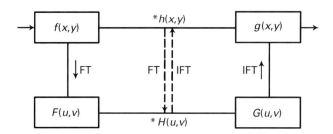

Figure 7.14

$$f(x, y) * h(x, y) \leftrightarrow F(u, v)H(u, v) \qquad (7.7a)$$

and

$$f(x, y)h(x, y) \leftrightarrow F(u, v) * H(u, v) \qquad (7.7b)$$

Instead of processing an image by convolving it with a mask or kernel, for smoothing or sharpening, the Fourier transform of the image can be multiplied by the corresponding filter in the frequency domain and the inverse Fourier transform taken (Fig. 7.14) to give the same result. Although the latter pathway comprises more steps, it is usually more computationally efficient because the speed of the algorithms used to compute the Fourier transform and inverse Fourier transform more than compensate for the complexity of convolution.

Fast Fourier transform (FFT) algorithms are efficient implementations of the discrete Fourier transform, and have proven essential in its development as a practical tool for the analysis of digital images. One of the most common fast Fourier transform algorithms recursively subdivides an image into smaller images, which are transformed and subsequently recombined. If the image is divided into smaller images of size $N/2$ at each step, the algorithm is limited in application to square images whose sides are integral powers of two; for images that do not meet this requirement, either a square, power-of-two sized region can be selected, or the image can be extended by padding out with zero values to the next square, power-of-two size. There are however many other algorithms that are not limited to square, power-of-two size images. The gain in computational efficiency in using a fast Fourier transform algorithm is considerable; for an image of length $N (=2^n)$ the saving in time over direct computation of the discrete Fourier transform is of the order of $2^n/n$. Activity 7.3 explores the accuracy of a fast Fourier transform algorithm by taking a Fourier transform and then its inverse, and comparing the result with the original image.

(viii) *Projection* The one-dimensional Fourier transform of a projection of a two-dimensional function at an angle φ forms a line in the two-dimensional Fourier space of the image at the same angle. This is known as the *Central Slice Theorem*, and is the basis of the *Radon Transform* used in the reconstruction of tomographic images by backprojection.

(ix) *Energy*   The energy of an image is given by the sum of the squares of its pixels. Since the frequency domain images, both magnitude and phase, are an equivalent representation, the energy can also be found by taking the square of the magnitude of the Fourier coefficients in reciprocal space. This is referred to as *Rayleigh's Energy theorem* or *Parseval's theorem*:

$$P(u, v) = \sum |f(x, y)|^2 = \sum |F(u, v)|^2 \tag{7.8}$$

where the summation is over all pixels. The power terms are obtained by multiplying the respective complex amplitude and its complex conjugate.

Activity 7.4 explores some of the properties of the discrete Fourier transform.

7.4   Sampling

Figure 7.15(i) illustrates a one-dimensional analog waveform and its (analog) Fourier amplitude spectrum. Digitizing an analog signal involves sampling it at a number of equally spaced positions, and quantizing those values to form discrete pixel values. The distance between samples constitutes the pixel size and determines the smallest detail that can be seen in the digitized image, i.e. the spatial resolution. Intensity quantization limits the number of gray values in the digital image, e.g. using 8 bits for each pixel value limits the number of gray levels resolution to 256.

The regularly spaced samples are obtained by multiplying the analog image by a *comb function* or *infinite impulse train*, $III(x)$, composed of an infinite grid of infinitely narrow and infinitely tall spikes (impulses or δ-functions), the area underneath each being unity and their separation, Δx, being equal to the linear pixel size (Fig. 7.15(ii)). This represents the ideal *sampling* process. The result of the multiplication is that the spikes are scaled by the sample values (Fig. 7.15(iii)). It is interesting to consider the effect of sampling in the frequency domain. Since multiplication in one domain, spatial or frequency, is equivalent to convolution in the other, the spectral shape of the analog signal in the frequency domain is convolved with another comb function (recall that the Fourier transform of a comb function is another comb function (Fig. 7.4), whose separations are inversely related to the separations in the spatial domain); this gives rise to a periodic *replication* of the spectral shapes centered on frequencies of $\pm n/\Delta x$, where Δx is the sample spacing in the spatial domain (Fig. 7.15(iii)). The inverse of the sample spacing, $1/\Delta x$, can be identified as the sampling frequency, f_s. For example if the samples were taken 0.002 inches apart, the sampling frequency would be 500 samples per inch, often denoted as 500 dpi (dots per inch).

In fact the sampling comb function is infinite. In order to make it finite, we need to truncate it by multiplying it by a rectangular or *box-car* function, $rect(x)$ (Fig. 7.15(iv)), whose length is equal to the linear size, L, of the waveform, which is an integral number of pixels, $N\Delta x$. The rect function in the spatial domain is a "do nothing" window, in that it truncates the spatial data to the physical size of the waveform but does not modify the data values within the waveform. However it modifies the frequency spectrum somewhat (Fig. 7.15(v)) due to convolution with its Fourier transform, a narrow sinc function, $sinc(f)$.

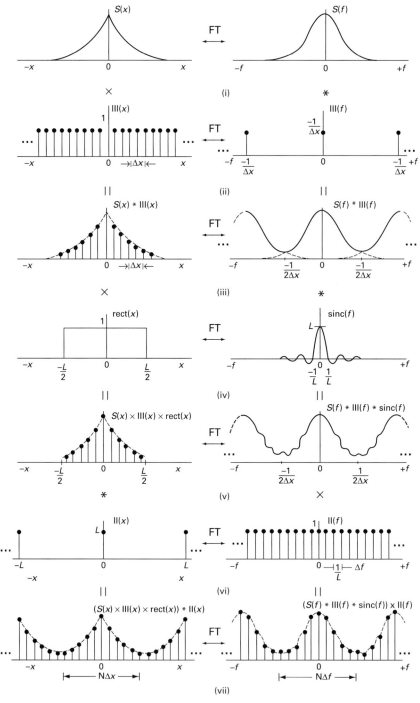

Figure 7.15   The process of image digitization shown in the spatial and frequency domains: (i) the analog image; (ii) comb function for sampling in the spatial domain; (iii) effect of sampling; (iv) truncation function; (v) effect of truncation; (vi) comb function for sampling in the frequency domain; (vii) effect of sampling in the frequency domain – the discrete Fourier transform.

The holding of the values in the spatial domain between samples can be represented by convolving the sampled points with a narrow rectangular function, whose width equals the distance between sampling points, i.e. the pixel size. This is equivalent to multiplication in the frequency domain of the replicated spectrum by a wide sinc function, which is the Fourier transform of the rectangular hold function. This suppresses the Fourier magnitudes of the replicated spectrum at higher spatial frequencies, resulting in a blurring of the sampled function and is the cause of the *partial volume* effect in computed tomography (CT) and other digital modalities. We have not shown this additional effect in Figure 7.15.

Computation of the Fourier transform requires evaluation at discrete frequencies, the discrete Fourier transform (DFT). These frequencies are chosen to be N values sampled at equal intervals over the periodicity of the frequency domain (Fig. 7.15(vi)). Thus,

$$\triangle f = 1/(N \triangle x) = 1/L \qquad (7.9)$$

The process of multiplying the Fourier transform by this comb function, $\text{II}(f)$, is to convolve its spatial domain equivalent by a wide comb function to give a periodic, discrete spatial function (Fig. 7.15(vii)). Thus calculating the discrete Fourier transform implies that the spatial domain image itself is periodic.

For real data, the discrete Fourier transform produces N complex values, whose real parts are an even function of frequency and whose imaginary parts are an odd function of frequency. This results in the amplitude image having even symmetry and the phase image having odd symmetry.

In a practical digital system, the heights of the digitized samples (i.e. pixel value) are also quantized; they are limited to a discrete set of 2^n values for n-bit quantization. If the sampled height falls between two of these discrete values it is approximated to the closer of the values. This results in an approximation known as quantization error (see Section 2.4.2).

7.4.1 Window functions

Due to the periodic assumption implicit in the discrete Fourier transform of an image, the image frame wraps from its right edge around to its left edge, and from its bottom edge around to its top edge (Fig. 7.16). If there are significant differences between the right and left edges, or between the top and bottom edges, the Fourier transform sees abrupt spatial

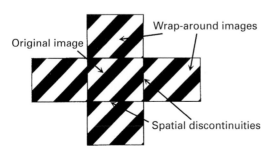

Figure 7.16   The Fourier transform sees the original image as though it were periodic. This introduces spatial discontinuities at the edges of the original image which the Fourier transform tries to model, causing erroneous frequency components to be introduced.

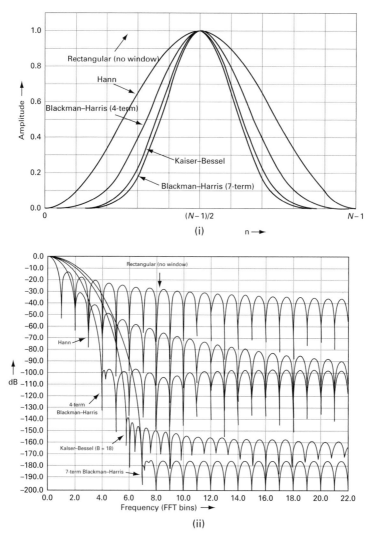

Figure 7.17   (i) Profiles of several commonly used window functions and (ii) their Fourier transforms. See also color plate.

discontinuities in the image which it attempts to model. When the frequency image is transformed back to the spatial domain, it contains spatial distortion artifacts because of the attempt to model discontinuities that did not really exist in the original image.

Let us consider this in more detail. In the frequency domain the actual image can be extracted from the infinitely repeating image by multiplying the latter by a two-dimensional rect (or box-car) function. However, the inverse Fourier transform of this product introduces *ringing* in the spatial domain because of convolution with the lobes of the sinc function, which is the Fourier transform of the rect function. Both the ringing and the wrap-around effect can be minimized by pre-multiplying the sampled image in the frequency domain by a tapering *window* function, which rolls off smoothly from unity in the center to zero at both ends (Fig. 7.17(i)). The narrowest windows in the

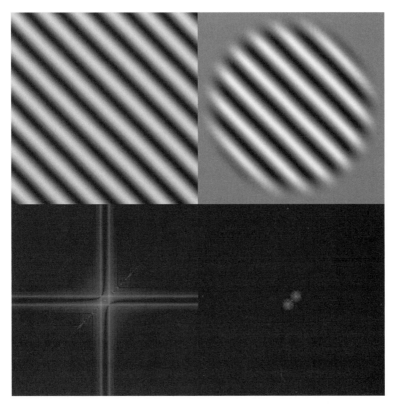

Figure 7.18   Image and windowed version of image (top), and their respective Fourier (power) images (bottom).

frequency domain will have the widest main lobes in the time domain, and vice versa (Fig. 7.17(ii)). In general, window functions can be applied either in the spatial or frequency domains. Selecting the best window is not a simple task, since each is a compromise between having a narrow main lobe (for good resolution) and having small secondary side lobes (to minimize ringing). The four-term Blackman–Harris window function is a good general purpose window, having a moderately narrow main lobe and a side lobe rejection of about 100 dB.

The discrete Fourier transforms of both an image and a windowed version of the same image are shown in Figure 7.18. Clearly the streaking of the spots in the Fourier transform is significantly reduced by windowing.

7.4.2   Aliasing

The sampling process can introduce *aliasing*, which results in false low-frequency signals, if the sampling frequency is not sufficiently high, i.e. the pixel size is not sufficiently small. It is possible for adjacent copies, or *aliases*, of the replicated signal, which are separated by $1/\Delta x$, to overlap in the frequency domain if they contain

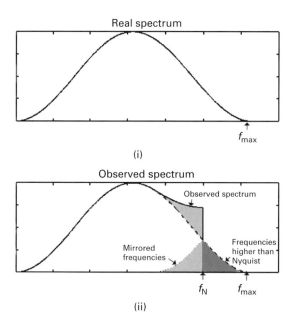

Real spectrum

(i)

Observed spectrum

Observed spectrum

Mirrored
frequencies

Frequencies
higher than
Nyquist

f_N f_{max}

(ii)

Figure 7.19   (i) Real frequency spectrum of a waveform. (ii) Observed spectrum after aliasing.

frequencies greater than $1/2\Delta x$. This overlap can be seen to happen in Figure 7.15(iii). The frequency at which aliasing begins is known as the Nyquist frequency, f_N (=$1/2\Delta x$), and is equal to one-half of the sampling frequency, f_S (=$1/\Delta x$). To avoid aliasing, samples must be taken such that the Nyquist frequency is equal to, or greater than, the highest frequency within the signal (or, equivalently, the sampling frequency must be greater than twice the maximum frequency within the signal). This is known as the *Nyquist–Shannon sampling criterion* (see Chapter 2.4.1). Failure to meet this condition results in corruption of the sampled signal, such that the original analog signal cannot be exactly recovered by an inverse transform. Instead of disappearing, frequencies higher than the Nyquist frequency reappear at lower frequencies mirrored about the Nyquist frequency and then add to the frequencies already there. Figure 7.19(i) shows the real frequency spectrum of a waveform sampled at a sampling frequency higher than twice the maximum frequency in the signal (the *Nyquist–Shannon sampling criterion*). Figure 7.19(ii) illustrates the effect of sampling when the sampling frequency does not meet this condition. The effect is to mirror the power above the Nyquist frequency, f_N, down into the Nyquist range, irreversibly corrupting the shape of the observed spectrum.

In order to avoid aliasing, the highest frequencies in the analog signal should be removed by a low-pass filter prior to sampling. This necessarily limits the bandwidth of the digitized image, but it ensures that the digitized image is not corrupted by mirrored frequencies.

Insufficient sampling of the high spatial frequencies adjacent to borders of abrupt intensity change can produce aliasing artifacts in the form of lower-frequency lines that

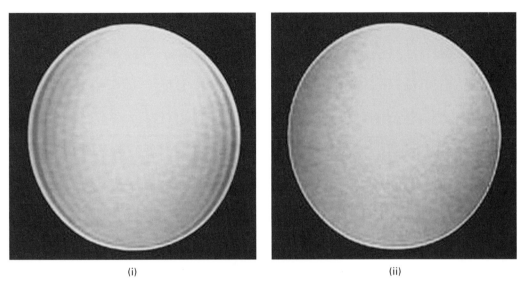

(i)	(ii)

Figure 7.20 MRI image of a water phantom using (i) 128 samples in the horizontal direction and 256 samples in the vertical direction and (ii) 256 samples in both directions.

run parallel and adjacent to the borders. Figure 7.20 shows axial images of a phantom containing water, surrounded by air. The artifacts are related to the finite number of samples used to reconstruct an image; the more samples during reconstruction, the less intense and narrower the artifacts.

A wrap-around artifact in MRI can occur when the field of view (FoV) is smaller than the object being imaged (Fig. 7.21). Parts of the object that lie beyond the field of view are seen at the edge of the image, as if folded back into the image, or wrapped around the entire image to appear on the opposite side of the image. The wrap-around artifact occurs primarily in the phase-encoding direction, and is caused by the circularity of phase space. *Oversampling* in Fourier space (i.e. using a sampling rate significantly higher than twice the highest frequency of any details in the image) can obviate the effect, although there is a time penalty for doing this since acquisition time is proportional to the number of phase-encoding steps). Many newer MR imaging systems employ a combination of over-sampling, digital filtering, and decimation (i.e. reduction of data – the opposite of interpolation) to eliminate the wrap-around artifact. Oversampling creates a larger field of view, but generates too much data to be conveniently stored. Digital filtering elim-inates the high-frequency components from the data, and decimation reduces the size of the data set.

7.4.3 Sub-sampling

Sub-sampling (or down-sampling) an image can result in aliasing. Figure 7.22(i) shows a 256×256 axial image of the brain acquired by MRI, whose Fourier transform is shown in Figure 7.22(ii). If the spatial image is sub-sampled by multiplying it by a comb function

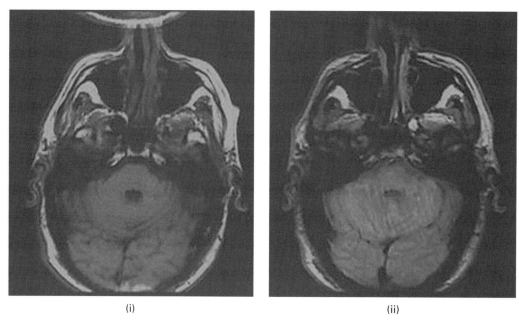

(i)   (ii)

Figure 7.21   Axial images of the brain showing (i) wrap-around of the back of the head on to the front of
the head and (ii) reduced wrap-around due to oversampling.

(Fig. 7.22(iii)), which samples every eighth pixel in either direction, the result is a very
sparse copy of the image (Fig. 7.22(iv)). The Fourier transform of this image comprises
many small regions, each 32×32 pixels and containing what seems to be the Fourier
transform of the original image (Fig. 7.22(v)). By increasing the sample spacing in the
spatial domain, the periodicity of the frequency image was reduced. Unfortunately,
however, the Fourier transform of the original image extends to higher frequencies
than are available in these small regions, and aliasing of the spectra occurred as they
were folded back into the regions resulting in very severe corruption of the data. This can
be seen if one of these small regions is isolated (Fig. 7.22(vi)), and its inverse Fourier
transform taken (Fig. 7.22(vii)). Aliasing has severely corrupted the resulting spatial
image. This effect is very different from low-pass filtering the original image (Fig. 7.22
(viii)). The visual appearance of aliasing artifacts depends on the original image, but
generally results in new patterns where none should exist. The way to avoid such aliasing
would have been to filter out the high frequencies in the original image prior to sub-
sampling.

Activity 7.5 has examples of images which exhibit aliasing when sub-sampled.

7.4.4   Reconstruction from samples

Once the analog image has been sampled, the information between sampled points has
been lost. A very practical question then arises as to whether the original analog image
can be recovered completely and exactly from the sampled points, for example when we

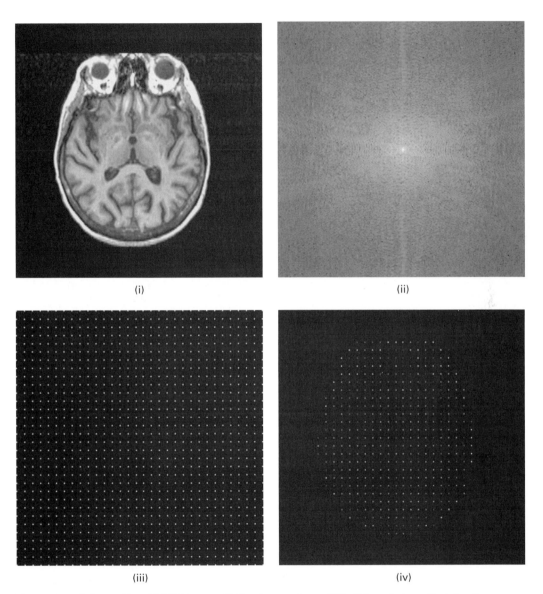

(i)   (ii)

(iii)   (iv)

Figure 7.22   Sub-sampling. (i) MRI image; (ii) Fourier transform of (i); (iii) comb (sampling) function; (iv) sub-sampled image.

want to display a digital image, after processing perhaps, on an analog computer monitor or print it on film or paper. Reconstruction requires a suitable interpolation of the sampled points.

Consider the situation in the frequency domain in one dimension, using the right-hand half of Figure 7.23. In the absence of aliasing, multiplying the sampled spectrum (Fig. 7.23(i), right) with a rectangular function that is non-zero for

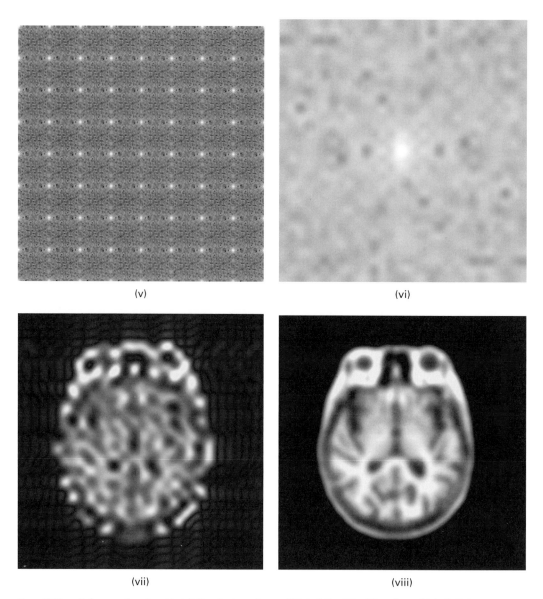

(v)

(vi)

(vii)

(viii)

Figure 7.22 Sub-sampling (cont.). (v) Fourier transform of (iv); (vi) a 32 × 32 region of (v); (vii) inverse Fourier transform of (vi); (viii) low-pass filtered version of image (i).

$-1/(2\Delta x) \leq u \leq 1/(2\Delta x)$ (Fig. 7.23(ii), right), where Δx is the spacing between samples, isolates the original analog spectrum (Fig. 7.23(iii), right) from its replicas. This is equivalent to convolution of the sampled points in the spatial domain (Fig. 7.23(i), left) with a sinc function (Fig. 7.23(ii), left), sometimes referred to as *sinc interpolation*. The resulting profile in the spatial domain (Fig. 7.23(iii), left) is an analog signal, equal to the original analog profile filtered by an ideal low-pass filter (Section 7.7.1).

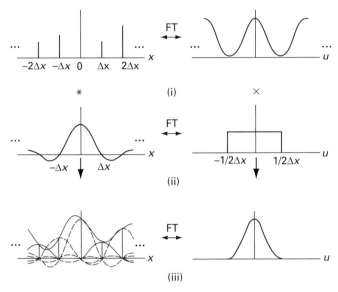

Figure 7.23 Sinc interpolation: the analog signal is recovered by convolving the sampled values (i) by scaled sinc functions (ii), as indicated by the dashed lines in (iii), as shown in the sketches on the left-hand side. The equivalent frequency domain sketches are shown on the right-hand side.

7.5 Cross-correlation and autocorrelation

Cross-correlation is a standard method of estimating the degree to which two sets of numbers are related. One set, often referred to as a mask, is slid past a reference set and a sum-of-products calculated at each position; high output values indicate where the two sets are similar, and low values where they are dissimilar. The process is similar to convolution, except that the mask is not rotated by 180° prior to calculating the sum-of-products; indeed if the mask is symmetric, then both processes are identical. For two images, f and h, each output pixel of the cross-correlation image is given by

$$g(i,j) = \sum_{m=-a}^{a} \sum_{n=-a}^{a} f(m,n)h\,(m-i,n-j) \qquad (7.10)$$

where $a = (k-1)/2$. This equation should be compared with Equation (6.12), the defining equation for convolution. We can express this cross-correlation function (CCF) in terms of the convolution operation as

$$\text{CCF} = f(x,y) * h^*(x,y) \qquad (7.11)$$

where $h^*(x, y)$ is the complex conjugate of $h(x, y)$, formed by rotating it by 180° or equivalently by flipping its rows and columns.

When the two functions (images) are identical, the term *autocorrelation function, ACF*, is used. The ACF indicates how the values of an image at a particular spatial location are statistically related to the values of the same image at other shifted locations, and can be used to detect periodicities in the image. Since the product of two quantities in one domain is equal to the Fourier transform of their convolution product in the other, then the Fourier transform of the autocorrelation function of an image is equal to its power spectrum

$$\text{FT}[f(x, y) * f^*(x, y)] = F(u, v)F^*(u, v) = |F(u, v)|^2 = P(u, v) \qquad (7.12)$$

or, equivalently, the Fourier transform of the power spectrum is the autocorrelation function. More succinctly, the power spectrum and the autocorrelation function are Fourier transform pairs. This is known as the *Weiner–Khinchin* relationship. Because of the efficiency of *fast Fourier transform* algorithms, it is generally quicker to obtain the power spectrum of an image and then compute its Fourier transform than calculate the autocorrelation function directly in the spatial domain.

When the images are different, i.e. cross-correlation, the following relationship holds:

$$\text{FT}[f(x, y) * g^*(x, y)] = F(u, v)G^*(u, v) \qquad (7.13)$$

Cross-correlation in the spatial domain can be obtained from the (inverse) Fourier transform of $F(u, v) \, G^*(u, v)$, the cross power, where $G^*(u, v)$ is the complex conjugate of $G(u, v)$.

Cross-correlation can be used for template matching (i.e. finding whether an image contains an object or template) and in spatially registering similar images (e.g. from different imaging modalities). In both cases, the peak of the cross-correlation function is sought. In practice, the images may need to be normalized to the same intensity range to avoid an uneven background in the correlation image, and the computation performed in the frequency domain.

In Figure 7.24, the normalized cross-correlation function of a template and a reference image is displayed as a surface plot. The peak indicates where the two images are best correlated, and its location indicates the offset or translation between them. A problem that affects the matching, whether it is implemented in the spatial or frequency domain, is that correlation is neither *rotation-* nor *scale*-invariant; the process does not work well unless the template is the same size as the feature in the reference image, and is similarly oriented.

Cross-correlation by itself works poorly as a template matcher. The mask and reference images need to be pre-processed to remove low frequencies and to enhance features such as edges. Activity 7.6 explores a practical example of template matching.

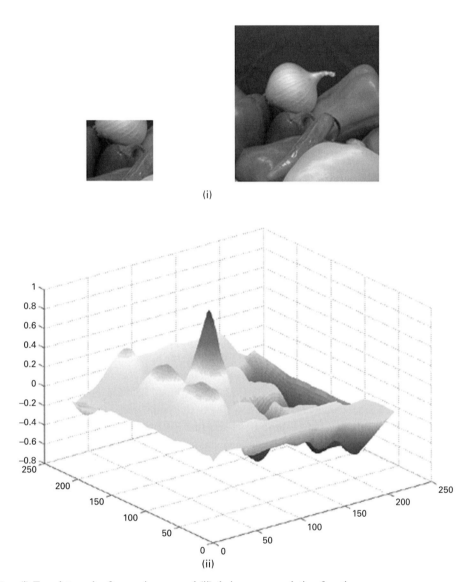

Figure 7.24 (i) Template and reference images and (ii) their cross-correlation function.

7.6 Imaging systems – point spread function and optical transfer function

A linear, shift-invariant (LSI) imaging system is characterized by a point spread function (PSF) or impulse response function, $h(x, y)$, which describes how it blurs a point (Section 2.2.2). The full width at half maximum height, FWHM, of the point spread function is taken as a measure of its width and therefore of the resolution of the system. The point spread function of most imaging systems can often be approximated by a radially symmetric Gaussian shape. The imaging process comprises the input

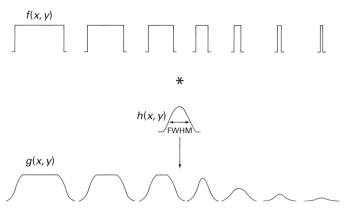

Figure 7.25   The effects of imaging sharp-edged features of various sizes. For large features the image contrast is unchanged but the edges are rendered unsharp. When the features are small their contrast is reduced, but their size remains fixed at the FWHM of the point spread function.

or object being convolved with the point spread function to give the output or image (Section 6.4).

Large features in the object experience some blurring of their edges. For features of a size similar to or smaller than the FWHM of the point spread function, the contrast of the corresponding images progressively decreases with the object size, and the image size retains the size of the point spread function (Fig. 7.25). The convolution process ensures that features smaller than the FWHM of the point spread function never appear in the image. Instead, they appear as wide as the FWHM, but with reduced contrast because convolution preserves the area under a profile. Thus, the point spread function, characterized by its FWHM, determines the size of the smallest feature seen by the system. The loss of contrast becomes progressively worse for smaller features, i.e. higher spatial frequencies.

Limited spatial resolution causes difficulties in the measurement of the thickness and brightness of thin structures. Convolution by the point spread function causes the image to be wider and less bright than the object, and the effect is increasingly significant for object sizes smaller than about twice the FWHM of the point spread function. The phenomenon is exacerbated in digital systems due to the inherent finite sampling, especially when a coarse raster is used such as in nuclear medicine imaging. The resulting overestimation of thickness and underestimation of density can be modeled by convolution with a Gaussian point spread function (Fig. 7.26). Accurate estimates of thickness, for example cardiac wall thickness in SPECT images, can be obtained by deconvolving the image with the point spread function of the imaging system.

Since convolution in one domain is equivalent to multiplication in the other, convolutional blurring can also be described by the multiplication of the Fourier transform of the image by the Fourier transform of the point spread function. The Fourier transform of the point spread function is known as the (*optical*) *transfer function,* OTF, of the imaging system. The optical transfer function is a complex function which determines the amplitude and phase of the output relative to the input. Imaging can therefore be

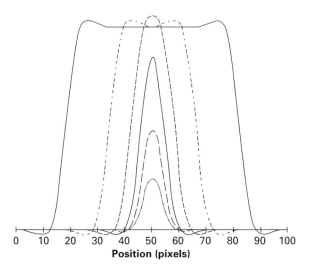

Figure 7.26 Image profiles from rectangular object features of widths 64, 32, 16, 8, 4 and 2 pixels after convolution with a Gaussian point spread function (FWHM = 8.8 pixels).

considered using two equivalent methods, according to the schema of Figure 7.14, where $h(x, y)$ and $H(u, v)$ are identified as the point spread function and the optical transfer function, respectively, of the imaging system rather than specific processing masks or filters. Thus, the point spread function and the optical transfer functions are equivalent characterizations of the imaging system response. A good imaging system has a narrow point spread function, i.e. it adds little spatial blurring, which gives rise to a wide optical transfer function in the Fourier domain, indicating that it produces a faithful image up to high spatial frequencies.

In general, the optical transfer function, OTF, can be described as

$$\text{OTF} = \text{MTF } e^{i\varphi} \tag{7.14}$$

where its modulus (magnitude) is the modulation transfer function, MTF (i.e. the frequency response of the imaging system) and the phase term ($e^{i\varphi}$) is the phase transfer function, PTF (i.e. the phase response of the imaging system). A perfect imaging system would have a modulation transfer function of unity and a phase transfer function of zero at all spatial frequencies.

In general, the modulation transfer function alone is not a complete descriptor of the imaging system because it excludes phase information. However, if the point spread function, $h(x, y)$, is real and symmetrical, which is generally true for x-ray imaging systems, then the optical transfer function is real rather than complex, and the modulation transfer function can be used interchangeably with it.

Figure 7.27 illustrates the relationship between the point spread function and the modulation transfer function. They are Fourier transform pairs. A perfect x-ray imaging system would have a point spread function of zero width, and a modulation transfer function of

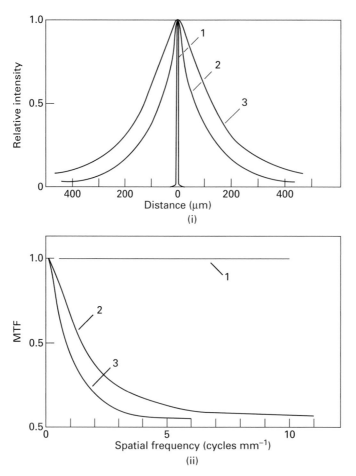

Figure 7.27　　The relationship between (i) the point spread function, PSF, and (ii) the modulation transfer function, MTF.

unity at all spatial frequencies. The FWHM of the point spread function, taken as the spatial resolution of the system, corresponds to a width on the modulation transfer function plot that defines the highest frequency that is resolvable and is the frequency where the modulation transfer function is approximately 0.1 (i.e. 10%). This contrast level broadly corresponds to the *minimum threshold of visibility.* (Indeed a modulation transfer function of 9% is implied in the definition of the *Rayleigh criterion* for the resolution of two diffraction-limited point sources.)

If a sinusoidal test pattern is imaged, then the ratio of the amplitude of the image profile to the amplitude of the object profile gives the value of the modulation transfer function at the spatial frequency of the grating. For a sinusoidal test pattern whose spatial frequency changes continuously across it (Fig. 7.28), the modulation transfer function can be computed directly at different spatial frequencies (Fig. 7.29). The MTF at low frequencies is close to unity, but decreases at higher spatial frequencies indicating the increased difficulty of accurately imaging small objects.

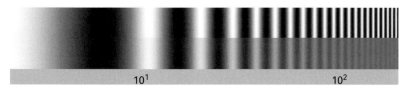

Figure 7.28 (Top) A sinusoidal test pattern of uniform contrast with spatial frequencies from 2 to 200 lp mm^{-1} and (bottom) the image formed by a certain imaging system. The modulation transfer function of the system drops to 0.5 (50%) at $\sim$42 lp mm^{-1} and to 0.1 (10%) at $\sim$126 lp mm^{-1}.

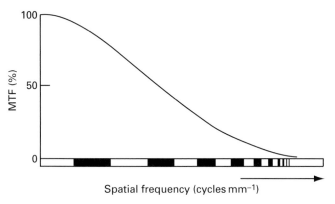

Figure 7.29 Modulation transfer function (MTF) as a function of the spatial frequencies being imaged.

The modulation transfer function is such a convenient descriptor of system performance because the total modulation transfer function of a system is the product of the modulation transfer functions of all its constituent stages. On the other hand, the total point spread function of a system is the convolution product of all the constituent point spread functions which is a much more complicated relationship.

7.7 Frequency domain filters

Convolution with a linear mask in the spatial domain can be equivalently performed by multiplication with a filter, the Fourier transform of the mask, in the frequency domain (Fig. 7.14). However this does not apply to non-linear masks, such as the median mask, which cannot be transformed directly into filters in the frequency domain.

7.7.1 Low-pass or smoothing filters

The ideal low-pass filter is a "brick-wall" filter which passes all frequencies up to a certain cut-off, k_0, and removes all frequencies beyond that. It is described by

$$
\begin{aligned}
H(k) &= 1 \quad \text{if} \quad k \le k_0 \\
&= 0 \quad \text{if} \quad k > k_0
\end{aligned}
\tag{7.15}
$$

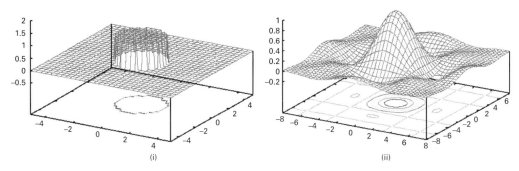

Figure 7.30   (i) Low-pass "brick wall" filter and (ii) its Fourier transform.

and is shown in Figure 7.30(i). Multiplying the transform of an image, $F(u, v)$ or $F(k)$, by such a filter preserves the low frequencies and removes the high frequencies, which contain information on the sharp edges, thus producing a smoothing effect.

The Fourier transform of an MRI image of the brain (Fig. 7.31(i)) has a Fourier transform extending to high spatial frequencies (Fig. 7.32(ii)). When the latter is multiplied by a low-pass brick-wall filter, frequencies beyond the cut-off frequency of the filter are removed (Fig. 7.31(iii)). After an inverse Fourier transform, the recovered image (Fig. 7.31(iv)) is blurred due to the loss of high frequencies and there are ringing artifacts around sharp edges in the recovered image. These result from the sharp discontinuities in the "brick-wall" filter. Its Fourier transform is a sinc function mask (not shown), whose side lobes produce the ringing artifact along intensity edges. The narrower the filter, the more severe is the resulting blurring and ringing.

Filters with a Gaussian, or near Gaussian, profile have a gradual roll-off in both domains (Fig. 7.32) and no discontinuities. They do not produce ringing artifacts, and therefore are preferred for smoothing noisy images. The standard deviation of the Gaussian in the frequency domain is the inverse of the standard deviation of the mask in the spatial domain, and vice versa. The mask profile is that of a weighted average.

Another example of a filter with a gradually tapering shape is the low-pass Butterworth filter, whose shape is given by

$$H(k) = \frac{1}{(1 + k/k_0)^{2n}} \tag{7.16}$$

where n is the *order* of the filter and k_0 is the cut-off frequency, at which the value of the transfer function falls to 0.5 (Fig. 7.33). As n increases the filter becomes sharper, with increased ringing in the spatial domain as a consequence. A filter with $n = 1$ produces no ringing, and ringing is generally imperceptible with $n = 2$, but it becomes significant for higher orders.

Low-pass filtering is used to reduce noise and produce a smoother image. This can make it easier to recognize features in an image by blurring small gaps and grayscale variations within them.

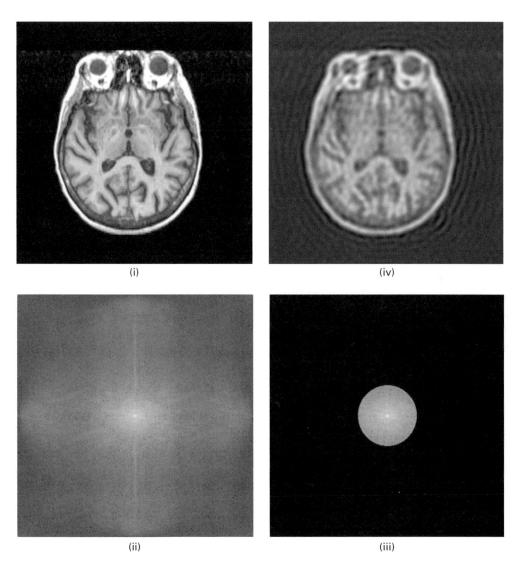

(i)   (iv)

(ii)   (iii)

Figure 7.31   (i) Axial brain MRI image (512×512 pixels). (ii) Fourier transform of (i). (iii) Image (ii) multiplied by a low-pass brick-wall filter of radius 64 pixels. (iv) Inverse Fourier transform of (iii).

7.7.2   High-pass or sharpening filters

The ideal high-pass filter is a "brick-wall" filter which passes all frequencies higher than a certain cut-off frequency, k_0, and removes all frequencies below that. It is described by

$$
\begin{aligned}
H(k) &= 0 \quad \text{if} \quad k \leq k_0 \\
&= 1 \quad \text{if} \quad k > k_0
\end{aligned}
\tag{7.17}
$$

Again, because of its sharp discontinuity, it produces unwanted ringing.

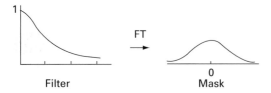

Figure 7.32   Gaussian filter and its Fourier transform, the Gaussian mask.

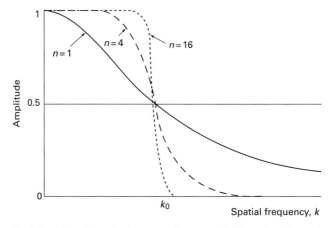

Figure 7.33   Radial profiles through a low-pass Butterworth filter, for values of order n of 1, 4 and 16.

When the Fourier transform of an image (Fig. 7.34(ii)) is multiplied by a high-pass brick-wall filter, frequencies below the cut-off frequency of the filter are removed (Fig. 7.34(iii)). After an inverse Fourier transform, the recovered image (Fig. 7.34(iv)) shows only the edges of the original image, and these edges are corrupted by ringing artifacts, which are severe in this example. Since a high-pass filter eliminates the zero-frequency (d.c.) component in an image, the average background of the filtered image is near black, but it is generally raised to mid-gray by adding an offset. The resulting image generally has poor contrast. A useful strategy to combat this is to add the result of the high-pass filtering to a portion of the original image, using higher bit-bit arithmetic to avoid overflow. This approach, known as *high-boost filtering*, is a generalization of unsharp masking (Section 6.4.2). The image is similar to the result of Sobel masking in the spatial domain. In general, (spatial) masks are more commonly used for edge detection while (frequency) filters are more often used for high-frequency boosting.

A high-pass Butterworth filter with a gradually tapering shape has a transfer function given by

$$H(k) = \frac{1}{\left(1 + k_0/k\right)^{2n}} \qquad (7.18)$$

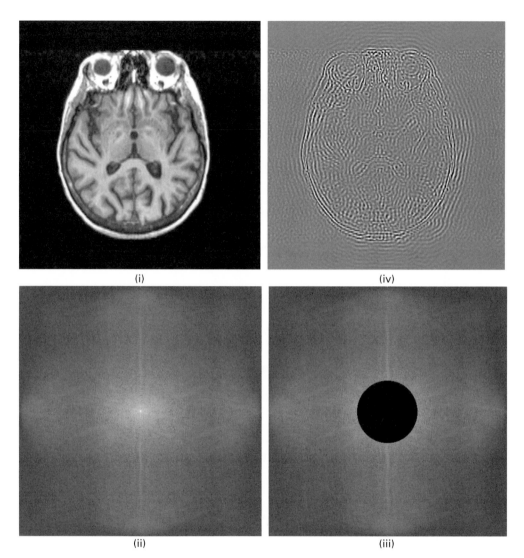

Figure 7.34   (i) Axial brain MRI image (512×512 pixels). (ii) Fourier transform of (i). (iii) Image (ii) multiplied by a high-pass brick-wall filter of radius 64 pixels. (iv) Inverse Fourier transform of (iii).

and is shown in Figure 7.35. The order determines the sharpness of the cut-off and the amount of ringing.

Figure 7.36 shows a typical high-pass filter and its Fourier transform mask, which characteristically has a large positive term in the center surrounded by smaller negative terms. There are a number of computer exercises involving various filters in Activity 7.7.

7.7.3   Band-pass and band-reject filters

Band-pass filters are a combination of both low-pass and high-pass filters. They attenuate all frequencies smaller than a frequency k_{low} and higher than a frequency k_{high}, while the

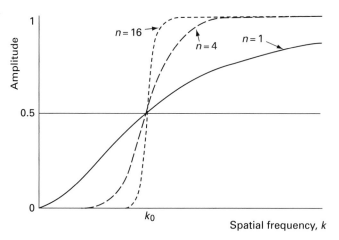

Figure 7.35 Radial profiles through a high-pass Butterworth filter, for values of order n of 1, 4 and 16.

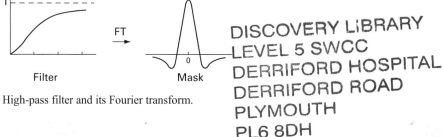

Figure 7.36 High-pass filter and its Fourier transform.

frequencies in a pass band between the two cut-offs remain in the resulting output image (Fig. 7.37). They can be constructed by multiplying a low-pass and a high-pass filter in the frequency domain, where the cut-off frequency of the low-pass filter is higher than that of the high-pass filter.

The difference of Gaussians (DoG) mask (Fig. 6.23) is equivalent to a band-pass filter. It involves the subtraction of one blurred version of an original grayscale image from another, less blurred version of the original. In the frequency domain the blurred images are obtained by multiplying the original grayscale image with low-pass Gaussian filters of differing widths. Subtracting one image from the other preserves spatial information that lies between the ranges of frequencies that are preserved in the two blurred images. It is useful for enhancing edges in noisy images.

A filter with an inverse frequency response to the band-pass filter is the *band-reject filter*. If the reject band is narrow, the filter is known as a *notch filter*. It is useful in removing a periodic signal of clearly defined frequency, such as interference patterns that can arise from pick-up of mains frequency in electronic components. The notch filter multiplies that particular frequency by zero, eliminating it in the Fourier domain; the inverse Fourier transformed image no longer contains the interfering pattern, but legitimate spatial details at that frequency are also removed which may cause some slight visual degradation. Figure 7.38(i) shows a chest radiograph contaminated by a periodic diagonal stripe. Its Fourier transform (Fig. 7.38(ii)) shows the

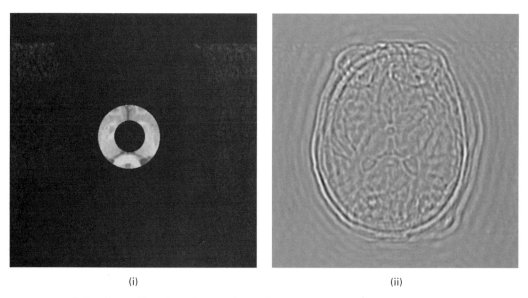

Figure 7.37   (i) Band-pass filtered Fourier transform (of the image in Fig. 7.31(i)). (ii) Inverse Fourier transform of (i).

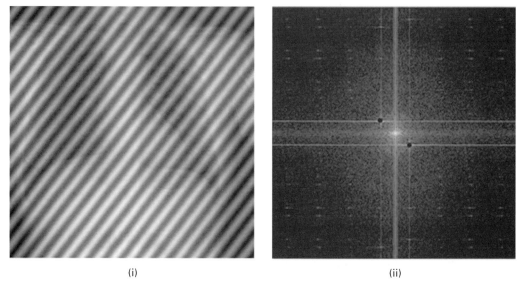

Figure 7.38   (i) Chest radiograph contaminated by periodic diagonal stripe and (ii) its Fourier transform. (iii) Result of multiplying by a notch filter and (iv) inverse Fourier transform of (iii).

frequency of the stripe, which can be removed (Fig. 7.38(iii)) by a notch filter. The inverse Fourier transform (Fig. 7.38(iv)) contains the major features of the radiograph without the contaminating stripe. Activity 7.8 considers both band-pass and notch filters.

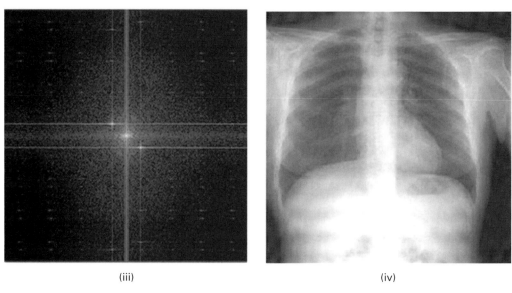

(iii)   (iv)

Figure 7.38   (cont.)

7.7.4   Homomorphic filters

Homomorphic filtering (Fig. 7.39) is a generalized technique for improving the appearance of an image by simultaneously normalizing its brightness and increasing its contrast. An image, $f(x, y)$, can be expressed as the product of illumination, $i(x, y)$, and reflectance, $r(x, y)$ components:

$$f(x, y) = i(x, y) \cdot r(x, y) \tag{7.19}$$

but these are not separable in the Fourier domain. However if the pixel-by-pixel logarithm of the image is taken, then this new image is separable in the Fourier domain:

$$\begin{aligned} F(z(x, y)) &= F(\ln f(x, y)) \\ &= F(\ln i(x, y) + \ln r(x, y)) \end{aligned} \tag{7.20}$$

This separates the illumination and reflectance components, and a filter function $H(u, v)$ can now operate on them separately. The illumination component is characterized by slow spatial variations and hence low frequencies; while the reflectance component tends to change abruptly at edges and is characterized by high frequencies. A filter function can be chosen to attenuate the low frequencies, compressing the dynamic range, and amplify the high frequencies, enhancing the contrast.

Homomorphic filtering has been used to reduce tissue intensity variation in MRI images due to inhomogeneity of the radiofrequency pulses.

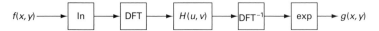

Figure 7.39 Schematic for homomorphic filtering. (DFT^{-1} indicates the inverse discrete Fourier transform.)

7.7.5 Spatial masks vs. frequency filters

Equivalent results can be obtained by processing an image in the spatial domain using convolution masks, or by Fourier transformation and multiplication in the frequency domain using the corresponding filters, but there are computational trade-offs. Generally, for small masks of size up to about 9×9, which are typical, convolution masking is efficient, but for larger masks it becomes more computationally advantageous to filter in the frequency domain.

7.8 Tomographic reconstruction

An important application of Fourier transforms in medical imaging is in the reconstruction of tomographic images. Computed tomography, as used in x-ray CT, MRI, SPECT and PET, creates two-dimensional images of the human body in different planes by recording projections at many angles around it. Fourier theory gives us an insight into the means of reconstructing images from the acquired projections.

There are a number of algorithms which can be used to reconstruct images from projections. The two most common, backprojection (and filtered backprojection) in x-ray CT and PET and SPECT, and direct Fourier reconstruction in MRI, can be understood using Fourier techniques.

7.8.1 Backprojection

Backprojection is the classical image reconstruction method. One-dimensional projections are collected along various directions, each providing information on the total attenuation along those paths, and these are projected back (i.e. back projected) and added to reconstruct the original image (Fig. 3.29).

Figure 7.40 shows a two-dimensional slice of an object, illuminated by a uniform beam of x-rays, at an angle θ to a reference coordinate system (x, y); the measured projection is denoted $p\,(r, \theta)$, and projections are acquired at different values of θ from $0°$ to $360°$.

The Radon transform describes a function in terms of its projections. The mapping from the function to the projections is the Radon transform, and the reconstruction of the function from the projections is the inverse Radon transform. The Radon transform, $\mathbf{R}\{f(x, y)\}$, of an object function $f(x, y)$ in the spatial domain is defined by the projection $p(r, \theta)$ in the polar coordinate system (r, θ) as

$$p(r,\theta) = \mathbf{R}\{f(x,y)\} = \int_{L} f(x,y)\mathrm{d}l \qquad (7.21)$$

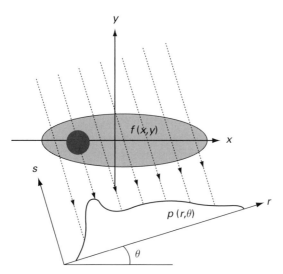

Figure 7.40   A line integral projection, $p(r, \theta)$, obtained at an angle θ.

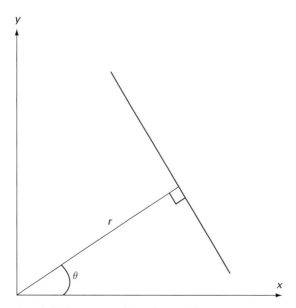

Figure 7.41   A straight line expressed in polar coordinates.

where the line integral $\int_{L}$ is taken along a line in the x–y plane given by

$$x \cos \theta + y \sin \theta = r \qquad (7.22)$$

This is the equation of a line in polar coordinates, where r is the perpendicular distance from the origin and θ is the angle with the normal (Fig. 7.41). Figure 7.40 shows the line integral projection $p(r, \theta)$ of the Radon transform. A set of projections can be obtained for different angles θ, and comprises the (two-dimensional) Radon transform.

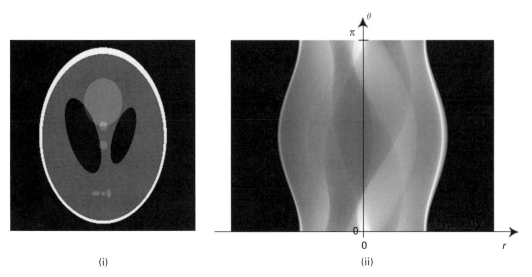

(i)   (ii)

Figure 7.42   (i) A head phantom and (ii) its corresponding (parallel-beam) sinogram.

Projections are measured as a collection of line integrals of the linear attenuation coefficient, $\mu(x, y, z)$, within a transverse cross-section. Given a set of projections at different angles θ, i.e. the Radon transform of the cross-section, the problem is to reconstruct the cross-section itself in terms of the attenuation coefficients, which is the transverse image. This is achieved by taking the inverse Radon transform, equivalent to backprojection, of the set of projections.

A line in the (x, y) plane maps to a point in (r, θ) space. A particular point (x_1, y_1) has many lines that can pass through it, each of which results in a point in (r, θ) space and satisfies Equation (7.22) with x_1 and y_1 as constants. The locus of all such points is a sinusoid, so that a point in (x, y) space corresponds to a sinusoid in (r, θ) space, i.e. in the projection or Radon domain. A real object, comprising a collection of points in the spatial domain, appears as a superposition of sinusoids with different amplitudes and phases in the projection domain. If the one-dimensional projections are stacked on top of each other, so that r and θ are displayed as rectilinear or Cartesian coordinates, they appear as a collection of overlapping sinusoids called a sinogram. A CT image of a head phantom, and its corresponding sinogram, is shown in Figure 7.42. The bottom row of the sinogram corresponds to the projection of the object at $\theta = 0°$, and the top row to the projection just short of $180°$. Beyond that the sinogram is periodic in θ.

It is possible to visualize this reconstruction simply as backprojection and superpositioning of the acquired projections, formally known as the *Linear Superpositioning of Back Projections* (LSBP) but frequently referred to as (simple) backprojection. This corresponds to a direct implementation of the inverse *Radon transform*. The projections are projected back along the directions from which they came, giving each pixel in the path the full value of each point in the projection, instead of trying to partition it between the pixels; the values are then summed to give pixel intensities, $f(x, y)$:

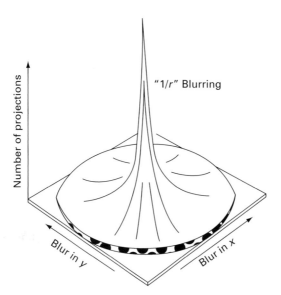

Figure 7.43   The "1/r" blurring function, i.e. the PSF of the simple back projection algorithm.

$$f(x, y) = \sum_{j=1}^{n} p(r, \theta_j) \tag{7.23}$$

and reduced in a final step.

Simple backprojection gives an approximate reconstruction of the original object, with the approximation improving as the number of projections is increased. However, even with an infinite number of projections, there is residual blurring of the reconstructed image (Fig. 3.29). The blurring is an artifact of the backprojection algorithm, often referred to as the *star artifact*, and is essentially the point spread function of the backprojection or inverse Radon transform algorithm (Fig. 7.43). It shows how the blurring is symmetric about the x and y directions, and how it reduces as the number of scans is increased; because of its characteristic shape, the blurring is also known as "1/r" *blurring*. A more sophisticated algorithm, *filtered backprojection*, is required to reduce this effect; it consists of applying a filter to each projection before backprojection.

The acquired projections, $p_a(x, y)$, suffer blurring during simple backprojection. They can be related to a notional "ideal" projection, $p(x, y)$, that would not suffer blurring, convolved with the PSF of the backprojection algorithm, the 1/r blurring function. Thus,

$$p_a(x, y) = p(x, y) * s(r) \tag{7.24}$$

where $s(r) = 1/r$, the blurring function. Transforming this relationship to the frequency domain simplifies the convolution operation to a multiply operation

$$P_a(u, v) = P(u, v) \times S(k) \tag{7.25}$$

where capitalization indicates the Fourier transform, and u and v are the components of the spatial frequency, k.

Rearranging,

$$P(u, v) = \frac{P_a(u, v)}{S(k)} \tag{7.26}$$

The Fourier transform of $1/r$ is $1/k$, so that this becomes

$$P(u, v) = P_a(u, v) \times k \tag{7.27}$$

i.e. the Fourier transform of the acquired projection should be *filtered* by multiplying with a filter which is proportional to frequency, a *ramp* filter, in order to give the Fourier transform of the "ideal" projection. The "ideal" projections are then back projected and superposed to give an image of the original object with little or no blurring. The ramp filter does not need to be implemented beyond the Nyquist frequency, $1/2a$, where "a" is the sampling distance, i.e. the distance between the centers of adjacent detectors. Indeed it is advantageous not to continue beyond this frequency, since only noise will be amplified. The ramp filter amplifies the high spatial frequencies in the image, resulting in a sharper, but noisier, final image, counteracting the "$1/r$" blurring. In order to reduce ringing artifacts and improve the noise performance of the filter, the amplification of high spatial frequencies can be reduced somewhat by using a filter such as the Shepp–Logan, low-pass cosine, or Hamming instead (Fig. 7.44). CT scanners allow the user to select from a menu of such filters during reconstruction; the most appropriate filter to use depends on the anatomy being displayed. "Smooth" or "soft tissue" filters are more rounded, with some loss of spatial resolution from residual blurring. "Sharp" or "bone" filters are close to the truncated ramp, providing more enhancement of the edges but also a noisier image.

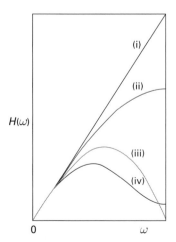

Figure 7.44 Common filters used in filtered backprojection: (i) ramp, (ii) Shepp–Logan, (iii) cosine, (iv) Hamming.

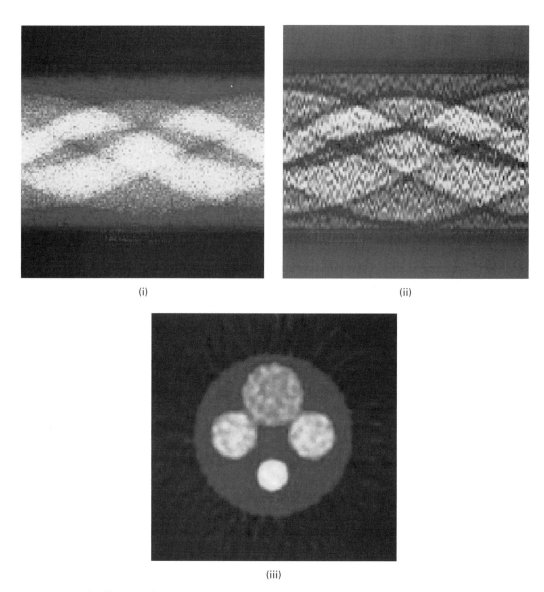

(i)   (ii)

(iii)

Figure 7.45   The direct Fourier reconstruction method used for two-dimensional image reconstruction from projections. See also color plate.

Figure 7.45 shows an example of an acquired sinogram, its appearance after filtering, and the reconstructed image using the filtered sinogram. There are computer exercises on filtered backprojection in Activity 7.9. The backprojection process is depicted in the mpeg movie `filtback` in the accompanying material for Chapter 7; it can be viewed with Windows Media Player.

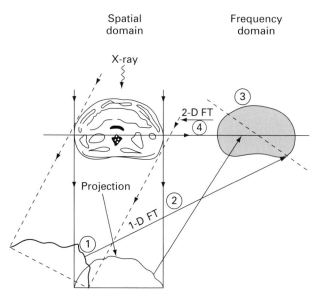

Spatial domain   Frequency domain

X-ray

2-D FT

Projection

1-D FT

Figure 7.46   The direct Fourier reconstruction method used for two-dimensional image reconstruction from projections.

7.8.2   Direct Fourier reconstruction

The Central Slice theorem establishes the connection between the slice and its projections. It shows that the one-dimensional Fourier transforms of the projections are equivalent to the values of the two-dimensional Fourier transform of the image, measured on lines through the origin of frequency space at the same angles as the original projections were acquired (Fig. 7.46). Thus, a two-dimensional Fourier transform in polar co-ordinates can be assembled from the one-dimensional Fourier transforms of many projections. After a polar to Cartesian interpolation, an inverse two-dimensional Fourier transform gives the image reconstruction of the axial (i.e. cross-sectional) slice in the spatial domain. Interpolation of the data on to a rectangular grid prior to taking the inverse transform is necessary. The two-dimensional interpolation is computer intensive unless a large number of projections are acquired, and this limits the utility of the method for x-ray CT. In MRI imaging, however, where the measured data are already obtained in terms of frequencies, the direct Fourier reconstruction technique is more attractive.

Computer-based activities

Activity 7.1 Fourier spectra

Open the Fourier applet by opening **Fourier applet/Fourier.htm**. Click the sine box at the top right to see a sine wave at the top, and Fourier "magnitude" and "phase" spectra below. The sine wave consists of a single magnitude term, the $n = 1$ term. Click the next box down to see a triangular wave. Its magnitude components are labeled from the left, $n = 0, 1, 2, 3, \ldots$ The zero-frequency, $n = 0$, term has zero magnitude. Position the mouse on the $n = 1$ magnitude term to see its contribution. The second harmonic, $n = 2$, term is also zero, indicating that it is not present in the triangular wave. The third harmonic, $n = 3$, term is present but its contribution, given by its height in the Fourier magnitude spectrum, is much smaller than the first harmonic term. All the *odd* harmonics, $n = 1, 3, 5, 7, \ldots$, are present; but all the *even* harmonics, $n = 2, 4, 6, 8, 10, \ldots$, are absent. Because the triangular wave is so similar to a sinusoid, the first harmonic predominates and the higher, odd harmonics just moderate the shape of the sinusoid slightly. The triangular wave is composed of a linear sum of odd harmonics, with weights given by the heights in the Fourier magnitude spectrum. The weights, or *Fourier coefficients*, decrease with increasing harmonics as $1/n^2$, that is, 1, 1/9, 1/25, \ldots

Look at the sawtooth shape. It is composed of a sum of all harmonics, both odd and even; and the Fourier coefficients go as $1/n$, that is 1, 1/2, 1/3, 1/4, \ldots The phases alternate between $90°$ and $-90°$, determining whether the term is a sine or a cosine.

Look at the square wave. It is composed of odd harmonics only, with Fourier coefficients that go as $1/n$. Reduce the number of terms shown using the slider, and then increase them slowly to see how the additional terms contribute to the shape of the square.

The noise button shows the randomness of white noise, which comprises a random mixture of magnitudes and phases. Each time it is pressed a different random mixture is shown. Unlike the other shapes, the Fourier coefficients do not become smaller at higher frequencies. Instead they fluctuate about a constant value.

Explore the effects of rectifying and full-wave rectifying a sinusoid. Note the constant zero-frequency term in each case. For full-wave rectification the first harmonic term is absent and the second harmonic is the dominant term, so that the process essentially doubles the frequency of the original signal.

Activity 7.2 Fourier transforms of images

Open in ImageJ the images **horiz stripe<n>** and **vert stripe<n>**, where **<n>** is 2, 4, 8, 16, 32 and 64, and indicates the number of pixels per wavelength in the image. Choose the straight line selection and plot a profile through each image (**Analyze/Plot Profile**) to check that the stripes have sinusoidal profiles; using a short line may be advantageous. Take the Fourier transform of each image (**Process/FFT/FFT**). **Horiz stripe2** has a wavelength of 2 pixels. This corresponds to the narrowest stripes and the highest frequency. In the Fourier image, the two spots are at the edge of the image corresponding to the *Nyquist frequency.*

Fourier magnitude spectra have very large dynamic ranges ($\geq 10^6$). With a linear LUT the brightest pixels would dominate, and the lower values would not be seen. Most software, ImageJ included, scales the pixel values by applying a log transformation prior to displaying the transform. This reduces the dynamic range, and allows more details to be displayed. However, if we want just to see the bright details we could reverse this transformation by applying an inverse log LUT to the image. Import the inverse LUT (**File/Import/LUT ...** and choose `invlogLUT.txt`) to view the transform of `stripe 45`. All that remains visible is the strong center component and the very strong spots at 45°.

Add two images, for example `vert stripe16` and `horiz stripe4`, using **Process/Image Calculator ... Add**. Create the sum of the images in a new window, and make it 32-bit to avoid overflow. Obtain the Fourier magnitude image, and use the inverse log LUT to view the strong spots.

Open `horiz stripe16`, and threshold it (**Image/Adjust/Threshold...**) at pixel value 128 to form an image with a square profile. Take its Fourier magnitude transform and note the additional spots. Are their positions where you expect them to be, given the Fourier series of a square wave?

Take `horiz stripe32` and subtract 128 from all its pixels (using **Process/Math/Subtract ...**), and then multiply its pixels by two (using **Process/Math/Multiply**). What is the shape of the horizontal profile through this image? It should be *half-wave rectified* (have a look at the image `rectified`). Take its Fourier magnitude transform; is this what you expect?

Make a horizontal stripe pattern with a profile showing *full wave rectification*. (Invert `horiz stripe32`, subtract 128 and multiply by 2, and then add the result to the half-wave rectified image from the last paragraph.) Does the Fourier magnitude transform show spots where you expect?

Take the Fourier magnitude transform of `house`, and explain the origin of the various spots.

Activity 7.3 Accuracy of the fast Fourier transform (FFT) algorithm

Apply the Fourier transform to the `house` image using the **FFTDirect** plugin in ImageJ, obtaining both magnitude and phase images. Use these images and the **FFTInverse** plugin to reconstruct the original image. The (direct) FFT and inverse FFT algorithms use 32-bit floating-point arithmetic to provide the necessary accuracy. The reconstructed image looks identical to the original image to the human eye, but compute the difference image between them using **Process/Image Calculator** and obtain a 32-bit difference image. The pixels in the image are small but not completely zero. Use **Analyze/Set Measurements** and check Mean Gray Value and Standard Deviation to six decimal places, then **Analyze/Measure**. The sizes of these parameters indicate the level of the errors involved in the FFT and inverse FFT calculations.

Activity 7.4 Properties of the Fourier transform

Find the Fourier magnitude images of `car1` and `car1 translated` using the **FFTDirect** plugin in ImageJ (in **Plugins/Ch.7 Plugins**), and compare them. What property of the Fourier transform can you deduce from the result? Which features in the transform images arise from the cars, and which from the textured surface below them? Find the Fourier magnitude images of `car2` and `car2 rotated` using **FFTDirect**, and compare them. What property of the Fourier transform can you deduce from this result?

Open **fourier**, and use the **FFTDirect** plugin, selecting **Magnitude**, to get the Fourier amplitude image, and select **Phase**, to get the Fourier phase image. You can use these two transform images in **FFTInverse** to recover the original image. Instead use the amplitude image only (enter it both as the magnitude and phase image), and observe the result of the inverse Fourier transform. Then use the phase image only and observe the result of the inverse Fourier transform. You may have to adjust the brightness and contrast of the resulting images. What does this suggest about the relative importance of the Fourier amplitude (magnitude) and phase images?

Open **lena** and obtain the Fourier amplitude and phase images. Reconstruct a new spatial image using **FFTInverse** (in **Plugins/Ch.7 Plugins**) to combine the amplitude image from the **fourier** image with the phase image from **lena**. Then combine the phase image from **fourier** with the amplitude image from **lena**. What do you conclude?

The crucial importance of the phase information is not intuitively obvious. While the amplitude spectrum specifies *how much* of each frequency component is present, the phase spectrum specifies *where* each component resides in the image. Evidently, as long as the components are kept in position, their amplitudes appear to be less critical to the integrity of the image. For this reason, most practical filters operating in the frequency domain are designed to affect the amplitude only, and preserve the phase information. They are known as *zero phase* filters and introduce no phase distortion.

Take the Fourier transform of **grid**. Note how the closely spaced pattern along the *x* axis is transformed to widely separated spots, and how the widely spaced pattern along the *y* axis is transformed to closely separated spots.

Activity 7.5 Aliasing

Open **radial lines** and use **Image/Scale ...** and a scale of 0.5 to sub-sample, then a scale of 2.0 to re-sample the image. Uncheck **Interpolate** each time. Note the loss of high frequencies in the re-sampled image. Repeat using **radial resolution** and the video test pattern, **test pattern**; note the characteristic *Moiré* pattern.

Do the same with **diagonal**; the aliasing effect is manifested as "jaggies" on the diagonal stripes, which are more prominent the larger the sub-sampling.

Activity 7.6 Template matching

Open the images **mask** and **reference** in ImageJ. The task is to find all locations of **mask**, the letter X, within the **reference** image. Go to **Process/FFT/FD Math**, enter the image names in the boxes, choose **Correlate** and check **Do Inverse Transform**. The two images are cross-correlated. Threshold the image (**Image/Adjust/Threshold ...**) to find the highest pixel values, which indicate the locations in the image which match the mask well. The location of X in the **reference** image is identified, although there is also a fairly good match at the similarly shaped letters K and N. Note that the final image suffered a fixed shift from the original **reference** image. The shift between the position of the letter in the original and its response in the processed image results from changing the phase during the multiplication of the two complex images.

Activity 7.7 Frequency domain filtering

Open **axialbrainMRI** and the low-pass "brick-wall" filter, **low-pass filter**, in ImageJ. Highlight **axialbrainMRI**, go to **Process/FFT/Custom Filter...** and choose **low-pass filter** as the filter. The resulting filtered image has less noise, but is somewhat blurred. Its contrast can be increased by stretching (**Process/Enhance Contrast ... Normalize**). Note the ringing around prominent edges. Open **Gaussian lp filter** and use it to filter the original image; observe that the filtered image has reduced the noise, and that there is no visible ringing artifact.

Use the high-pass "brick-wall" filter, **high-pass filter**, to filter the original **axialbrainMRI** image. As a result of blocking the low frequencies, areas of constant intensity in the original image become zero. The edges, containing the high frequencies, have positive and negative intensity values in the filtered image. In order to display the image on the screen, an offset is added to the output in the spatial domain and the image intensities are scaled. This results in a middle gray value for low-frequency areas and dark and light values for the edges. Note the ringing artifact. Open **Gaussian hp filter** and use it to filter **axialbrainMRI**. Compare the result. Try low- and high-pass filtering with the **skull** image.

Add the result of the Gaussian high-pass filtering to the original image, using 32-bit arithmetic (using **Process/Image Calculator** and checking Create New Window and 32-bit Result), and enhance its contrast (**Process/Enhance Contrast/Normalize**, with 5% saturated pixels). This image has sharper edges, and the process is known as *high-boost filtering*. Compare the result with Sobel masking (use **Process/Sharpen**) in the spatial domain.

Activity 7.8 Band-pass and notch filters

Band-pass filters can be obtained using **Process/FFT/Bandpass Filter ...** Both the low and high frequencies defining the pass band need to be specified, but start with the default values. Band-pass filter **axialbrainMRI**, after converting it to a 32-bit image; use various pass bands. Check **Display Filter** to see the filter used in each case.

Open **striped lena**, and take the fast Fourier transform – both magnitude and phase (**Plugins/Ch.7 Plugins/FFTDirect**). Using the Paintbrush from the Tools menu, paint the two diagonal spots in the magnitude image that correspond to the diagonal stripes to black, and take the inverse transform (**Plugins/Ch.7 Plugins/ FFTInverse**). Note how most of the stripes have been removed from the spatial image. There are still remnants close to the periphery of the picture. Remove these by painting out the streaks that pass through the diagonal spots in the Fourier transform magnitude image. Take the inverse Fourier transform and confirm the removal of the remnants.

Activity 7.9 Simulating filtered backprojection

CTSim is an open-source computer program (© 1983–2001 Kevin M. Rosenberg, MD) that simulates the process of transmitting x-rays through phantom objects. (V.3.0.3 operates directly in Windows XP, or it can be run on a Mac computer using the Leopard OS. A separate download is available for Unix/Linux.) It reconstructs the original phantom image from the projections using filtered back-projection; it also has a wide array of image analysis and image processing functions.

It is available at http://ctsim.org/download.html. Alternatively, a copy is available for download from the textbook site. Double-click **ctsim-installer-win32-3.0.3. exe** and follow the instructions to install it in your computer.

The fastest way to put CTSim through its basic operation is as follows.

(1) File – Create Phantom …
   This creates a window with the geometric phantom. Choose the Herman head phantom.
(2) Process – Rasterize …
   This creates an image file of the phantom by converting it from a geometric definition into a rasterized image. Use the defaults shown in the dialog box.
(3) View – Display Scale Auto …
   Use this command on the new rasterized image window. This optimizes the intensity scale for viewing the soft-tissue details of the phantom. Select the median center and a standard deviation factor of 0.1.
(4) Process Projections …
   Use this command on the geometric phantom window. This simulates the collection of x-ray data. Use the defaults shown in the dialog box. Turn on Trace Level – Projections to watch the x-ray data being simulated, and then collected to form a sinogram. Note that you can pause the simulations, and then step through them slowly.
(5) Reconstruction – Filtered Backprojection …
   Use this command on the projection window. This reconstructs an image from the projections. Use the defaults shown in the dialog box, except switch the Trace Level to Full to see the backprojections building up to the final reconstructed image. Again, you can pause this process and then step through each (filtered) backprojection individually.
(6) View Auto …
   Use this command on the new, reconstructed image window. This optimizes the intensity scale for viewing the soft-tissue details of the reconstruction. Select the median center and a standard deviation factor of 0.1.
(7) Analyze – Compare Images …
   Use this command on the rasterized phantom image window. This will bring up a dialog box asking for the comparison image. Select the reconstruction image that you have just made and also select the "Make difference image" check box. You will then see the image distance measurements and also a new window, with the difference between the rasterized phantom and the reconstruction.

By varying the parameters of the rasterization, projection and reconstructions you can perform endless computed tomography experiments.

Vary the number of acquisition views used in projection (starting from the default value of 320, then 160, and then 80). Keep all other parameters fixed at the default values. Describe the differences in the quality of the reconstructed images in these three cases.

Save the Herman head phantom as **herman.phm**, and open it with Wordpad to see its contents. Each line in the text file describes an element of the phantom. You can see the form of each line at www.ctsim.org/manual/ctsim7.html#phantomfile and can then build up a phantom of your own design.

Activity 7.10 Filtered backprojection

Open **phantom** in ImageJ. Choose **Ch.7 Plugins/Radon Transform** and click Calculate to open the corresponding set of projection data or sinogram. With the "ramp" filter selected, click Reconstruct to do filtered backprojection. Repeat the reconstruction step using the Shepp–Logan, cosine and Hamming filters in turn. Compare the results to the original **phantom** image in terms of image quality.

From the **Radon Transform** plugin, click Import Data and import **SLsinogram2** (whose data bins are stored in columns); this is a sinogram of the same phantom image but with fewer projections taken (30, instead of 180). Reconstruct a phantom image from this sinogram image using the four different filters as before. Compare the results with the previous reconstructions.

Exercises

7.1 What are the typical units for the variables (x, y) and (u, v) used in representing images in the spatial and frequency domains?

7.2 Show that the Fourier transform and its inverse are linear processes.

7.3 Draw schematic diagrams of the Fourier spectra of the following images:
   (i) a rectangle with horizontal side twice the length of the vertical side;
   (ii) the rectangle in (i) rotated 45° clockwise;
   (iii) the rectangle in (i) scaled down by a factor of two.

7.4 What is the Fourier transform of the one-dimensional rect function

$$\text{rect}(x) = 1, \quad \text{for} \quad |x| \leq \frac{1}{2},$$
$$= 0, \quad \text{for} \quad |x| > \frac{1}{2}? \text{ (requires integration)}$$

7.5 Consider an image that is black except for a single pixel wide stripe from the top left to the bottom right (Fig. E7.1, top left). Can you explain its Fourier transform (Fig. E7.1, bottom left)? Also, consider an image of noise (Fig. E7.1, top right), i.e. every pixel has a random value, independent of all other pixels. Can you explain its Fourier transform (Fig. E7.1, bottom right)? What does the bright spot in the middle

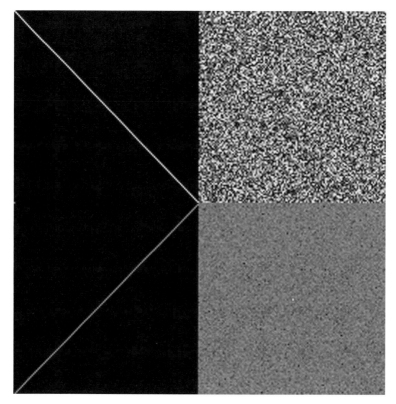

Figure E7.1   Stripe and noise, and their Fourier transforms.

of the noise Fourier transform image represent? Why does the Fourier transform of the noise appear dark gray?

7.6 What is the result of performing a Fourier transform on the Fourier transform of an image? Try it out. Can you explain the result?

7.7 What increase in speed can be expected in using a fast Fourier transform algorithm rather than direct arithmetic to compute the Fourier transform of an image of size 1024×1024?

7.8 During digitization samples are taken a distance Δx apart. What is the highest frequency allowed in the image to avoid aliasing?

7.9 A medical imaging system takes samples at intervals of Δx in both the x and y directions. What is the highest frequency permitted in the images so that the sampling is free of aliasing?

7.10 What sampling frequency should be used to avoid aliasing if the full width at half maximum, FWHM, of the point spread function is 5 mm?

7.11 A computed tomography imaging system has a point spread function with a full width at half maximum, FWHM, of 2 mm. How small do the image pixels have to be to avoid aliasing problems? For a field of view of 50 cm how many pixels are required along each side of the image?

7.12 How can an analog image be recovered from its sampled (digitized) version? Describe the operations required in (i) the spatial domain and (ii) the frequency domain. Comment on the conditions to be met for accurate recovery of the analog image.

7.13 Explain the relationship between convolution and correlation. Under what circumstances are they identical?

7.14 Using the equation of a Gaussian, show that its full width at half maximum, FWHM, is 2.36 times its width parameter, σ, or standard deviation.

7.15 The point spread function of a medical imaging system is given by

$$h(x, y) = e^{-(|x|+|y|)}$$

Is the point spread function separable? Is it circularly symmetric? What is the modulation transfer function, MTF, of the system?

7.16 Why are smoothing and sharpening of images important operations in medical image processing and analysis? Give some specific examples to illustrate your answer.

7.17 How would filtering with an averaging mask affect the output of a Fourier transform? Choose an image, and compare its Fourier transform with that of the image after filtering with a 5×5 averaging mask. Explain the result. What is the effect of increasing the size of the averaging mask?

7.18 How does a set of projections at different viewing angles relate to the Fourier transform of an object?

7.19 Why is there a need for filtering when reconstructing an image using backprojection? What are the necessary properties of such a filter? Compare three different filters and indicate for which anatomies they may be most effective.

7.20 Describe a direct Fourier reconstruction method using the Central Slice theorem.

8 Image restoration

Overview

An image is never an exact representation of the object under observation; it is always corrupted by degradations during acquisition and within the imaging system itself. These include noise, blurring and distortion. Image restoration removes or reduces these degradations. The point spread function (PSF) or the modulation transfer function (MTF) provides a complete, quantitative description of an imaging system and directly characterizes the image degradation within the system and can be used to restore the fine detail in images. The problem is more complicated if the image is also degraded by significant amounts of noise. Restoration techniques attempt to model the degradation and apply the inverse process to recover the original image. They are most effective when the point spread function or modulation transfer function is known and the nature of the blurring and noise are well understood. Geometric distortions can be reversed using inverse bilinear equations and gray-level interpolation.

Learning objectives

After reading this chapter you will be able to:

- identify the main sources of image noise and discuss their characteristics;
- choose appropriate general strategies for minimizing the effects of noise;
- discuss the advantages of adaptive filtering;
- model image degradation comprising blur and additive noise;
- employ suitable values to Wiener filter a noisy, blurred image;
- compare the performance of inverse filtering with Wiener filtering;
- explain how distortion can be removed from images.

8.1 Image degradation

Images can be degraded by a number of different mechanisms, including noise, blurring and distortion. Noise is present because any imaging device must use a finite exposure (or integration) time, which introduces stochastic noise from the random arrival of photons. Optical imperfections and instrumentation noise (for example, thermal noise in CCD devices) result in more noise. Sampling causes noise due to aliasing of high-frequency signal components, and digitization produces quantization errors. Further noise can be introduced by communication errors and compression. Blurring is present in any imaging system which uses electromagnetic radiation (for example, visible light and x-rays). Diffraction limits the resolution of an imaging device to features on the order of the illuminating wavelength. Scattering of light between the target object and imaging system (for example, by the atmosphere) introduces additional blurring. Lenses and mirrors cause blurring because they have limited spatial extent and optical imperfections. Discretization results in yet more blurring because devices such as CCDs average illumination over regions rather than sampling it at discrete points. Distortion arises from unequal magnification within the field of view.

The goal of image restoration is to reconstruct the original image from its degraded version. It is essentially an *inverse* problem, where we apply the inverse of the transformation that caused the degradation. The better we can model the degradation, the better we are able to find its inverse. In many cases, however, we will only have limited statistical knowledge of the degradation, and the inverse transform will be correspondingly *ill-conditioned*.

8.2   Noise

Noise is unwanted fluctuation in the pixel values of an image. It results in a degradation of the image quality. Since it is a random or *stochastic* process it is not possible to predict its values precisely, but it is possible to determine its statistical properties. Figure 8.1 shows part of a profile through a noisy (analog) image. Although it is not possible to write a mathematical expression to describe the complete profile, it is possible to quantify the noise in terms of various average properties such as its mean value, its mean square value and its probability density function.

The simplest way of characterizing a random variable is in terms of its expected value and variance. The expected value of a variable is the long-run average value of that variable. If a is a random variable the *expected value* (*expectation* or *mean*) of a is denoted as either μ_a or $E\{a\}$. It represents the (probability-weighted) average value for the random variable.

If a is taken to be the pixel value (or pixel amplitude) in an image, its mean value, $\bar{a}$, can be obtained either by integrating the profile (i.e. finding the area under it) and dividing by the distance in that direction, L, where the distance L should be long, preferably infinitely long,

$$\bar{a} = \lim_{L \to \infty} 1/L \int_0^L a(x)\,dx \tag{8.1a}$$

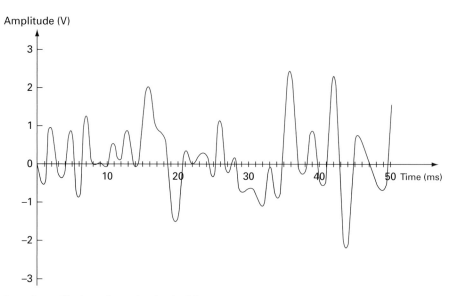

Figure 8.1   Part of a profile through a noisy (analog) image.

or, if the probability density function, $p(a)$, of the noise (the probability of having a particular value a) is known, by using

$$E\{a\} = \bar{a} = \int\limits_{-\infty}^{\infty} ap(a)\mathrm{d}a \qquad (8.1b)$$

Both methods are equivalent and are illustrated in Figure 8.2.

Figure 8.3 shows two profiles, each of which has random noise with a mean of zero. In order to distinguish them, their mean square value could be taken, using either

$$\overline{a^2} = 1/L \int a^2(x)\mathrm{d}x \qquad (8.2a)$$

or

$$E\{a^2\} = \overline{a^2} = \int a^2 p(a)\mathrm{d}a \qquad (8.2b)$$

The link between $\bar{a}$ and $\overline{a^2}$ is provided by the variance, σ^2, defined as

$$\begin{aligned}
\sigma^2 &= \int (a - \bar{a})^2 p(a)\mathrm{d}a \\
&= E\{|\Box a|^2\} = E\{|a - E\{a\}|^2\} \\
&= E[a^2 - 2aE\{a\} + E^2\{a\}] = E\{a^2\} - |E\{a\}|^2 \\
&= \overline{a^2} - (\bar{a})^2 \qquad (8.3)
\end{aligned}$$

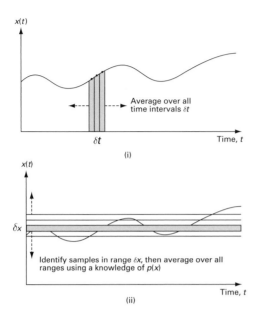

Figure 8.2   Alternative methods of finding the mean value of noise.

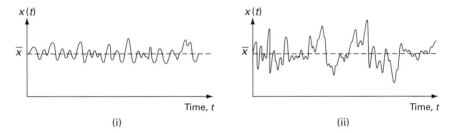

Figure 8.3   Two different profiles both with zero mean noise components.

In terms of an image with an additive noise component, the mean total power, the mean square amplitude ($\overline{a^2}$ or $E\{a^2\}$), is given by the sum of the d.c. power in the signal, the square of the mean amplitude (($\overline{a^2}$) or $|E\{a^2\}|$), and the mean power in the noise, the variance or σ^2.

The signal-to-noise ratio, SNR, of the image, is given by

$$\mathrm{SNR} = |E\{a\}|^2/\sigma^2 \tag{8.4}$$

Noise in imaging systems can be either *independent* of the signal (i.e. the image pixels), and can often be described as additive,

$$g(x, y) = f(x, y) * h(x, y) + n(x, y) \tag{8.5}$$

or it can be *dependent* noise, a function of the signal strength or pixel value, in which case it is simulated using a more complicated multiplicative model:

$$g(x, y) = [f(x, y) + n(x, y) \cdot f(x, y)] * h(x, y)$$
$$= [f(x, y) + (1 + n(x, y))] * h(x, y)$$
$$\approx [f(x, y) \cdot n(x, y)] * h(x, y) \tag{8.6}$$

Quantum noise and film grain noise are actually multiplicative, whereas electronic noise is additive. For most image restoration processes the noise is considered to be additive.

8.2.1   Types of noise

Noise is always present in images to some extent. Different types of noise can be identified according to their origin. Any imaging device must use a finite exposure (or integration) time, which introduces stochastic noise from the random arrival of photons. Optical imperfections and instrumentation noise (for example, thermal noise in semiconductor devices) can result in further noise. Sampling causes noise due to aliasing of high-frequency signal components, and digitization produces quantization errors. Additional noise can be introduced by communication errors and compression.

White noise

This is noise with a constant power spectrum, i.e. its power spectral density, often referred to as its *noise power spectrum* (NPS), is constant with frequency. Theoretically, the spectrum would extend to infinite frequency and therefore the total noise power would be infinite; in practice, the spectrum of any naturally occurring white noise falls off at sufficiently high frequencies. The terminology is derived from an analogy with white light, which contains nearly all the frequencies in the visible spectrum in equal proportions.

White noise is totally uncorrelated, i.e. each pixel value is unrelated to neighboring pixel values. This implies that its autocorrelation function is zero. However, being uncorrelated does not restrict the values a signal can take; any distribution of values is possible. For example, a binary signal which can only take on the values 1 or 0 is "white" if the sequence of zeros and ones is statistically uncorrelated. Noise having a continuous distribution, such as a normal distribution, can also be white.

Colored noise

Pink noise, 1/f noise or *flicker noise* has a power spectral density that is proportional to the reciprocal of the frequency. Over an *octave*, a doubling of frequency, it drops to half power, i.e. it drops off at 3 dB per octave. *Brown noise, Brownian noise* or *red noise* has a power spectral density that is proportional to the reciprocal of the square of the frequency. Over an *octave* it drops to one-quarter of its power, i.e. it drops off at 6 dB per octave. Graphically, Brown noise mimics Brownian motion, the random movement of particles suspended in a fluid. Brown noise can be produced by integrating white noise.

Periodic noise

This arises typically from electrical interference, especially in the presence of a strong mains power signal during image acquisition. It is spatially dependent and generally sinusoidal at multiples of a specific frequency. It is recognizable as pairs of conjugate spots in the frequency domain, and can be conveniently removed either manually or by using a *notch* (narrow band reject) filter.

Gaussian noise

Gaussian noise has a probability density function, or normalized histogram, given by

$$p(a) = \sqrt{(1/2\pi\sigma^2)} \, \exp(-(a-\mu)^2/2\sigma^2) \tag{8.7}$$

where a is the gray value, μ is the average gray value and σ is its standard deviation. Approximately 70% of its pixel values are in the range $[(\mu-\sigma), (\mu+\sigma)]$. It is a particularly attractive model since it can be analytically integrated, which may explain its over-use. It also conveniently has the same spectral shape in the frequency domain. Gaussian noise comes from many natural sources, such as the thermal vibrations of atoms in antennas (referred to as thermal noise or Johnson noise) and black body radiation from warm objects.

It is often incorrectly assumed that Gaussian noise is necessarily white noise. However, neither property implies the other. Being Gaussian refers to the way gray values are distributed, while the term "white" refers to the lack of correlation between pixel values, and this randomness results in all frequencies being present in the same amounts, i.e. a flat power spectrum. Gaussian white noise is a good approximation of many real-world situations and generates mathematically tractable models.

Impulse (or salt-and-pepper) noise

Another common form of noise is *data drop-out* noise, commonly referred to as *impulse noise* or *salt-and-pepper noise*. Here, the noise is caused by errors in data transmission. Corrupted pixels are either set to the maximum value or to zero, giving the image a "salt and pepper" like appearance. Unaffected pixels remain unchanged. The noise is usually quantified by the percentage of pixels which are corrupted.

Quantization noise

Quantization noise is inherent in the amplitude quantization process and occurs in the analog-to-digital converter, ADC, when sampled values are fitted to a finite number of levels. The noise is additive and independent of the signal when the number of bits $n \geq 4$.

For a digitized signal that is *bounded* with a minimum and maximum pixel value, a_{min} and a_{max}, respectively, the signal-to-noise ratio, SNR, is given by

$$\text{SNR} = 20 \log_{10}(a_{max} - a_{min})/\sigma_n \tag{8.8}$$

where σ_n is the standard deviation of the noise. When the input signal is a full-amplitude sine wave it can be shown (see Exercise 8.1) that the SNR becomes

$$\text{SNR} = 6n + 1.76 \, \text{dB} \tag{8.9}$$

Quantization noise can usually be ignored as the total signal-to-noise ratio of a complete system is typically dominated by the smallest signal-to-noise ratio of a component of the system, i.e. the largest noise. In semiconductor detectors this is photon noise.

Photon noise (also called quantum noise or shot noise)

Photon noise results from the statistical nature of electromagnetic waves, which include visible light, x-rays and γ-rays: all are emitted as packets of energy, photons, with a probability distribution that is a Poisson distribution. Its average level is $\sqrt{N}$, where N is the signal average, so that it is not independent of the signal nor is it additive. However, when N is large Poisson statistics become binomial, or Gaussian if we have so many bins that the distribution is essentially continuous: this is the Central Limit theorem.

Speckle (or multiplicative) noise

Although Gaussian noise and speckle noise can appear superficially similar in an image, they are a result of different processes and require different approaches for their removal. Whereas Gaussian noise can be modeled by random values added to the pixel values of an image, speckle noise is modeled by random values which are multiplied by the pixel values. Speckle noise is a major problem in some radar applications.

8.3   Noise-reduction filters

If the only degradation present in an image, $g(x, y)$, is additive noise then

$$g(x, y) = f(x, y) + n(x, y) \tag{8.10}$$

where $f(x, y)$ is the original, undegraded image and $n(x, y)$ is the noise; and in the frequency domain

$$G(u, v) = F(u, v) + N(u, v) \tag{8.11}$$

In the case of periodic noise, which gives rise to particular frequencies in the Fourier domain, it can be readily removed using a narrow *band-reject filter* known as a *notch filter* (see Activity 7.8). Figure 8.4(i) shows an image degraded by periodic noise. This noise can be mostly removed by filtering out the relevant spots in the Fourier domain (Fig. 8.4(ii)), and taking the inverse Fourier transform (Fig. 8.4(iii)).

Noise is more commonly present over a range of frequencies, whereas frequently an image has the majority of its energy at low and mid frequencies. Thus, low-pass filters (Section 6.4.1) that reduce the amplitude of high-frequency components can be used to reduce the noise, although in practice it is difficult to achieve much noise reduction without blurring the edges in an image. Sometimes these operations are best implemented in the frequency domain, as filters, and sometimes more conveniently in the spatial domain, as masks. Global averaging masks, whether uniform or weighted, produce significant blurring of edges, but median masks, which are non-linear in operation, preserve edges and do not blur them. Median masks are particularly efficient at removing impulse or salt-and-pepper noise. Figure 8.5(i) shows an image degraded by

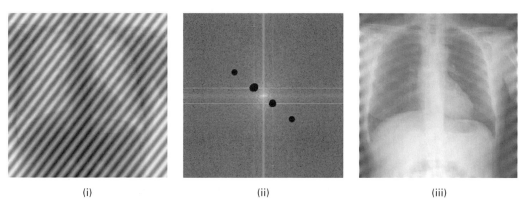

(i)   (ii)   (iii)

Figure 8.4   (i) An image degraded by periodic noise. (ii) Removal of the corresponding frequencies in the Fourier transform. (iii) Inverse Fourier transform of (ii).

salt-and-pepper noise. A median mask successfully removes this type of noise (Fig. 8.5(ii)). An averaging mask of the same size blurs the noise but also the underlying image (Fig. 8.5(iii); a larger averaging mask reduces the appearance of the salt-and-pepper noise but blurs the underlying image even more (Fig. 8.5(iv)).

Figure 8.6 illustrates how neither a median nor an averaging mask is able to remove Gaussian noise successfully.

When an image, $f(x, y)$, is contaminated by multiplicative or speckle noise

$$g(x, y) = f(x, y) * n(x, y) \tag{8.12}$$

then *homomorphic* filtering can be used. This comprises taking the logarithm of the image to yield an additive linear result

$$\log\{g(x, y)\} = \log\{f(x, y)\} + \log\{n(x, y)\} \tag{8.13}$$

followed by conventional linear filtering to reduce the log noise component, and then taking the exponential after filtering.

8.3.1   Adaptive filters

Adaptive masks are a class of masks which change their behavior based on the statistics of the pixels within a defined local neighborhood for each pixel. They are inherently non-linear masks. Their performance in reducing noise is superior to that of global masks, but there is an increase in filter complexity.

Consider the case of additive, Gaussian noise where the variance of the noise corrupting an image $f(x, y)$ to form the noisy image $g(x, y)$ is σ_N^2, and can be estimated from the noisy image. Once a neighborhood size is chosen, the mean, m_L, and variance, σ_L^2, of the pixels within each neighborhood can be calculated. An adaptive mask would then produce an estimate, $\hat{f}(x, y)$, of the original image pixels using

$$\hat{f}(x, y) = g(x, y) - (\sigma_N^2/\sigma_L^2)(g(x, y)) - m_L \tag{8.14}$$

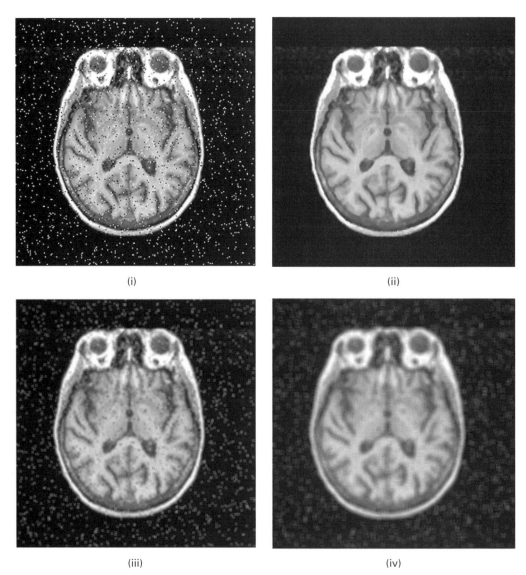

Figure 8.5   (i) A 256×256 image with salt-and-pepper noise and the effect of convolution with (ii) a 3×3 median mask, (iii) a 3×3 averaging mask and (iv) a 5×5 averaging mask.

This produces an output close to $g(x, y)$ if the local variance is high; this is appropriate because high variance implies changes such as edges, which should be preserved. Conversely, if the local variance is low (i.e. approaching σ_N^2), such as in background areas of the image, the output will be close to the local mean value, m_L. This reduces noise while preserving edges. This particular mask is known as the *minimum mean square error* (MMSE) mask.

    Another example of an adaptive mask is where the neighborhood size changes to meet some criterion. An example of this type of mask is the Kuwahara mask. Although it can

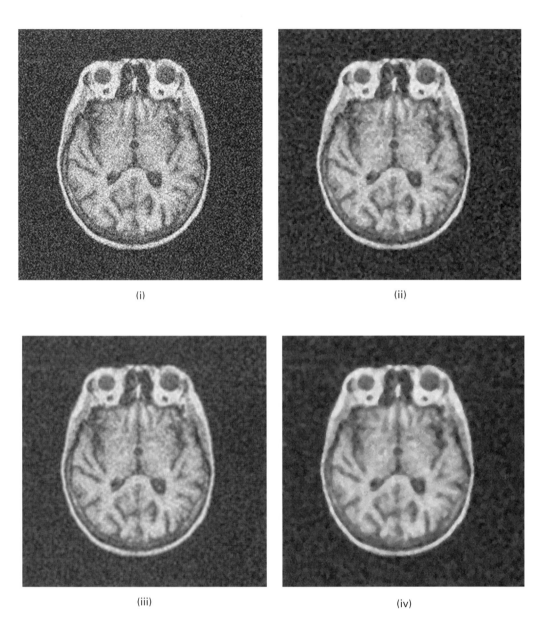

(i)

(ii)

(iii)

(iv)

Figure 8.6 (i) An image degraded by Gaussian noise ($\sigma = 40$) and the effect of convolution with (ii) a 3×3 median mask, (iii) a 5×5 median mask, (iv) a 3×3 averaging mask and (v) a 5×5 averaging mask.

be implemented for a variety of different neighborhood shapes, we will describe it for a square neighborhood of size $J = K = 4L + 1$, where L is an integer. The window is partitioned into four overlapping sub-neighborhoods ($i = 1, 2, 3, 4$) as shown in Figure 8.7. The mean brightness, m_i, and the variance, σ_i^2, are measured in each of the four regions. The output value of the center pixel in the window is then set to the mean value of the

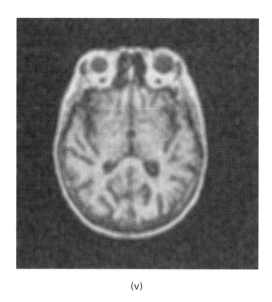

(v)

Figure 8.6   (cont.)

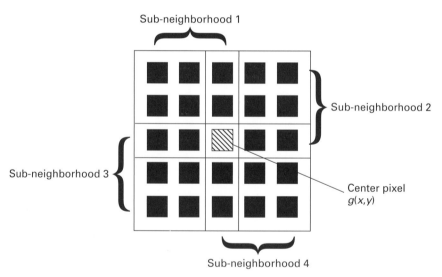

Figure 8.7   Four square regions defined for the Kuwahara filter. In this example $L = 1$ and thus $J = K = 5$. Each region is $[(J+1)/2] \times [(K+1)/2]$. (After Young, Gerbrands and van Vliet, 1998, fig. 29.)

sub-neighborhood which has the smallest variance. Thus the noise is reduced, while the edges are enhanced (Fig. 8.8).

An adaptive median mask can be constructed for improved performance in removing salt-and-pepper noise. One way would be to detect pixels that differ from those in the chosen neighborhood window by more than a given multiple of the neighborhood's standard deviation, and to replace only these pixels by the median value of the

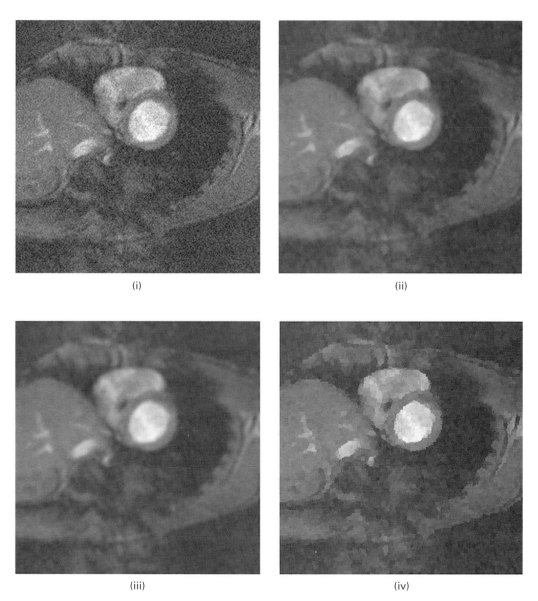

(i)

(ii)

(iii)

(iv)

Figure 8.8 (i) A noisy image and the effect of convolution with (ii) a 5×5 median mask, (iii) a 5×5 averaging mask and (iv) a 5×5 Kuwahara mask.

neighborhood. The principle behind this mask is that if adequate sampling was chosen upon acquisition, no such outlying (extreme value) pixels should be found. Figure 8.9 shows the effect of such a filter on an image contaminated with salt-and-pepper noise. The result (Fig. 8.9(ii)) should be compared with the result of applying a global 3×3 median mask (Fig. 8.6(ii)). The difference between these two results (Fig. 8.9(iii)) is not great, but it is real. Activity 8.1 provides practice with this type of adaptive median mask.

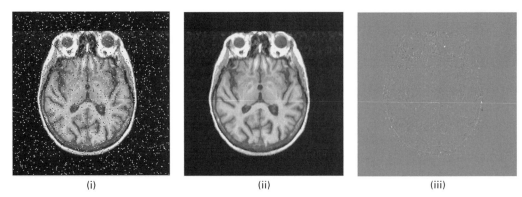

(i)   (ii)   (iii)

Figure 8.9   (i) A 256 × 256 image with salt-and-pepper noise (identical to Fig. 8.2(i)). (ii) The effect of convolution with an adaptive median filter (using a multiple (see text) of 1.0). (iii) The difference between the image in (ii) and the image in Fig. 8.2(ii).

Another type of adaptive median mask would be one where the actual size of the neighborhood changes (increases from a nominal value) during operation depending on the statistics of the pixel values in the neighborhood of the pixel under consideration. For example, the neighborhood size could be increased if the range of pixel values is lower than a certain chosen level; the neighborhood size would then be reset prior to considering the next pixel.

8.4   Blurring

Blurring is characterized by the point spread function, PSF, or impulse response of the system, which is the output of the imaging system for an input point source. Most blurring processes can be considered as linear and can therefore be described by convolution using a spatially invariant point spread function. It is as if there is an internal blurring mask within the system that blurs the incoming signals. This internal mask, or point spread function, is often represented by a Gaussian. The blurring produced by gamma cameras in nuclear medicine imaging is notably different; it is non-linear, although it is often simulated assuming a symmetric, stationary tomographic point spread function.

Equivalent to convolution in the spatial domain, blurring can also be described by multiplication with the (optical) transfer function, OTF, of the blurring process or its magnitude, the modulation transfer function, MTF, in the frequency domain (Fig. 8.10).

With visible light diffraction limits the resolution of an imaging device to features on the order of the illuminating wavelength, scattering introduces additional blurring, and lenses and mirrors have optical imperfections. In simple projection x-ray systems the focal spot intensity distribution and beam-limiting apertures result in a finite point spread function. In x-ray fluoroscopy the finite size of the iodide crystals in the input fluorescent screen and shortcomings in the focusing of electrons within the image intensifier (II) tube contribute to the point spread function. In direct or digital radiography, the size of the

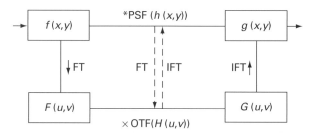

Figure 8.10 Imaging by an imperfect imaging system involves convolution with the system PSF or, alternatively, multiplication in the frequency domain by its MTF.

semiconductor-based detectors introduces blurring because they average illumination over regions rather than sampling it at discrete points.

8.4.1 Deblurring

It is possible to recover an image that has been blurred by an imaging system by modeling the blurring and applying the inverse process to recover the original image. The output or blurred image, $g(x, y)$, is obtained by convolving the input image, $f(x, y)$, which may be the object scene or an intermediate image of it, with the point spread function, $h(x, y)$, of the imaging system:

$$g(x, y) = f(x, y) * h(x, y) \qquad (8.15)$$

In principle, if the point spread function of the system, $h(x, y)$, is known, then the original input image can be easily recovered from the blurred image by *inverse filtering* or *deconvolution*. The equivalent frequency domain representation of the degradation process is

$$G(u, v) = F(u, v) \cdot H(u, v) \qquad (8.16)$$

where G, F and H are the Fourier transforms of f, g and h, respectively. ($H(u, v)$ is the modulation transfer function of the imaging system.) Division in the frequency domain gives $F(u, v)$,

$$F(u, v) = G(u, v)/H(u, v) \qquad (8.17)$$

from which the original image can be obtained by inverse Fourier transform; thus deconvolution achieves *deblurring* by division of the blurred image by the modulation transfer function of the imaging system.

The result of deconvolution is usually disappointing (Fig. 8.11), even for Gaussian point spread functions. Small values in the modulation transfer function produce very large values during division, which then dominate the deconvolved image. This effect can be seen in Activity 8.2.

In practice, the image is also degraded by noise as well as blurring. Image restoration in the presence of noise is difficult since it is an *ill-posed inverse problem*: there is not enough information in the degraded image to determine the original image unambiguously.

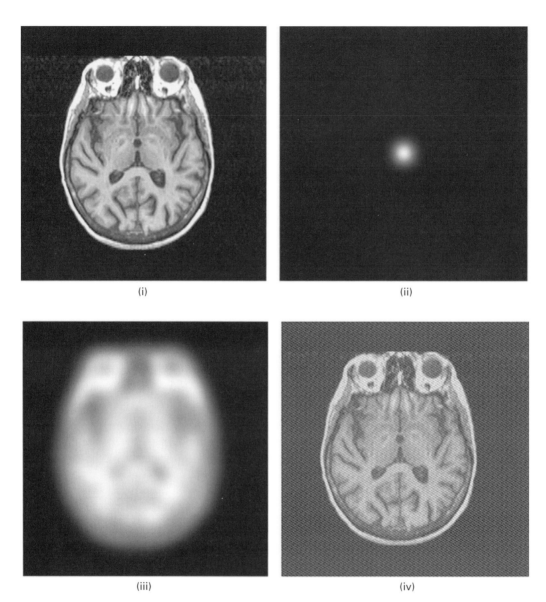

(i)   (ii)

(iii)   (iv)

Figure 8.11   (i) An image. (ii) A Gaussian blurring or point spread function. (iii) The result of convolving (i) with (ii). (iv) The result of deconvolving (iii) with (ii).

8.5   Modeling image degradation

If the noise is additive (Fig. 8.12), then the degraded image from a linear, space-invariant (LSI) imaging system is given by

$$g(x, y) = f(x, y) * h(x, y) + n(x, y)$$

which is Equation (8.5).

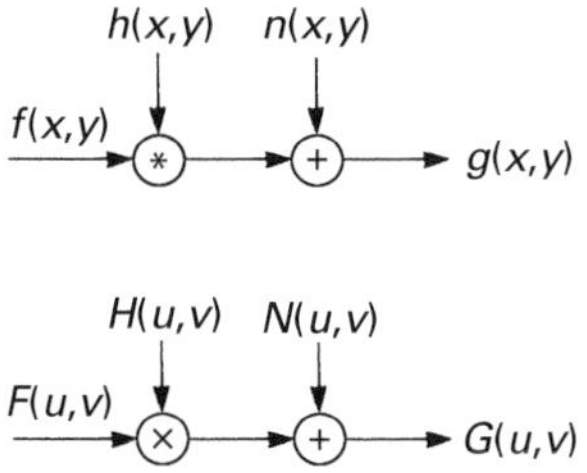

Figure 8.12 Imaging by an imperfect, but linear, imaging system which adds noise as well as blurring, as seen in both the spatial (top) and frequency (bottom) domains.

Taking the Fourier transform of this yields

$$G(u, v) = F(u, v) \cdot H(u, v) + N(u, v) \tag{8.18}$$

which can be re-arranged to give

$$F(u, v) = G(u, v)/H(u, v) - N(u, v)/H(u, v) \tag{8.19}$$

from which the original undegraded image could be recovered, in theory at least, by inverse Fourier transform.

This process of removing both the noise and the blurring is known as (*direct*) *inverse filtering*. However, the term involving the noise is problematic; noise is random and generally broadband, while the modulation transfer function of the imaging system, $H(u, v)$, falls to zero beyond its cut-off frequency. The outcome is that the noise dominates the restoration for spatial frequencies beyond the system cut-off, even when the noise power is small, and numerical overflow results from divisions by zero. In practice this results in very poor performance.

8.5.1 Wiener filters

The classic remedy is to employ Wiener filtering in the frequency domain, to remove those frequencies which would be dominated by noise. The Wiener filter is an optimal filter in the sense that it delivers the best estimate of the original, undegraded image in a least squares sense for additive Gaussian noise, i.e. it finds an estimate, $\hat{f}(x, y)$, of the uncorrupted image, $f(x, y)$, such that the mean square error between them is minimized. It is in fact the adaptive mask we introduced in Section 8.2.1, the *minimum mean square error* (MMSE) mask. This error measure is given by

$$e^2 = E\{(f(x, y) - \hat{f}(x, y))^2\} \tag{8.20}$$

where $E\{.\}$ is the expected value of the argument. However, in order to realize the *minimum mean square error* estimate strictly the signal-to-noise ratio needs to be known precisely at every frequency:

$$\hat{F}(u, v) = \frac{1}{[H(u, v)]} \cdot \frac{[|H(u, v)|^2]}{[|H(u, v)|^2 + (|N(u, v)|^2/|F(u, v)|^2)]} \cdot G(u, v) \tag{8.21}$$

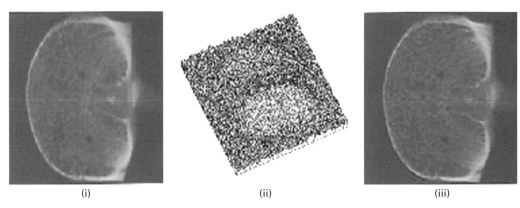

(i)   (ii)   (iii)

Figure 8.13   (i) Image of a transverse section of vertebral bone. (ii) Plot of the point spread function of the x-ray imaging system, showing the intensity of a pinhole image of the x-ray source. (iii) The restored image using Wiener filtering, with $K = 10$. (With permission, from *Radiography*, 2001, 7, 255–62.)

where $|N(u, v)|^2$, $|F(u, v)|^2$ are the power spectra of the noise and the undegraded image, respectively. (Comparison of Equations (8.20) and (8.19) shows that the former does not blow up to infinity unless both $H(u, v)$ and $|N(u, v)|^2$ are zero for the same value(s) of u and v.) Fortunately, even crude approximations often work extremely well: for example

$$F(u, v) = \frac{1}{[H(u, v)]} \cdot \frac{[|H(u, v)|^2]}{[|H(u, v)|^2 + K]} \cdot G(u, v) \qquad (8.22)$$

where K is the inverse of the signal-to-noise ratio of the image averaged over all frequencies. More conveniently, K can be considered as an adjustable empirical parameter chosen to balance sharpness against noise. The restored images using Wiener filtering are much superior to those using direct inverse filtering.

Wiener filtering can be used to restore projection radiographs of vertebral bone, using the pinhole image of the focal spot in the image plane as the point spread function, PSF (Fig. 8.13). Activity 8.3 provides exercises in Wiener filtering.

Wiener filtering is a rather conservative process, emphasizing noise reduction over image reconstruction. This is a by-product of it minimizing mean square error. Classical Wiener deconvolution can only handle linear, spatially invariant systems with additive noise, although this may be a reasonable approximation for many types of degradation. Spatially variant processes, on the other hand, including motion blur that involves rotation, and processes such as coma, astigmatism and curvature of field, are even more challenging.

Another problem is that most images are highly *non-stationary*, i.e. the signal varies considerably throughout the image. In some regions of the image there are details and edges and therefore high-frequency components; in other regions there are relatively constant gray values and therefore low-frequency components. The noise content, too, may be non-stationary. The net result is that there is not a global signal-to-noise ratio applicable throughout the image, as assumed in Equation (8.23), and this confounds the Wiener filter. If the restoring point spread function is relatively small compared to the size of the image, which is generally the case, then signal-to-noise ratios may be obtained for various regions of the image and used to restore those regions only. However, the computational expense of such a scheme is relatively high. An alternative method is *constrained* least squares filtering, in which an attempt is made to control the noise sensitivity problem by imposing a constraint on the smoothness of the restored image. However, despite the more rigorous mathematical basis, the results of constrained least squares filtering are not always visually superior to classical Wiener filtering with a manual adjustment of the parameter K.

8.5.2   Other filters

Wiener filtering can be generalized somewhat to give the *geometric mean filter*

$$\hat{F}(u, v) = \frac{[H^*(u, v)]^\alpha}{[|H(u, v)|^2]} \cdot \frac{[H^*(u, v)]^{1-\alpha}}{[|H(u, v)|^2 + \beta(|N(u, v)|^2 / |F(u, v)|^2)]} \cdot G(u, v) \qquad (8.23)$$

where α and β are two positive, real constants. This represents a family of filters.

- When $\alpha = 1$ this reduces to the inverse filter.
- When $\alpha = 0$ it becomes the *parametric Wiener filter*, which reduces to the standard Wiener filter when $\beta = 1$.
- When $\alpha = 1/2$ and $\beta = 1$ it is commonly called the *spectrum equalization filter*.

Various iterative deconvolution methods perform even better than the Wiener filters and their variants with images of low signal-to-noise ratio, but they cannot readily be implemented using standard imaging software without custom programming.

8.5.3   Blind image restoration

Most image restoration methods are based on knowledge of the imaging system, e.g. its point spread function, and the noise power spectrum. If these are not known, and information on the degradation must be extracted from the observed image itself, then the task is known as *blind image restoration*. The system point spread function can be estimated by isolating a small object in the image, suspected to have arisen from a point source, or a suspected sharp edge. The noise covariance function can be estimated by measuring the image covariance over a region of relatively constant background, and its Fourier transform (FT) taken to give the noise power spectrum.

8.6   Geometric degradations

An image can be geometrically distorted within an imaging system, due to unequal magnification within the field of view. If the magnification is smaller off-axis than along

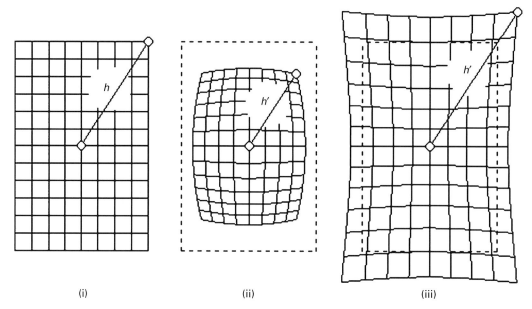

(i)   (ii)   (iii)

Figure 8.14   (i) Original object; (ii) image showing barrel distortion; and (iii) image showing pincushion distortion.

the axes, barrel distortion results; if it is greater off-axis than along the axes, pincushion distortion results (Fig. 8.14).

The amount of distortion can be expressed as

$$(\text{percentage})\text{distortion} = ((D_2/(nD_1)) - 1) \times 100\% \tag{8.24}$$

where D_1 is the length of the diagonal of the small central square in the image, D_2 is the length of the diagonal of the largest square in the image, and n is the ratio of their sizes in the object.

Pincushion distortion is often evident in fluoroscopic images (Fig. 8.15). Off-axis electrons tend to flare out from their ideal course, resulting in larger off-axis magnification of the image.

By convention, in still photography, the normal lens for a particular format has a focal length approximately equal to the length of the diagonal of the image frame or digital photosensor. For a full-frame 35 mm camera with a 36 mm by 24 mm format, the diagonal measures 43.3 mm, and by custom the normal lens adopted by most manufacturers is 50 mm. Wide-angle lenses have shorter focal lengths, and many produce a more or less rectilinear image at the film plane, although often with some degree of barrel distortion where the image appears to be mapped around all or part of a spherical object (Fig. 8.16 (i)). Extreme wide-angle lenses that do not produce a rectilinear image are called fish-eye lenses (Fig. 8.17), and produce very significant barrel distortion. There are two types of fish-eye lens. The first has a 180° field of view in all directions and results in a circular image on 35 mm film; these lenses typically have a focal length around 8 mm. The second, more common, type of fish-eye lens is known as a "full frame fish-eye" and

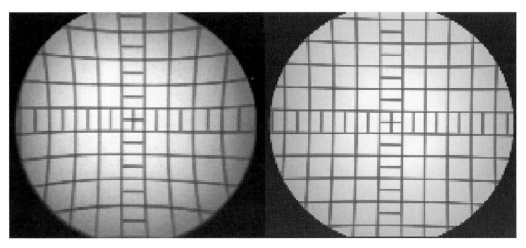

Figure 8.15   Images subject to pincushion distortion; the image on the left has sustained more distortion than the image on the right.

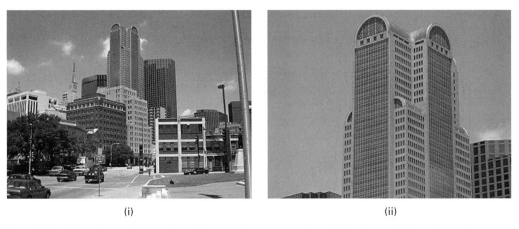

(i)   (ii)

Figure 8.16   (i) An image taken with a wide-angle lens showing barrel distortion and (ii) an image taken with a telephoto lens showing slight pincushion distortion. See also color plate.

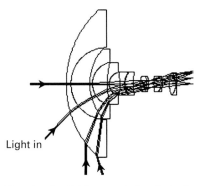

Light in

Figure 8.17   Showing the light rays entering the bottom half of a fish-eye lens.

it has a 180° diagonal field of view. (Typically, horizontal coverage is about 140° and vertical coverage is about 90°, and they have a focal length of about 16 mm.) Fish-eye lenses are often installed as security devices inside the front door of a house to show a wide field of view. On the other hand, long focal length or telephoto lenses tend to exhibit pincushion distortion (Fig. 8.16(ii)).

Barrel and pincushion distortions are the inverse of each other. We could correct the barrel distortion in an image by viewing it or projecting it with a lens that introduced an equal amount of pincushion distortion.

The general affine transformation can be used to model simple spatial transformations such as scaling, rotation and translation (Section 6.3), combinations of which can produce an image-shearing operation (Fig. 8.18(ii)). Parallel lines remain parallel, and straight lines remain straight, but angles and shapes are not preserved. The general affine transform

$$\begin{bmatrix} x' \\ y' \\ 1 \end{bmatrix} = A \begin{bmatrix} x \\ y \\ 1 \end{bmatrix} = \begin{bmatrix} a_{xx} & a_{xy} & b_x \\ a_{yx} & a_{yy} & b_y \\ 0 & 0 & 1 \end{bmatrix} \begin{bmatrix} x \\ y \\ 1 \end{bmatrix} \tag{8.25}$$

describes the transform of points (x, y) into (x', y') using a matrix A. To recover the original points (x, y) from (x', y') it is necessary to find the inverse of the matrix, A^{-1}. The geometric transform can be specified by using a few selected *control points*, whose location in the distorted and undistorted images is known. For the affine transform three pairs of corresponding points are sufficient to find the six coefficients.

The general affine transform can be extended to projective transforms (where straight lines remain straight, but parallel lines do not remain parallel) as in map projections (Fig. 8.18(iii)). Further generalization provides non-linear spatial warping of an image, where the transform may be described by a polynomial (Fig. 8.18 (iv)). In the case where the

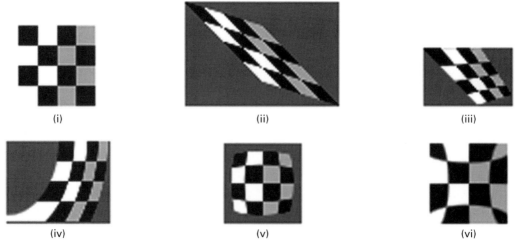

(i)   (ii)   (iii)

(iv)   (v)   (vi)

Figure 8.18   (i) Original image; (ii) affine transform; (iii) projective transform; (iv) second-order polynomial transform; (v) barrel transform; and (vi) pincushion transform.

distortion/warping process within the region bounded by the control points can be modeled by a pair of bilinear equations

$$x' = c_0 + c_1 x + c_2 y + c_3 xy \tag{8.26}$$

and

$$y' = d_0 + d_1 x + d_2 y + d_3 xy \tag{8.27}$$

the coefficients can be calculated if four corresponding control points in each image are known. The coefficients can then be used to transform *all* the pixels within the quadrilateral bounded by the control points and recover the corrected (undistorted) image. Second-order polynomial warping is described by

$$x' = c_0 + c_1 x + c_2 y + c_3 xy + c_4 x^2 + c_5 y^2 \tag{8.28}$$

$$y' = d_0 + d_1 x + d_2 y + d_3 xy + d_4 x^2 + d_5 y^2 \tag{8.29}$$

A cubic term is involved in barrel (Fig. 8.18(v)) and pincushion (Fig. 8.18(vi)) distortion.

Reverse address computation usually results in non-integer values for x' and y', and *gray-level interpolation* (Section 6.3) is required to find the pixel values at integer coordinate locations for the corrected image. The simplest solution would be to adopt the pixel value of the nearest reverse address to the integral locations, *nearest-neighbor* or *zero-order interpolation*. While computationally simple, it has the disadvantage of producing undesirable artifacts such as the distortion of straight edges in high-resolution images. This error can be significantly reduced by using *bilinear interpolation*, where the values at the integer positions are computed from a weighted average of the four nearest non-integer positions obtained from the reverse transform. More sophisticated techniques, such as *bicubic* or *cubic B-spline* interpolation, can be used at significantly higher computational cost.

Correcting for geometric distortion, *unwarping*, is often used as a prequel to registering images obtained from different imaging modalities. Figure 8.19 shows the result of unwarping and registering an image that had been subject to pincushion distortion.

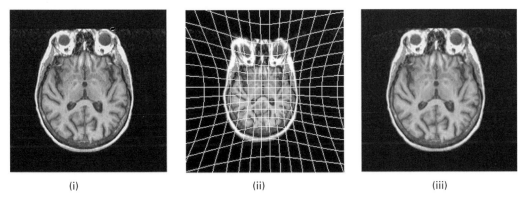

(i)   (ii)   (iii)

Figure 8.19   (i) A target image used to define the unwarping. (ii) The warped (source) image, with calculated distortion lines. (iii) The result of unwarping image (ii).

Computer-based activities

Activity 8.1 Adaptive median mask

Open image `salt-and-pepper1` in ImageJ, and use a 3×3 median mask (**Process/ Filter/ Median ...** with a radius of 1 pixel) to reduce its salt-and-pepper noise. Now use an adaptive median mask (**Plugins/ Ch.8 Plugins/ Adaptive_Median**, set k1, k2 and k3 all equal to zero, check on **Salt-and-Pepper Noise removal**, and enter 1.0 as the multiple for standard deviation) on the original image. Compare the two results and see whether a different multiple might result in a superior result for the adaptive median mask.

Repeat with image `salt-and-pepper 2`.

Activity 8.2 Deconvolution

Open `axialbrainMRI` in ImageJ. We can simulate a poor imaging system by convolving this with a Gaussian point spread function. Open `Gaussian5x5. txt`, which is a 5×5 Gaussian with $\sigma = 0.625$, and view its terms. `Gaussian blur` is an image with these terms embedded in the center; open it in ImageJ and observe it with **Analyze/Surface Plot ...**, checking Draw Wireframe. Use **Process/FFT/FD Math ...**, choose `axialbrainMRI` and `Gaussian blur`, **Convolve** as the operation, and check Do Inverse Transform. The resulting image, `Result`, is a noticeably blurred image.

We can attempt to recover the original image by using deconvolution. Using **Process/FFT/FD Math ...**, choose `Result` and `Gaussian blur` as the images, **Deconvolve** as the operation, check Do Inverse Transform and call the result `Result2`. Compare `Result2` with the original image, by subtracting 32-bit versions of them (**Image/Type/32-bit**, then **Process/Image calculator** and subtract).

Repeat the exercise using `bigGaussian`, which has a wider point spread function, to obtain `Result3`. Compare the result of deconvolution with the original image. Is the process more or less successful than with `Gaussian blur`? Why? Compare the Fourier transforms of the original image, `axialbrainMRI`, and `Result3`; what is the difference?

Activity 8.3 Wiener filtering

Open `blurred` in ImageJ. The image is (motion) blurred; we will try to restore it so as to try to read the license plate. Let's model the blurring as a radially symmetric uniform averaging filter of radius 7 pixels: open `pillbox`. Try to recover the original image by using deconvolution using **Process/FFT/FD Math**, and confirm that it is not successful.

Instead we will use Wiener filtering. Use the **SNR** plugin (in **Ch.5 Plugins**) to estimate the value of the SNR of the `blurred` image, and hence its inverse, K. Click **Plugins/ Ch.8 Plugins/ Wiener_filter**, and specify the images, the output precision (32-bit) and the complex number precision (double precision). Choose a value for the inverse of the SNR, K (called the Regularization parameter in this plugin) and click OK. If too small a value of K is used the effect of the Wiener filter is too small, and if too large a value is used the noise is sharpened. Try various values of K to find which allows you to read the license plate most clearly. You may have to enhance the contrast of the resulting image. Note that it is the K value that primarily determines the noise reduction, and the size of the blurring function that determines the amount of deblurring.

The ringing pattern around the edges of the resulting image is due to the sharp discontinuity in the de-blurring PSF, i.e. the **pillbox** image. Try Wiener filtering with **bigGaussian**, which does not have sharp discontinuities. The result may be disappointing, indicating that it does not model the original blurring well.

Images **brainGB2** and **boneGB2** have both been subject to Gaussian blur with a radius of 2 pixels. Construct a suitable PSF to model this blur and use Wiener filtering to remove it.

Activity 8.4 Unwarping and registering

Open the distorted (and rotated) image **distortbrain** and the original image **axialbrainMRI**. The plugin **UnwarpJ** (Biomedical Imaging Group, Swiss Federal Institute of Technology, Lausanne (Sorzano *et al.*, 2005)) uses cubic B-spline interpolation to unwarp a "source" image and register it to a "target" image. It runs in fully automatic mode without relying on control points chosen by the operator. In **Plugins/Ch.8 Plugins/UnwarpJ** choose the distorted image as the source and the undistorted image as the target. Click "Done" and observe, during the registration process, the current difference image and a mapping of the grid from the target image on to the source image. When the unwarping and registration is complete, the result is a stack of three images comprising (i) the source image unwarped and registered to fit the target image, (ii) the target image and (iii) the source mask with the same deformation as the source image.

Repeat using the distorted image **distortbarium** and the original image **barium**.

Exercises

8.1 The array below represents a small grayscale image. Calculate the 4×4 image that would result if the middle 16 pixels were transformed using (i) a 3×3 averaging mask and (ii) a 3×3 median mask.

17	51	97	125	34	23
35	96	228	245	85	47
56	128	205	245	118	58
85	230	254	202	186	86
188	240	210	150	122	96
96	105	204	88	56	11

8.2 The signal-to-noise ratio due to quantization, SNR_q, is generally calculated using a sinusoidal input spanning the full range of the analog-to-digital converter (ADC). The error involved in placing a sampled value on the nearest available level, the quantization error, can be anywhere between zero, when the sampled value just happens to correspond to one of the levels, and a maximum size of $\pm q/2$, when the sampled value falls mid-way between two levels, separated by q. Find the SNR (in dB) as a function of the number of bits of the ADC, and identify SNR_q. (Hints: The mean square signal is $A^2/2$, where A is the amplitude of the sinusoid. The mean square noise is $q^2/12$ (draw the distribution of errors, square it, and find the mean).)

8.3 An amateur photographer chances upon a bank robbery. As the robbers' van speeds past him he takes a photograph of the side of the van. Unfortunately the photograph is blurred because he forgot to "pan" with the moving van, and the sign on the van cannot be read. Suggest a method for restoring the image. What blurring function should be used? Can it be estimated from the image itself?

8.4 Consider the problem of image blurring due to uniform acceleration in the x direction. If the image is at rest at position x_0 at time $t=0$ and accelerates with a uniform acceleration a, then its position at time $t=T$ is given by $x=x_0+(1/2)\,aT^2$. Find the blurring function. (Assume that the shutter opening and closing times are negligible.)

8.5 You are working with a noisy video camera and digitizer, and observe that the standard deviation of the noise is about twelve gray levels. You have detail in the image which requires better than five gray levels of precision to be sure of resolving it. How many images would you need to average to see this detail?

Part III

Image analysis

9 Morphological image processing

Overview

Morphological image processing is a tool for extracting or modifying information on the shape and structure of objects within an image. Morphological operators, such as dilation, erosion and skeletonization, are particularly useful for the analysis of binary images, although they can be extended for use with grayscale images. Morphological operators are non-linear, and common usages include filtering, edge detection, feature detection, counting objects in an image, image segmentation, noise reduction and finding the mid-line of an object.

Learning objectives

After reading this chapter you will be able to:

- describe three different ways to define distance in a digital image;
- outline the algorithms for the main morphological operators;
- choose the appropriate morphological operator, or series of operators, to perform certain processing tasks, such as noise reduction and object separation;
- use the appropriate structuring elements in a hit-or-miss transform to detect simple shapes;
- distinguish between skeletonization and the medial axis transform;
- discuss the applications of morphological processing to grayscale images;
- implement the appropriate morphological operations for various processing tasks.

9.1 Mathematical morphology

The field of mathematical morphology contributes a wide range of operators to image processing, all based around a few simple mathematical concepts from *set theory* and, in the case of binary images, (*Boolean*) *logic* operations such as "AND," "OR," "XOR" (exclusive OR) and "NOT." The "union" operation, A∪B, for example, is equivalent to the "OR" operation for binary images; and the "intersection" operator, A∩B, is equivalent to the "AND" operation for binary images (Appendix B).

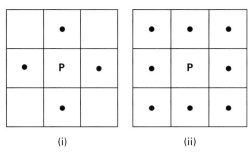

(i)   (ii)

Figure 9.1   Connectivity in two-dimensional images. (i) 4-connectivity – each pixel (P) has four connected neighbors (•). (ii) 8-connectivity – each pixel (P) has eight connected neighbors (•).

9.1.1   Connectivity

In binary images an object is defined as a *connected set* of pixels. With two-dimensional images *connectivity* can be either *4-connectivity* or *8-connectivity* (Fig. 9.1). In 4-connectivity, each pixel (P) has four connected neighbors (N) – top, bottom, right and left: the diagonally touching pixels are not considered to be connected. In 8-connectivity, each pixel (P) has eight connected neighbors (N) – including the diagonally touching pixels. For three-dimensional images neighborhoods can be 6-connected, 18-connected or 26-connected.

This leads to different ideas of distance. In a 4-connected neighborhood, N_4, the distance is known as the *city-block, taxicab* or *Manhattan distance* by analogy with a city based on an orthogonal grid of roads. It is the distance a taxicab would drive in Manhattan (if there were no one-way streets!). The distance in a 4-connected neighborhood is given by

$$d_4(x, y) = |x_1 - x_2| + |y_1 - y_2| \tag{9.1}$$

A diagonal step has a distance of two since it requires a horizontal and a vertical step. Equal distances from a certain position would form diamonds centered on it. In an 8-connected neighborhood, N_8, the distance is known as the *Chebyshev* or *chessboard distance*, by analogy with the moves available to a king in chess. The distance in an 8-connected neighborhood is given by

$$d_8(x, y) = \max\{|x_1 - x_2|, \ |y_1 - y_2|\} \tag{9.2}$$

A diagonal step has a distance of one, the same as a horizontal or vertical step. Equal distances from a certain position would form squares centered on it. Neither is the same as *Euclidean distance*, which is given by

$$d(x, y) = \sqrt{(x_1 - x_2)^2 + (y_1 - y_2)^2} \tag{9.3}$$

A diagonal step is given by a distance of $1/\sqrt{2}$, and equal distances from a certain position form circles centered on it. In physical space the Euclidean distance is the most natural distance, because the length of a rigid body does not change with rotation. Alternating the two metrics (N_4–N_8 or N_8–N_4) is an approximation to Euclidean distance.

9.2 Morphological operators

There are a number of morphological operators, but the two most fundamental operations are *dilation* and *erosion*; all other morphological operations are built from a combination of these two.

9.2.1 Dilation and erosion

In binary images dilation is an operation that increases the size of *foreground* objects, generally taken as white pixels, although in some implementations this convention is reversed. It can be defined in terms of set theory, although we will use a more intuitive algorithm. The connectivity needs to be established prior to operation, or a *structuring element* defined (Fig. 9.2).

The algorithm is as follows: superimpose the structuring element on top of each pixel of the input image so that the center of the structuring element coincides with the input pixel position. If *at least one* pixel in the structuring element coincides with a foreground pixel in the image underneath, including the pixel being tested, then set the output pixel in a new image to the foreground value. Thus, some of the background pixels in the input image become foreground pixels in the output image; those that were foreground pixels in the input image remain foreground pixels in the output image. In the case of 8-connectivity, if a background pixel has at least one foreground (white) neighbor then it becomes white: otherwise, it remains unchanged. The pixels which change from background to foreground are pixels which lie at the edges of foreground regions in the input image, so the consequence is that foreground regions grow in size, and foreground features tend to connect or merge (Fig. 9.3). Background features or holes inside a foreground region shrink due to the growth of the foreground, and sharp corners are smoothed (Fig. 9.4). Repeated dilation results in further growth of the foreground regions

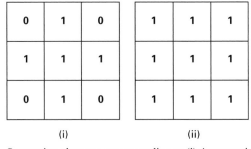

(i)   (ii)

Figure 9.2   Structuring elements corresponding to (i) 4-connectivity and (ii) 8-connectivity.

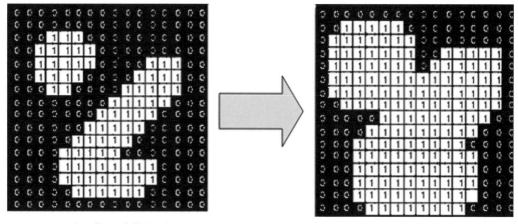

Figure 9.3   The effect of dilation in connecting foreground features, using a structuring element corresponding to 8-connectivity.

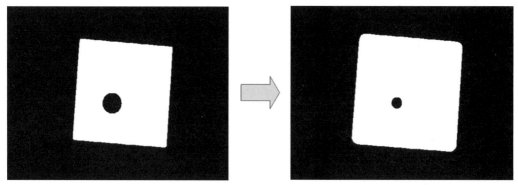

Figure 9.4   The effect of repeated dilation in shrinking background features and smoothing sharp corners, using a structuring element corresponding to 8-connectivity.

(Fig. 9.5). The pattern of growth depends on the structuring element used, as can be seen in Activity 9.1.

The structuring element can be considered analogous to a convolution mask, and the dilation process analogous to convolution, although dilation is based on set operations whereas convolution is based on arithmetic operations. After being reflected about its own origin, it slides over an image, pushing out the boundaries of the image where it overlaps with the image by at least one element. This growing effect is similar to the smearing or blurring effect of an averaging mask. One of the basic applications of dilation is to bridge gaps and connect objects: dilation with a 3×3 structuring element is able to bridge gaps of up to two pixels in length.

Dilation can be used to create the outline of features in an image (Fig. 9.6). If a binarized image is dilated once, and the original image subtracted pixel-by-pixel from the dilated image, the result is a one-pixel wide outline of the features in the original

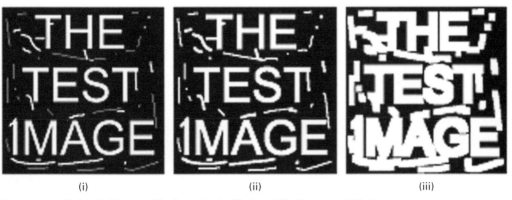

| (i) | (ii) | (iii) |

Figure 9.5   (i) Original image; (ii) after a single dilation; (iii) after several dilations.

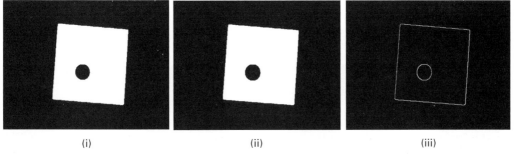

| (i) | (ii) | (iii) |

Figure 9.6   Outlining features in an image. (i) Original image; (ii) image dilated (once); (iii) result of subtracting image (i) from image (ii).

image. This operation tends to be more robust than most edge enhancement operations in the presence of image noise. The outline can be used in subsequent feature extraction operations to measure size, shape and orientation, for example, and these derived measurements can be used in feature classification (Chapter 11).

In contradistinction, erosion is an operation that increases the size of *background* objects (and shrinks the foreground objects) in binary images. In this case the structuring element is superimposed on each pixel of the input image, and if *at least one* pixel in the structuring element coincides with a background pixel in the image underneath, then the output pixel is set to the background value. Thus, some of the foreground pixels in the input image become background pixels in the output image; those that were background pixels in the input image remain background pixels in the output image. In the case of 8-connectivity, if a foreground pixel has at least one background (black) neighbor then it becomes black: otherwise, it remains unchanged. The pixels which change from foreground to background are pixels at the edges of background regions in the input image, so the consequence is that background regions grow in size, and foreground features tend to disconnect or further separate (Fig. 9.7). Background features or holes inside a foreground region grow, and corners are sharpened (Fig. 9.8). Further erosion results in further growth of the background, or shrinking of the foreground (Fig. 9.9).

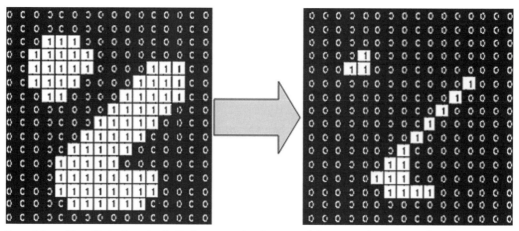

Figure 9.7   The effect of erosion in further separating foreground features, using a structuring element corresponding to 8-connectivity.

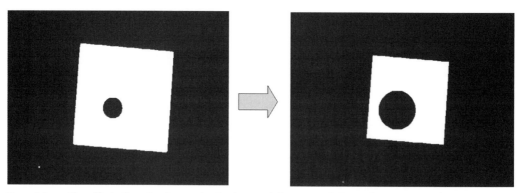

Figure 9.8   The effect of erosion in growing background features and sharpening corners, using a structuring element corresponding to 8-connectivity.

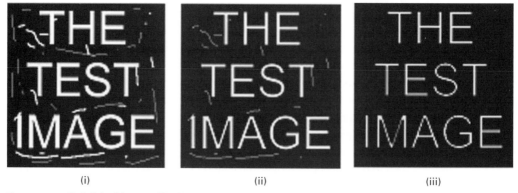

(i)   (ii)   (iii)

Figure 9.9   (i) Original image; (ii) after a single erosion; (iii) after two erosions.

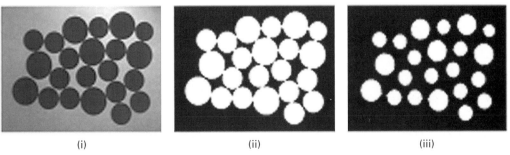

(i)   (ii)   (iii)

Figure 9.10   (i) Grayscale image with features that touch each other; (ii) the image after segmentation; (iii) erosion of image (ii).

Again erosion can be considered analogous to convolution. As the structuring element moves inside the image, the boundaries of the image are moved inwards because image foreground pixels in the image are changed to background pixels wherever the structuring element overlaps the background region by at least one element. One of the basic applications of erosion is to eliminate irrelevant detail, below a certain size, in an image. A structuring element eliminates detail smaller than about its own size. Erosion can be also used to create a one-pixel wide outline of the features in an image by subtracting the eroded image from the original image.

Erosion is the *dual* of dilation, i.e. eroding foreground pixels is equivalent to dilating background pixels. However, erosion of an image followed by dilation of the result, or vice versa, does not produce the original image; isolated foreground pixels removed during erosion, for example, are not re-instated during dilation.

Erosion can help in the counting of features which touch or overlap in an image (Fig. 9.10). The first stage in counting the features is to segment the image, i.e. simplify it by reducing it to black and white (see Chapter 10). If the features still touch each other, they can be separated by erosion (Activity 9.2).

It is possible to do a *constrained* or *conditional dilation*. An image, known as the *seed* image, is dilated but not allowed to dilate outside of a supplied *mask* image, i.e. the resulting features are never larger than the features in the mask image. This is illustrated in Activity 9.3. This can be a useful function in feature extraction and recognition (Chapter 11). An image (Fig. 9.11(i)) could be thresholded to give the mask image (Fig. 9.11(ii)), and then further processed to isolate parts of a certain sub-set of features (say, only those larger than a certain size) in a seed image (Fig. 9.11(iii)). The features can then be grown back to their original shape using the mask image to constrain the dilation (Fig. 9.11(iv)).

In a binary image, each feature is considered to be a connected set of pixels (either 4-connected or 8-connected). Before we can measure the properties of these features (for example, their areas), we need to *label* them. Labeling involves finding a foreground pixel in the image, giving it a label, and recursively giving the same label to all pixels that are connected to it or to its neighbors. This process is repeated until all the foreground pixels have been assigned to a feature and have a label; the label can be used to colorize

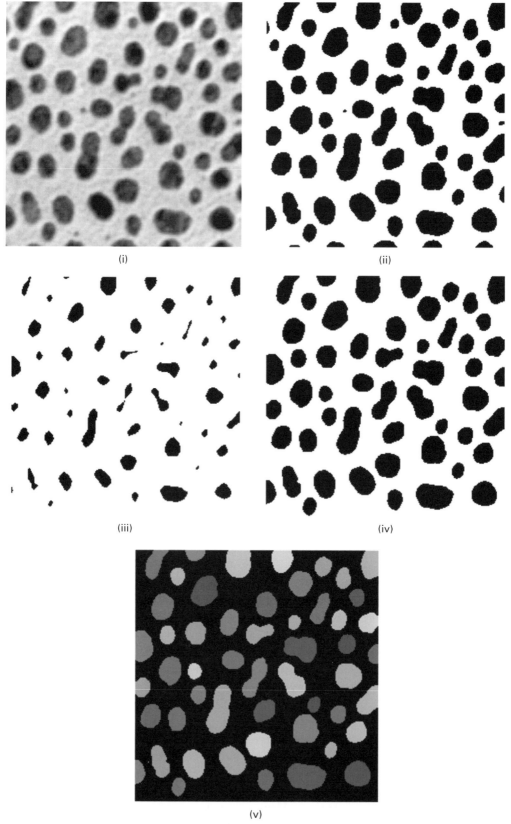

(i)

(ii)

(iii)

(iv)

(v)

Figure 9.11   (i) Original image; (ii) after thresholding; (iii) after 4 erosions; (iv) after 12 conditional dilations (the small objects have been removed); (v) after labeling and displaying each object in a different color. See also color plate.

the features (Fig. 9.11(v)). Labeling can be done in a two-pass process. The image is examined in raster order. When a foreground (ON) pixel is found, neighboring pixels are examined. (In 4-connectedness, it is sufficient to examine the pixel to the left and the pixel above it; in 8-connectedness the pixel on the top left diagonal should also be examined.) Four situations can occur. If none of these neighbors is ON, the current pixel is given a new label; if one of the neighbors is ON, the current pixel is given the same label; if more than one pixel is ON, and they are labeled similarly, the current pixel is given that same label; and if more than one pixel is ON, but they are labeled differently, the current pixel is given one of those labels and these labels are merged to a single label since they are connected and belong to the same feature. In the second pass the labels are reassigned sequentially. The properties of each individual feature can now be measured. For example, the area of a feature is the number of foreground pixels that have that particular label; when all the features are measured, their size distribution can be displayed.

9.2.2 Opening and closing

All the other mathematical morphology operators can be defined in terms of combinations of erosion and dilation along with set operators such as intersection and union. Some of the more important of these other operators are *opening*, *closing* and *skeletonization*.

Opening is defined as erosion followed by dilation using the same structuring element for both operations. The erosion part of it removes some foreground (bright) pixels from the edges of regions of foreground pixels, while the dilation part adds foreground pixels. The foreground features remain about the same size, but their contours are smoother. As with erosion itself, narrow isthmuses are broken and thin protrusions eliminated.

The effect of opening on a binary image depends on the shape of the structuring element: opening preserves foreground regions that have a similar shape to the structuring element, or that can completely contain the structuring element, while it tends to eliminate foreground regions of dissimilar shape. Thus binary opening can be used as a powerful shape detector to preserve certain shapes and eliminate others. The image in Figure 9.12(i) comprises a mixture of lines and circles, with the diameter of the circles being greater than the width of the lines. If a circular structuring element with a diameter just smaller than the diameter of the smallest circles is used to open this image, the resulting image (Fig. 9.12(ii)) contains just the circles and the lines have been eliminated. Activity 9.4 contains examples of opening used as a shape detector.

This is how to think of opening. Take the structuring element and slide it around *inside* each foreground object. Pixels which can be covered by the structuring element with it remaining entirely within the object are preserved. Foreground pixels which cannot be reached by the structuring element without it protruding outside the object are eroded away. When the structuring element is a circle, or a sphere in three dimensions, this operation is known as a *rolling ball*, and is useful for subtracting an uneven background from grayscale images.

Closing is defined as dilation followed by erosion using the same structuring element for both operations. Closing smoothes the contours of foreground objects but, in

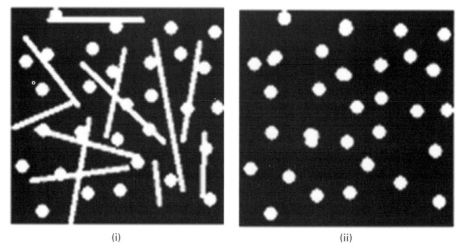

(i)   (ii)

Figure 9.12   Binary opening used as a shape detector. (i) An image comprising both lines and circles. (ii) The result after opening (i) with a circular structuring element.

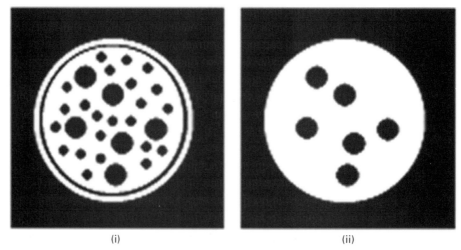

(i)   (ii)

Figure 9.13   (i) An image containing holes of two different sizes and (ii) the result of closing (i) with a circular structuring element mid-way in size between the two sets of holes.

contradistinction to opening, it merges narrow breaks or gaps and eliminates small holes. Figure 9.13 illustrates how closing can be used to eliminate the smaller holes in the image. A circular structural element of size mid-way between the diameter of the two sets of holes was used to close the image in Figure 9.13(i); the resulting image (Fig. 9.13(ii)) contains only the larger holes, since only they allow the structuring element to move freely inside them without protruding outside.

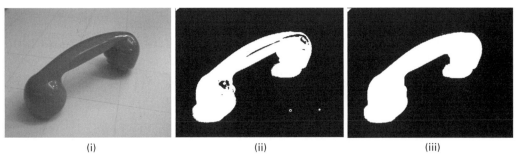

(i)   (ii)   (iii)

Figure 9.14   (i) Original grayscale image; (ii) segmented image showing various artifacts; (iii) the result of closing (ii) with a circular structuring element.

Opening and closing are frequently used to clean up artifacts in a segmented image prior to further analysis (Fig. 9.14). The choice of whether to use opening or closing, or a sequence of erosions and dilations, depends on the image and the objective. For example, opening is used when the image has foreground noise or when we want to eliminate long, thin features: it is not used when there is a chance that the initial erosion operation might disconnect regions. Closing is used when a region has become disconnected and we want to restore connectivity: it is not used when different regions are located closely such that the first iteration might connect them. Usually a compromise is determined between noise reduction and feature retention by testing representative images. You can practice using these operations in Activity 9.5.

As in the case of erosion and dilation, opening and closing are the duals of each other, i.e. opening the foreground pixels with a particular structuring element is equivalent to closing the background pixels with the same element. Opening and closing are also *idempotent* operations, i.e. repeated application of either of them has no further effect on an image.

9.2.3   Hit-or-miss transform

The hit-or-miss transform is a basic tool for shape detection or pattern recognition. Indeed almost all the other morphological operations can be derived from it.

The structuring element is an extension of those we have used before which contained only 1s and 0s: in this case it contains a pattern of 1s (foreground pixels), 0s (background pixels) and x's ("don't cares"). An example, used for finding a bottom left right-angle corner point, is shown in Figure 9.15.

The hit-or-miss operation is performed by translating the center of the structuring element to all points in the image, and then comparing the pixels of the structuring element with the underlying image pixels. If the pixels in the structuring element *exactly match* the pixels in the image, then the image pixel underneath the center of the structuring element is set to the foreground color, indicating a "hit." If the pixels do not match, then that pixel is set to the background color, indicating a "miss." The x's or "don't care" elements in the structuring element match with either 0s or 1s. When the

X	1	X
0	1	1
0	0	X

Figure 9.15   Example of the extended type of structuring element used in hit-or-miss operations.

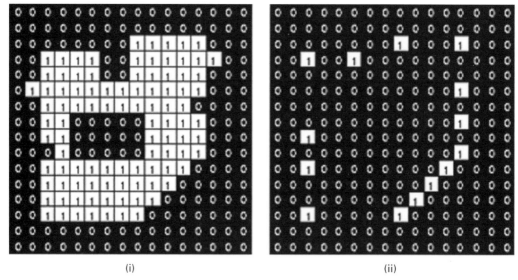

(i)   (ii)

Figure 9.16   (i) Image of a white feature and (ii) the final result, locating all the right-angle corners of the feature by combining the results of using the hit-or-miss transform with the four structuring elements of Figure 9.15.

structuring element overlaps the edge of an image, this would also generally be considered as a "miss." Look at the white pixel at the bottom left-hand corner of the feature in Figure 9.16, and imagine the structuring element of Figure 9.15 placed on it. This is recognized as a bottom left corner of the object because of the pattern of three 1s in the foreground, and the pattern of three 0s describing the background, which are matched in the structuring element. The other three neighboring pixels can be either 0s or 1s and this central pixel remains a corner point; hence they are designated x's (don't cares) in the structuring element.

In order to find all the corners in a binary image we need to run the hit-or-miss transform four times with four different structuring elements representing the four kinds of right-angle corners found in binary images (Fig. 9.17), and then combine the four results, using a logical "OR," to get the final result showing the locations of all right-angle corners in any orientation. Figure 9.16 shows the final result of locating all the

X	1	X
0	1	1
0	0	X

X	1	X
1	1	0
X	0	0

X	0	0
1	1	0
X	1	X

0	0	X
0	1	1
X	1	X

Figure 9.17 The four structuring elements used for finding corners in a binary image using the hit-or-miss transform. The leftmost one detects bottom left corners (as we saw in Fig. 9.15), and the others are derived from it with various rotations to detect the bottom right, top right and top left corners, respectively.

right-angle corners of a feature. Activity 9.6 illustrates other practical examples of using the hit-or-miss transform.

Different structuring elements can be used for locating other features within a binary image, for example isolated points in an image, or end points and junction points in a binary skeleton.

9.2.4   Thinning and skeletonization

Thinning is a morphological operation that successively erodes away foreground pixels from the boundary of binary images while preserving the end points of line segments. Thickening is the dual of thinning, i.e. thickening the foreground is equivalent to thinning the background.

The thinning operation is related to the hit-and-miss transform and can be expressed quite simply in terms of it. The thinning of an image I by a structuring element J is:

$$\text{thin}(I, J) = I - \text{hit-or-miss}(I, J) \tag{9.4}$$

where the subtraction is a *logical subtraction* defined by $X - Y = X \cap \text{NOT } Y$.

For example, the structuring element of Figure 9.18(i), and the three rotations of it by 90°, are essentially line detectors. If a hit-or-miss transform is applied to the rectangle of Figure 9.18(ii) using this structuring element, a pixel-wide line from the top surface of the rectangle is produced, which is one pixel short at both right and left ends. If the line is subtracted from the original image, the original rectangle is thinned slightly. Repeated thinning produces the image shown in Figure 9.18(iii). If this is continued, together with thinning by the other three rotations of the structuring element, the skeleton shown in Figure 9.18(iv) is produced.

Repeated thinning can be used to obtain a single-pixel wide *skeleton* or center line of an object. One of the most common uses of skeletonization is to reduce the thresholded output of an edge detector such as the Sobel operator to lines of a single pixel thickness. Skeletonization needs to be implemented as a two-step process that does not break the objects. The first step is normal thinning, but it is conditional; that is, pixels are marked as candidates for removal, but are not actually eliminated. In the second pass,

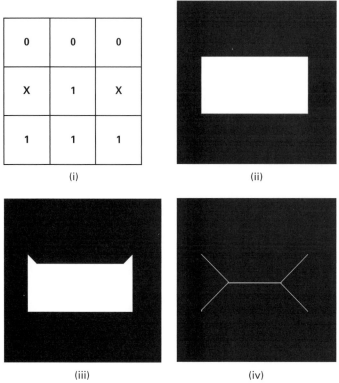

Figure 9.18   (i) Structural element for line detection; (ii) image of rectangle; (iii) image of rectangle after 12 iterations of thinning with the structural element of (i); (iv) thinning to convergence using the structural element of (i) and its three 90° rotations.

those candidates which can be removed without destroying connectivity are eliminated, while those that cannot are retained. The process is then repeated several times until no further change occurs, i.e. until *convergence*, and the skeleton is obtained. *Skeletonization* preserves the topology, i.e. the extent and connectivity, of an object. The skeleton should be minimally 8-connected, i.e. the resulting line segments should always contain the minimal number of pixels that maintain 8-connectness: and the approximate end-line locations should be maintained. Various implementations have been proposed; the algorithm of Zhang and Suen (Zhang and Suen, 1984) is probably the most widely used realization.

The skeleton is useful because it provides a simple and compact representation of the shape of an object. Thus, for instance, we can get a rough idea of the length of an object by finding the maximally separated pair of end points on the skeleton. Similarly, we can distinguish many qualitatively different shapes from one another on the basis of how many *junction points* there are, i.e. points where at least three branches of the skeleton meet. Although skeletonization can be applied to binary images containing regions of any shape, it is most suitable for elongated (Fig. 9.19), as opposed to convex or

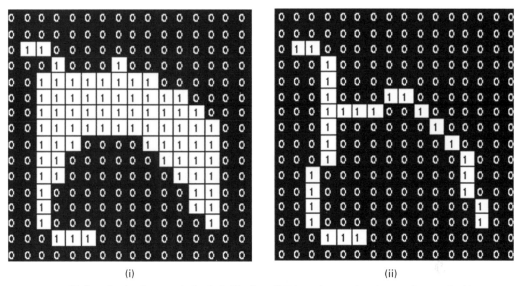

	(i)			(ii)

Figure 9.19 Skeletonization by morphological thinning. (i) Binary image showing an elongated white foreground object and (ii) its skeleton.

0	0	0		0	0	0
0	1	0		0	1	0
0	X	X		X	X	0

Figure 9.20 Structural elements used for pruning. At each iteration, each element must be used in each of its four 90° rotations.

blob-like, shapes. For example, it is useful for visualizing the center line of blood vessels in an angiogram and in automated recognition of hand-written characters.

Skeletons produced by this method tend to leave parasitic components or *spurs* as a result of small irregularities in the boundary of the original object. These spurs can be removed by a process called *pruning*, which is in fact just another form of thinning. The structuring element for this pruning operation is shown in Figure 9.20. Pruning is normally carried out for only a limited number of iterations to remove short spurs, since pruning until convergence actually removes all pixels except those that form closed loops (Activity 9.7).

Skeletonization can be understood in terms of the *prairie fire* analogy. Imagine that the foreground region in a binary image is made of some uniform slow-burning material such as dry grass on a bare dirt background. If fires were to be started simultaneously at all points along the boundary of the region, the fire would proceed to burn inwards towards

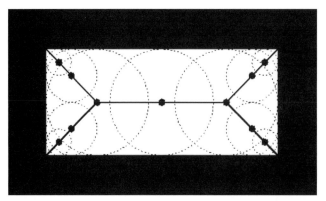

Figure 9.21   The skeleton of a rectangle defined in terms of bi-tangent circles.

the center of the region until all the grass was consumed. At points where the fire traveling from two different boundaries meets itself, the fire extinguishes itself and the points at which this happens form the so-called *quench line*. This line is the *skeleton*. Another way to think about the skeleton is as the loci of centers of bi-tangent circles that fit entirely within the foreground region being considered. Figure 9.21 illustrates this for a rectangular shape.

9.2.5   The medial axis transform and skeletonization

The terms *medial axis transform* (MAT) and skeletonization are often used interchangeably but they are different. Skeletonization produces a binary image showing the simple skeleton. The medial axis transform, on the other hand, produces a grayscale image where each point on the skeleton has an intensity which represents its distance to a boundary in the original object. Thus the medial axis transform (but not the skeleton) can be used to reconstruct the original shape exactly, which makes it useful for lossless image compression, by constructing circles of radius equal to the pixel value around each pixel. The skeleton is the medial axis transform, thresholded such that only the center pixels, one pixel in width, are above the threshold.

The medial axis transform is closely linked to the *distance transform*, which is the result of performing multiple successive erosions with a structuring element that depends on which distance metric has been chosen, until all foreground regions of the image have been eroded away, and labeling each pixel with the number of erosions that had to be performed before it disappeared (Fig. 9.22). The distance transform can also be used to derive various other symmetries from binary shapes. Although there are many different implementations, the medial axis transform is essentially the locus of slope discontinuities (i.e. the ridges) in the distance transform; if the distance transform is displayed as a three-dimensional surface plot with the third dimension representing the gray value, the medial axis transform can be imagined as the ridges on the three-dimensional surface.

The skeletons and the medial axial transforms, obtained from the distance transforms, of a number of images are compared in Figure 9.23.

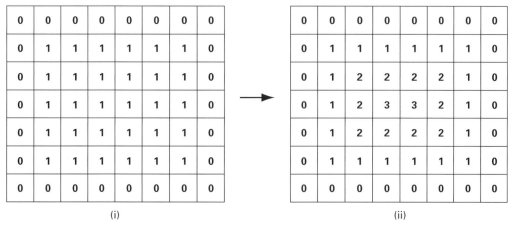

Figure 9.22 Schematics of (i) a binary image of a rectangle and (ii) its distance transform image (note we are using the N_8 distance metric).

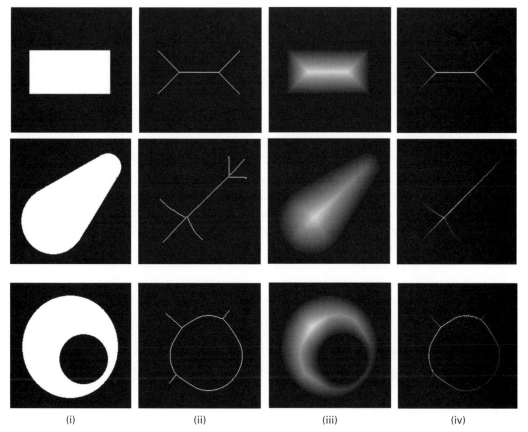

(i)   (ii)   (iii)   (iv)

Figure 9.23 (i) Original images; (ii) their skeletons; (iii) their Euclidean distance transforms (after contrast enhancement); and (iv) their medial axis transforms.

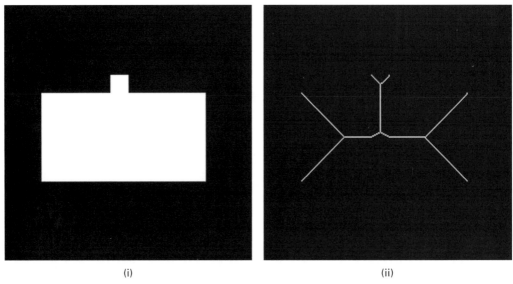

(i)   (ii)

Figure 9.24   (i) An image of a rectangle with a small change in its boundary; (ii) the result of skeletonizing image (i).

Both the skeleton and the medial axis transform are sensitive to small changes in the boundary of the object, which can produce artifactually more complex skeletons (Fig. 9.24; compare with Fig. 9.23(ii), top). The skeletonized image in Figure 9.25 shows the very complex skeleton produced by skeletonizing a thresholded image of a telephone receiver and the less complex skeleton, more representative of the true shape of the telephone receiver, produced when the thresholded image is closed prior to skeletonization. The skeleton can be further improved by pruning insignificant spur features. These examples indicate that additional processing may often be required prior to skeletonization.

Both skeletonization and the medial axis transform are also very sensitive to noise. If some "pepper noise" is added to the image of a white rectangle (Fig. 9.26(i)), the resulting skeleton (Fig. 9.26(ii)) connects each noise point to the skeleton obtained from the noise free image (see Fig. 9.23(ii), top).

Just as the skeleton of objects or features in an image can be determined, it is also possible to skeletonize the background. This gives the so-called "skiz" (skeleton of influence zone) image (Figs. 9.27 and 9.28). This effectively divides the image into regions or zones of influence around each feature. Discontinuous lines can be easily removed; starting at each end point (points with a single neighbor), connected pixels are eliminated until a node (a point with more than two neighbors) is reached. The skiz is actually the generalized Voronoi diagram (see Section 9.2.6).

9.2.6   The convex hull

The *convex hull* of a binary feature can be visualized quite easily by imagining stretching an elastic band around the feature. The elastic band follows the convex contours of the

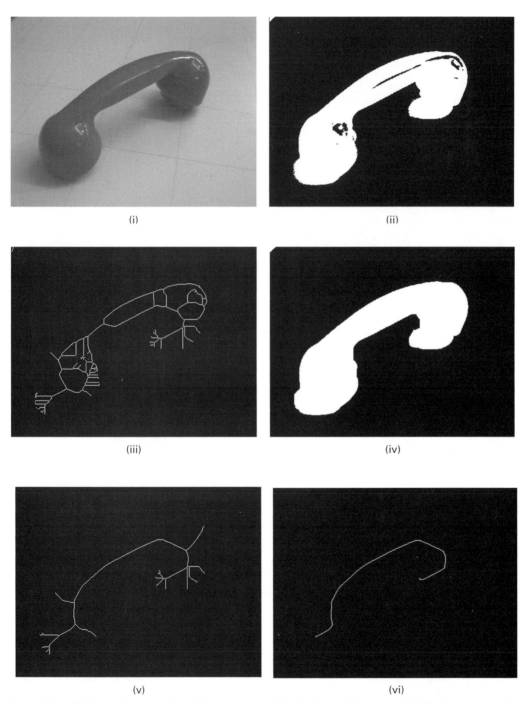

Figure 9.25 (i) Grayscale image of a telephone receiver; (ii) after thresholding image (i); (iii) after skeletonizing image (ii); (iv) after closing image (ii) with a circular structural element; (v) after skeletonizing image (iv); (vi) after pruning image (v).

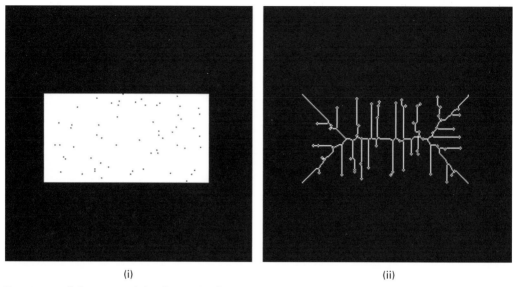

(i)   (ii)

Figure 9.26   (i) Image containing "pepper" noise and (ii) the resulting skeleton.

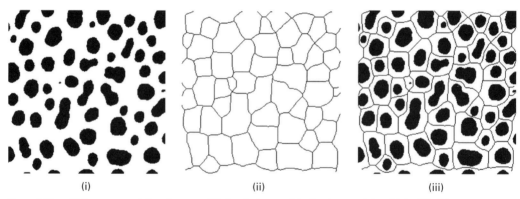

(i)   (ii)   (iii)

Figure 9.27   (i) Image containing features; (ii) the skeleton of the background (or skiz); (iii) skiz superimposed on original image to show zones of influence.

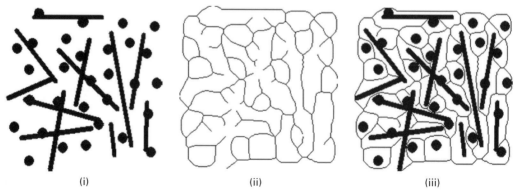

(i)   (ii)   (iii)

Figure 9.28   (i) Image containing features; (ii) the skeleton of the background, or skiz (note that there are some discontinuous lines which should be eliminated); (iii) skiz superimposed on original image to show zones of influence.

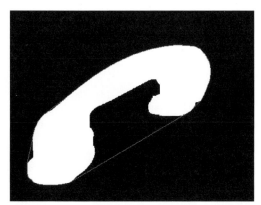

Figure 9.29   A feature enclosed by its convex hull (shown in red). See also color plate.

1	1	X
1	0	X
1	X	0

X	1	1
X	0	1
0	X	1

Figure 9.30   Structuring elements for determining the approximate convex hull using thickening. During each iteration, each structuring element should be used in turn, and then in each of their 90° rotations, giving eight effective structuring elements in total. The thickening is continued until no further changes occur.

feature, but "bridges" the concave contours. The resulting shape has no concavities and contains the original feature (Fig. 9.29). Where an image contains multiple disconnected features, the convex hull algorithm determines the convex hull of each of them, but does not connect disconnected features, unless their convex hulls happen to overlap.

The *convex hull* is the smallest convex polygon that contains the object in an image. Its simple shape often suffices to perform matching or recognition, and it delineates the *area of influence* of an object or region; if another region or its convex hull overlaps this convex hull, then it is said to encroach on the first region's area of influence.

An approximate convex hull can be computed using thickening with the structuring elements shown in Figure 9.30. The convex hull computed using this method is actually a "45° convex hull" approximation, in which the boundaries of the convex hull must have orientations that are multiples of 45°. Note that this computation can be *very* slow.

Figure 9.31(i) shows an image containing a number of cross-shaped binary objects. The 45° convex hull algorithm described above results in convex hulls which depend on

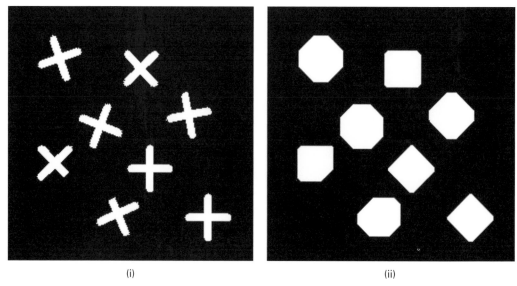

(i)   (ii)

Figure 9.31   (i) An image and (ii) its approximate (45°) convex hull.

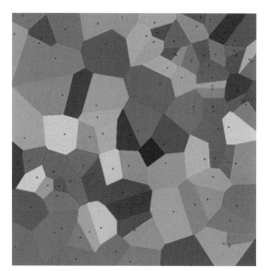

Figure 9.32   The Voronoi diagram of a set of points, showing the polygons of influence. See also color plate.

the orientation of the individual cross-shaped objects in the original image (Fig. 9.31(ii)). The process took a considerable amount of time – over one hundred thickening passes with *each* of the eight structuring elements!

Other more exact implementations of the complex hull exist, for example using angular sorting of the corners of an object (Graham scan), but they are beyond the scope of this text.

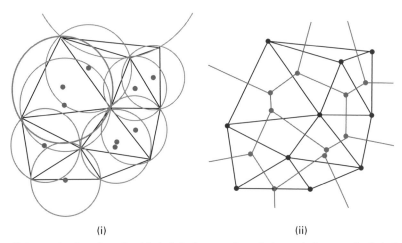

(i)   (ii)

Figure 9.33   (i) A set of points (in red) with their Delaunay triangulation and circumscribed circles. (ii) Connecting the centers of the circumscribed points produces the Voronoi diagram (in red). See also color plate.

For a set of points, the Voronoi diagram and its dual, the Delaunay triangulation, are mathematically related to the convex hull. The Voronoi diagram is obtained by drawing bisectors of the lines between points and connecting them to form convex polygons. These polygons are then the polygons of influence around the points (Fig. 9.32); they are not as general as the skiz where the zones of influence are not constrained to be polygons. The Delaunay triangulation is a set of triangles with the points as vertices, such that no point is inside the circumcircle of any of the triangles (Fig. 9.33). (Delaunay triangulations are often used to build meshes for the finite element method.) The outer boundary of the Voronoi diagram is the convex hull of all the points. Voronoi cells can also be defined by measuring distances to features that are not points. The Voronoi diagram with these cells is the medial axis.

9.3   Extension to grayscale images

The basic binary morphological operations can be extended to use with grayscale images; the results of such operations are grayscale images.

In grayscale dilation, for example, the structuring element is defined by a pattern of 1s and is superimposed on top of each pixel of the input image in turn. Only those pixels with a 1 on top of them are considered, and the output pixel, which replaces the central image pixel, is the *maximum* of the pixel values under consideration. For grayscale erosion, the image pixel is replaced by the *minimum* of the pixels considered by the structuring element. Thus dilation brightens and expands brighter areas of an image, and darkens and shrinks darker areas: erosion is the dual, and has the opposite effect.

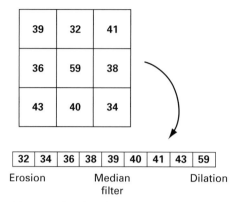

| 32 | 34 | 36 | 38 | 39 | 40 | 41 | 43 | 59 |

Erosion   Median   Dilation
                 filter

Figure 9.34   Schematic showing pixels in a 3×3 neighborhood being ranked, as a prelude to replacing the center pixel by the maximum, median or minimum value. Each option corresponds to grayscale dilation, median filtering and grayscale erosion, respectively.

Grayscale dilation and erosion are thus seen to be identical to convolution with the *maximum* and *minimum* rank masks, which operate like the median mask. The neighborhood around each pixel and the pixels are ordered by rank. If the center pixel is replaced by the maximum value in the neighborhood, grayscale dilation occurs. If the center pixel is replaced by the minimum value in the neighborhood, grayscale erosion occurs. And if the center pixel is replaced by the median value in the neighborhood, median filtering occurs (Fig. 9.34).

Grayscale opening and closing have the same form as their binary counterparts, i.e. grayscale opening is grayscale erosion followed by grayscale dilation, and grayscale closing is grayscale dilation followed by grayscale erosion:

$$\text{Open} = \text{Max}(\text{Min}(\text{Image})) \tag{9.5a}$$

$$\text{Close} = \text{Min}(\text{Max}(\text{Image})) \tag{9.5b}$$

Opening a grayscale image with a circular structuring element can be viewed as having the structuring roll under the profile of the image pushing up on the underside: the result of the opening is the surface of the highest points reached by any part of this *rolling ball* (Fig. 9.35). Conversely, grayscale erosion can be viewed as the rolling ball traversing the image profile and pressing down on it, with the result being the surface of the lowest points reached by any part of the rolling ball.

Properties such as duality and idempotence also apply to the grayscale operators.

9.3.1   Applications of grayscale morphological processing

Non-linear processing is often used to remove noise without blurring the edges in the image: recall how the median mask out-performed the linear averaging mask in removing salt-and-pepper noise. Morphological processing is often used because of its

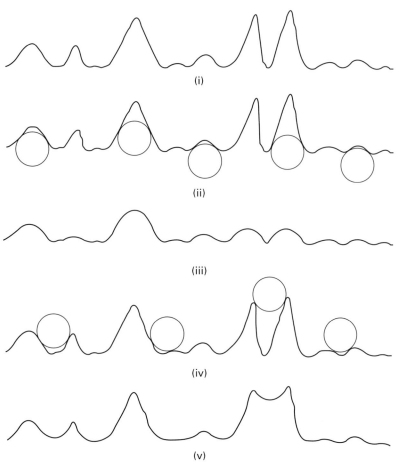

(i)

(ii)

(iii)

(iv)

(v)

Figure 9.35 (i) A grayscale image profile; (ii) positions of rolling ball for opening; (iii) result of opening; (iv) positions of rolling ball for closing; (v) result of closing. (After Gonzalez and Woods (2002).)

ability to distinguish objects based on their size, shape or contrast, namely whether they are lighter or darker than the background. It can remove certain objects and leave others intact, making it more sophisticated at image interpretation than most other image processing tools.

Grayscale opening smoothes an image from above the brightness surface, while grayscale closing smoothes it from below. They remove small local maxima or minima without affecting the gray values of larger objects. Grayscale opening can be used to select and preserve particular intensity patterns while attenuating others. Figure 9.36 illustrates the effect of grayscale opening with a flat 5×5 square structuring element. Bright features smaller than the structuring element are greatly reduced in intensity, while larger features remain more or less unchanged in intensity. Thus the fine-grained hair and whiskers in the original image are much reduced in intensity, while the nose region is still at much the same intensity as in the original. Note that the opened image does have a

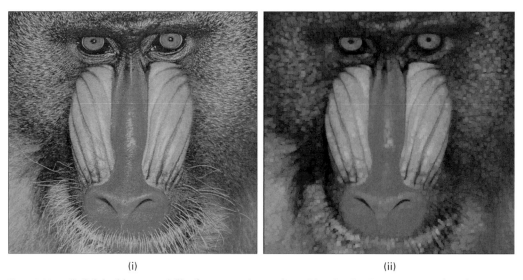

Figure 9.36   (i) Original image and (ii) after grayscale opening with a flat 5 × 5 square structuring element

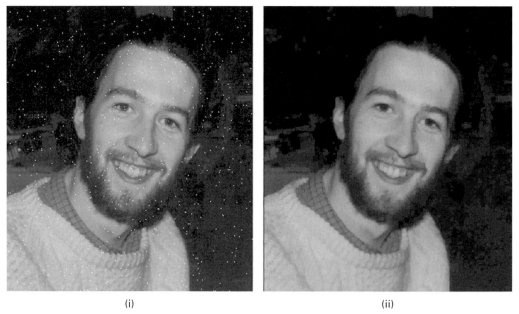

Figure 9.37   (i) Original image with "salt" noise and (ii) after grayscale opening with a flat 3 × 3 square structuring element.

more matt appearance than before since the opening has eliminated small fluctuations in texture.

Similarly, opening can be used to remove "salt noise" in grayscale images. Figure 9.37 shows an image containing salt noise, and the result of opening with a 3 × 3 square

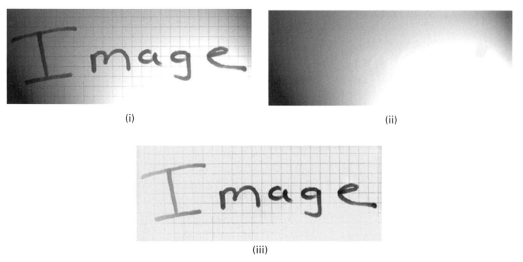

Figure 9.38 (i) Image of text on variable background; (ii) morphological thresholding produces variable background; (iii) subtraction of (ii) from (i) to separate text.

structuring element. The noise has been entirely removed with relatively little degradation of the underlying image.

A sequential combination of these two operations (open–close or close–open) is referred to as *morphological smoothing* and can be used to remove "salt-and-pepper" noise (see Activity 9.8).

In images with a variable background it is often difficult to separate features from the background. Adaptive processing is a possible solution. An alternative solution is so-called *morphological thresholding*, in which a morphologically smoothed image is used to produce an image of the variable background which can then be subtracted from the original image. The process is illustrated in Figure 9.38. Activity 9.9 contains several practice images.

Morphological sharpening can be implemented by the *morphological gradient*, MG, operation:

$$MG = \frac{1}{2} \left(Max(Image) - Min(Image) \right) \tag{9.6}$$

The effect of the morphological gradient on a one-dimensional gray-level profile is shown in Figure 9.39. The edges of the original image are replaced by peaks.

If a symmetrical structuring element is used, such sharpening is less dependent on edge directionality than using sharpening masks such as the Sobel masks.

The morphological *top hat* transformation, TH, is defined by

$$TH = Image - Open(Image) \tag{9.7}$$

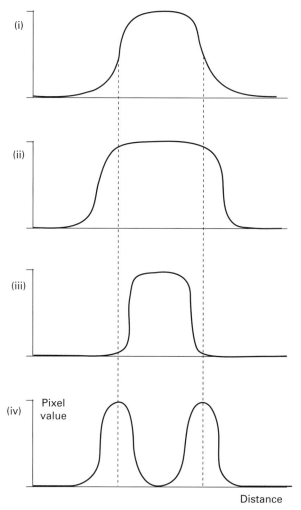

Figure 9.39 (i) Profile of gray-level image; (ii) profile of dilated image; (iii) profile of eroded image; (iv) profile of morphological gradient. (After Baxes, 1994.)

It is the analog of unsharp masking, and is useful for enhancing detail in the presence of shading.

In *local contrast stretching* the amount of stretching that is applied in a neighborhood is controlled by the original contrast in that neighborhood. It is implemented by

$$G = \frac{A - \text{Min}(A)}{\text{Max}(A) - \text{Min}(A)} \cdot \text{scale} \qquad (9.8)$$

The Max (dilate) and Min (erode) operations are taken over the structuring element: "scale" is a small number. This operation is an extended version of the *point* operation for contrast stretching presented in Equation (5.10).

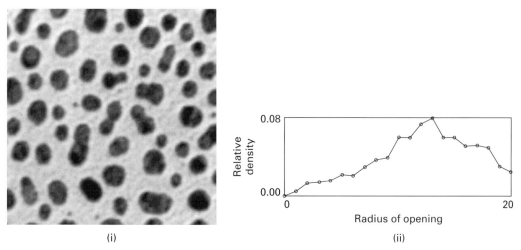

Figure 9.40   (i) Image containing features of different size and (ii) the histogram of feature-size distribution.

Granulometry is the name given to the determination of the size distribution of features within an image, particularly when they are predominantly circular in shape. Opening operations with structuring elements of increasing size can be used to construct a histogram of feature size, even when they overlap and are too cluttered to enable detection of individual features. The difference between the original image and its opening is computed after each pass. At the end of the process, these differences are normalized and used to construct a histogram of feature-size distribution. The resulting histogram is often referred to as the *pattern spectrum* of the image (Fig. 9.40 and Activity 9.10).

Computer-based activities

Activity 9.1 Neighborhood shapes

Open the image **deltaim**, which has a single white ("ON") pixel in the center of a 256^2 image, in ImageJ. Using **Plugins/Ch.9 Plugins/Morpho** plugin, set the operation to Max (equivalent to dilation), the number of iterations to 1 and the connectivity to 8. Repeat the dilation on the result, and then dilate again, and again. Observe how the point is dilated to show the neighborhood, using chessboard distances. Repeat with connectivity set to 4: observe how the 4-connected neighborhood is built up from city-block distances. The neighborhood shapes represent PSFs of different widths. Starting from **deltaim**, dilate using 4-connectivity, then 8-connectivity, then 4-connectivity, and so on. Note the shape of the neighborhood. What shape would result from Euclidean distances if it were possible to implement such a scheme? Which of the three schemes tested is closest to Euclidean?

Activity 9.2 Applications

Open `box` in ImageJ. Dilate the image using **Process/Binary/Dilate**, and subtract the original image (using **Process/Image Calculator**) from the result to obtain a one-pixel wide outline. You can also get edges by subtracting an eroded image from the original: the edges in both these images are one pixel shifted from each other. Repeat the outlining process using `mri`.

Open `objects` and threshold the image (**Image/Adjust/Threshold ...**). Note the gray-level histogram. A threshold between ~50 and ~80 separates the darker objects from the lighter background, but the objects remain connected in the thresholded image. Note that reducing the threshold value does not disconnect the objects: instead some of the objects begin to disappear. Why is this? It is often useful to smooth an object with a small (e.g. 3 × 3) median mask, which avoids blurring the edges, prior to thresholding. After choosing the threshold, apply it to the image (**Process/Binary/Make Binary**) to obtain a binary image (check its histogram using **Analyze/Histogram**). The objects in the resulting binary image *can* be disconnected using erosion (**Plugins/Binary/Erode**). The objects themselves are reduced in size, and you might then consider increasing them to their former size approximately by dilating them by the same number of iterations which it took to separate them.

Try to separate the individual cells in the image `cells`. Threshold and binarize as before. The cells are black on a white foreground: invert the image (**Edit/Invert**) to change to the more conventional situation of white (foreground) objects on a black background. Use erosions to disconnect the cells, but note that they become smaller and that the internal holes grow. You need to try to balance the erosions with dilations in an order that optimally disconnects the cells but preserves as much of their shape as possible. Determine whether 4-connectivity or 8-connectivity is better for this particular image.

Now try to separate the individual spots in the image `spots`.

Activity 9.3 Constrained/conditional dilation

Open `cermet` in ImageJ, smooth it slightly (**Process/Filters/Mean ...** and use a radius = 1), threshold it (**Image/Adjust/Threshold**) and save the result as `mask`. Make a duplicate (**Image/Duplicate ...**) of this image, erode it four times (**Process/Binary/Options**, set to 4 iterations, then **Process/Binary/Erode**) and save the new result as `seed`. Make a duplicate of `seed` and dilate it ten times (**Process/Binary/Options**, set to 10 iterations, then **Process/Binary/Dilate**). Note how the objects in the resulting image have grown much larger than those in the original thresholded image, `mask`.

Conditionally dilate (**Plugins/Ch.9 Plugins/BinaryConditionalDilate**) the `seed` image ten times with `seed` as the seed image and the thresholded image, `mask`, as the mask image, and the number of iterations set to 10. Compare the result with the earlier result using (unconditional) dilation: the objects in the (conditionally) dilated image are not allowed to grow bigger than their size in the mask image.

Delete all the open images and record all the previous steps in a macro. (Use **Plugins/ Macros/Record ...**, name the macro `ConDilate`, and proceed to work through the processing steps as before. Observe how they are recorded. When you have finished, click "Create.") The macro can be re-run at any time by **Plugins/ Macros/Run ...** and choosing `CondDilate.txt`.

Activity 9.4 Opening as a shape detector

Open **shapes** in ImageJ, and use the cursor to find the diameter of the circles. Open **Plugins/Ch.9 Plugins/Teacher Open** and choose "Disk" as the type of structuring element, and a size just smaller than the diameter of the smallest circles. ("Square" uses an N_8 neighborhood, "Cross" uses N_4 and "Disk" uses a structuring element as close to a circle as you can get using a square matrix.) Observe that the resulting image contains just the circles, i.e. you have used binary opening as a shape detector.

Open **mixed cells**. The image contains two kinds of cell: small black ones and larger gray ones. Threshold the image (**Image/Adjust/Threshold ...**) to separate the cells from the background. Use a circular structuring element (**Plugins/ Ch.9 Plugins /Teacher Open**) to remove the small cells and retain the larger cells. You should be able to do this fairly successfully by choosing an appropriate size of structuring element. (Note that it is not possible to isolate the small cells directly using this method.)

Activity 9.5 Applications of closing and opening

Open **holes** in ImageJ. Find the diameter of both the small holes and the large holes in the image using the cursor. Use **Plugins/Ch.9 Plugins/Teacher Close** with an appropriate structural element to eliminate the smaller holes.

Open **telephone** and threshold it (**Image/Adjust/Threshold ...**). The gray-level histogram is *bimodal*, showing two regions: the region with the lower pixel values roughly corresponds to the (dark) telephone receiver, and the other region corresponds to the background. Set the left-hand threshold to zero and the right-hand threshold to mid-way between the two regions. Note that the resulting thresholded image includes the dark shadows under the telephone, and that some pixels within the telephone appear white because they reflected more of the illuminating light. You can vary the right-hand threshold to minimize these effects. If you increase the threshold value the white area shrinks but the shadow area expands, and vice versa if you reduce the threshold value. Choose a value just below the mid-way value to minimize the shadow effect somewhat, and click "Apply." Since we consider the dark telephone as the object of interest, we do an opening to try to clean it up; remember that opening and closing are duals of each other. Use **Plugins/Ch.9 Plugins/Teacher Open** with a circular structuring element of size 9 pixels. Observe the result. Try to improve on it by using other sizes, or by using the "cross" structuring element (shaped like a "plus" sign) and various sizes.

Activity 9.6 Hit-or-miss transform

Open **rectangle** in ImageJ and use the hit-or-miss transform (**Plugins/Ch.9 Plugins/BinaryHitorMiss**) with a suitable structuring element (e.g. $\begin{smallmatrix} 2&1&2\\0&1&1\\0&0&2 \end{smallmatrix}$, where

0 indicates black, 1 is white and 2 is used to denote "don't care") to detect corners in the image. Choose 90° rotations and check white foreground. The result should be the four vertices of the rectangle.

Open **binaorta**, and use the hit-or-miss transform with a structuring element of $\frac{000}{111}$ and no rotations. Observe the result, which shows the positions at which this pattern was matched.

We would like to be able to detect junction points, either bifurcations (splittings) or vessel crossings, at all orientations in this image. Experiment with different structuring elements to try to achieve this, making use of the 45° rotation feature in the plugin. A limitation is that the plugin only uses 3×3 structuring elements.

Activity 9.7 Thinning and skeletonization

Open **rectangle** in ImageJ. The built-in skeletonization within ImageJ is not very reliable: invert the original image (**Edit/Invert**) and skeletonize it (**Process/ Binary/Skeletonize**).

Instead use a macro that makes use of an alternative binary thinning plugin. Open **rectangle** and run (**Plugins/Macros/Run**) the macro **skeleton1.txt**: the result is the 8-connected skeleton. Repeat with the macro **skeleton3.txt** to obtain the 4-connected skeleton. Repeat using **shape1**, **shape2** and **box2**.

Open **telephone** and smooth it (**Process/Smooth**) to reduce noise, which can confound successful thresholding. Threshold it (**Image/Adjust/Threshold**), minimizing the shadows; binarize the result (**Process/Binary/Make Binary**) and invert it (**Edit/Invert**). Open it (**Process/Binary/Open**) to remove the black holes in the white object, and then run (**Plugins/Macros/Run**) the macro **skeleton1.txt**. Prune the spurs in the resulting skeleton by stages using **Plugins/Macros/Run** and the macro **Prune1.txt** as often as required, or run **PruneAll.txt** to prune until convergence.

Skeletonization can be used to find the center line of blood vessels. Open **angio1**, an angiogram, and **angio2**, the image after thresholding. Binarize **angio2** (**Process/Binary/Make Binary**) and invert it (**Edit/Invert**). Run the 8-connectivity skeletonization macro (**skeleton1.txt**), followed by the stage-by-stage pruning (**Prune1.txt**). Compare your result with **angio3**.

Activity 9.8 Morphological smoothing

Open **salt and pepper** in ImageJ, and perform a grayscale opening (**Plugins/ Ch.9 Plugins/Teacher Open**) with a disk-shaped (circular) structural element of size 3 pixels. Note how the "salt" is removed from the image. Close this resulting image (**Plugins/Ch.9 Plugins/Teacher Close**) with a circular structural element to remove the "pepper." Compare the final result with **mri**, the original image before salt-and-pepper noise was added.

Activity 9.9 Morphological thresholding

Open **image** in ImageJ. The generally darker text appears on a lighter, but variable, background. However, simple thresholding (**Image/Adjust/Threshold ...**) is unable to separate the text from the background: try it!

Adaptive processing is a possible solution. Use **Plugins/Ch.9 Plugins/ Adaptive Threshold** and try different parameters. (A neighborhood/mask size of 11, constant of 3, and mean thresholding gives a reasonable result.) The text is separated from the variable background but the grid lines remain. They can be removed by opening **Process/Binary/Make Binary** then **Process/ Binary/Open**.

Morphological thresholding is an alternative solution. Use a sufficiently large structuring element and a close–open (**Plugins/Ch.9 Plugins/Teacher Close** followed by **Plugins/Ch.9 Plugins/Teacher Open** and a circular disk of size 15, say) to smooth out both the dark and light objects in the image, and produce an image of the variable background which can then be subtracted (**Process/Image Calculator ...** using "Subtract' and "32-bit Result") from the original image. This is similar to the effect of **Process/Subtract Background**; try different parameter values.

Use these different techniques on **yeast, uneven, sonnet** and the two mammographic images **lcc** (a left cranio-caudal view) and **rcc** (a right cranio-caudal view).

Activity 9.10 Granulometry

Open **cermet** in ImageJ, and start **Plugins/Ch.9 Plugins/Granulometry**. Choose the minimum and maximum radii as 0 and 20 pixels, respectively, and the step size as 1 pixel; check "yes" to view intermediate images. The density distribution or pattern spectrum takes a few iterations before it appears. What is the radius of the predominant particles within this image?

Exercises

9.1 Find the length of the shortest path from (a) $(1, 1)$ to $(5, 3)$ and (b) $(1, 6)$ to $(3, 1)$ using (i) 4-connectivity and (ii) 8-connectivity.

9.2 What is the difference between the result of opening performed once and twice? What is idempotency?

9.3 Sketch the structuring elements required for the hit-or-miss transform to locate (i) isolated points in an image, (ii) end points in a binary skeleton and (iii) junction points in a binary skeleton. Several structuring elements may be needed in some cases to locate all possible orientations.

9.4 How can the hit-or-miss transform be used to perform erosion? How can the hit-and-miss transform, together with the NOT (or inverse) operation, be used to perform dilation?

9.5 If an edge detector has produced long lines in its output that are approximately x pixels thick, what is the longest length spurious spur (prune) that you could expect to see after thinning to a single pixel thickness? Test your estimate on some real images. Hence, approximately how many iterations of pruning should be applied to remove spurious spurs from lines that were thinned down from a thickness of x pixels?

9.6 Sketch the skeleton of (i) a square, (ii) an equilateral triangle and (iii) a circle.

9.7 How can the medial axis transform be used to reconstruct the original shape of the region it was derived from?

9.8 What shape and size of structuring element would you need to use in order to detect just the horizontal lines in Figure E9.1?

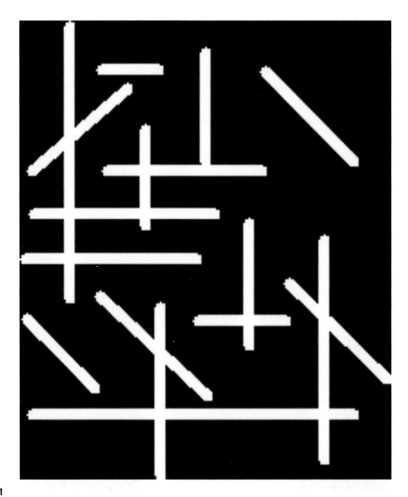

Figure E9.1

9.9 The features in the image shown in Figure E9.2(i) are flawed by small gaps, which have been removed in the image shown in Figure E9.2(ii). What processing operation would achieve this result? What size and shape of structuring element is required?

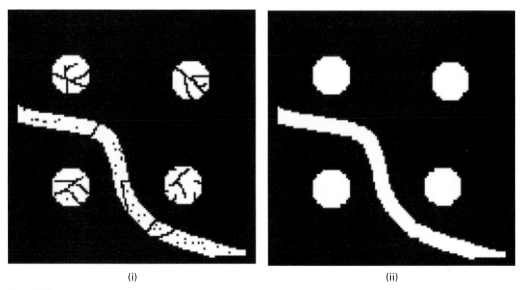

(i)   (ii)

Figure E9.2

9.10 What is (i) the skeleton and (ii) the medial transform of Figure E9.3?

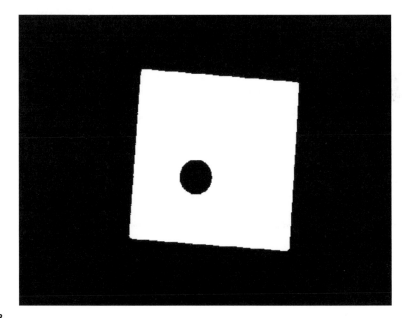

Figure E9.3

9.11 Which distance metric is used to obtain the distance transform in Figure 9.22?

9.12 Grayscale dilation and erosion are generalizations of binary dilation and erosion. Describe how they are implemented.

9.13 What is the top hat transformation and when is it used? Explain how the top hat transformation can help to segment dark characters on a light, but variable, background. Draw a one-dimensional profile through an image to illustrate your explanation.

9.14 Why is finding the approximate convex hull using thickening so slow?

9.15 What would be an effective way to remove "pepper" noise in a grayscale image? Explain.

10 Image segmentation

Overview

Image segmentation is a broad and active field, not only in medical imaging, but also in computer vision and satellite imagery. Its purpose is to divide an image into regions which are meaningful for a particular task. Various methods and approaches are used; the choice of a particular method depends on the characteristics of the problem to be solved and its place in a wider image analysis strategy. Segmentation is an essential step prior to the description, recognition or classification of an image or its constituents. There are two major approaches – region-based methods, in which similarities are detected, and boundary-based methods, in which discontinuities (edges) are detected and linked to form boundaries around regions. In order to develop robust interpretation systems, it is important to use as much relevant a priori information as possible during segmentation.

Learning objectives

After reading this chapter you will be able to:

- identify the main techniques used in region-based and boundary-based image segmentation;
- discuss the advantages and disadvantages of the different techniques;
- choose the most appropriate technique for a particular image;
- explain the basis for optimal segmentation;
- distinguish between bottom-up and top-down approaches;
- describe the algorithms for boundary-based segmentation;
- outline how the motion of an active contour (snake) is determined by an energy function, and distinguish between internal and external energy;
- illustrate the use of the morphological watershed.

10.1   What is segmentation?

Segmentation is the partitioning of an image into meaningful regions, most frequently to distinguish objects or regions of interest ("foreground") from everything else

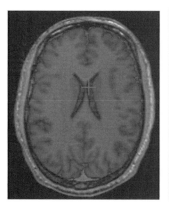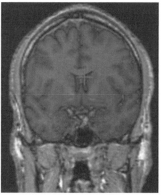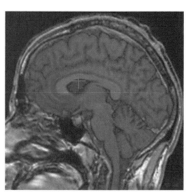

Figure 10.1   A characteristic shading has been added to the brain following segmentation. The three images show (from left to right) axial, coronal and saggital planes. A common point is marked in each image. See also color plate.

("background"). In the simplest cases, there would be only these two classes (foreground and background) and the segmented image would be a binary image. Segmentation is used, for example: for the detection of organs, such as the brain, heart, lungs or liver in CT or MR images; to distinguish pathological tissue, such as a tumor, from normal tissue; and in treatment planning. Psuedocolor can be added to the original image based on the extent of the segmented regions (Fig. 10.1). The most basic attribute used in defining the regions is image gray level or brightness, but other properties such as color or texture (Appendix C) can be used. Segmentation is often the first stage in pattern recognition systems; once the objects of interest are isolated from the rest of the image, certain characterizing measurements could be made (*feature extraction*), and this could be used to *classify* the objects into particular groups or classes.

There are many segmentation approaches, and they can be classified according to both the features and the techniques used. The features include gray values (brightness), texture and gradient magnitudes. Segmentation techniques can be classified as either contextual or non-contextual. *Non-contextual techniques* ignore the relationships that exist between features in an image; pixels are simply grouped together on the basis of some global attribute, such as gray level. Intensity-based thresholding, where each pixel is assigned to a particular region based on its gray value, is a non-contextual technique. *Contextual techniques* additionally exploit the relationships between image features. Thus, a contextual technique might group together pixels that have similar gray levels and are close to one another or have similar gradient values. Contextual techniques include: region-based techniques, such as region growing, where connected regions are found based on some similarity of the pixels within them; boundary-based techniques, where edge-based methods are used to delineate the boundaries between regions; and other methods, such as active contours and watershed segmentation.

10.2   Thresholding

Thresholding according to intensity/brightness is a simple technique for images which contain solid objects on a background of different, but uniform, brightness. Each pixel is compared to the threshold: if its value is higher than the threshold, the pixel is considered to be "foreground" and is set to white, and if it is less than or equal to the threshold it is considered "background" and set to black. The success of thresholding depends critically on the selection of an appropriate threshold (Fig. 10.2).

In the ideal case the gray-level histogram comprises two separate distributions, representing "foreground" objects and "background," with no overlap, and a single global

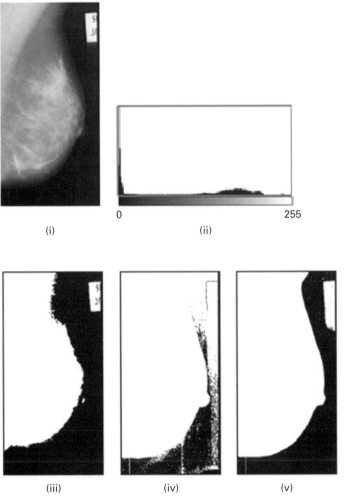

Figure 10.2   (i) An image, (ii) its histogram, and the image thresholded with a threshold that is (iii) too high, (iv) too low and (v) just right.

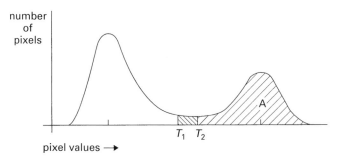

Figure 10.3   A bi-modal histogram showing the minimum sensitivity to threshold placement (between T_1 and T_2) at the valley between the peaks. The pixels in A, above the threshold (either T_1 and T_2) comprise the "foreground."

threshold, T, can be taken anywhere on the valley floor separating them. However, real images generally have a bi-modal gray-level histogram (Fig. 10.3) resulting from the overlapping of the two underlying distributions. Taking a value for the threshold at the bottom of the valley between the peaks or modes (between T_1 and T_2) is the "conventional" threshold, which minimizes the sensitivity to small errors in selecting the threshold.

A number of conditions can conspire to make global thresholding difficult. Poor image contrast can make it difficult to resolve foreground from background, resulting in overlapping peaks. A background of varying intensity can make it difficult or impossible to choose a single threshold that works well for the entire image. Poor spatial resolution, variable illumination and objects with varying levels of brightness can add to the difficulty. The variety of conditions under which segmentation is to be performed requires different approaches, some of which are described below, but often the decision on which approach is best can only be made by experimentation with the specific image.

10.2.1   Optimal thresholding

The bottom of the valley between peaks in the gray-level histogram is not the *optimal* threshold. *Optimal thresholding* considers the histogram of an image to be a weighted sum of two (or more) probability densities. The threshold is then set as the gray level which results in the smallest number of pixels being misclassified, i.e. background pixels being classified as foreground and vice versa. This corresponds to the intersection of the two normal distributions, and is not identical to the bottom of the valley between the two peaks, which is the conventional threshold (Fig. 10.4). (It is identical to the situation in diagnostic testing, when both normal and diseased patients produce a range of normally distributed test scores which overlap to some degree (Appendix B, Fig. B.8).)

Figure 10.5(i) shows a noisy image. The optimal threshold and conventional threshold are marked on its histogram (Fig. 10.5(ii)). Thresholding at the optimal threshold (Fig. 10.5(iii)) produces a better result than thresholding at the conventional threshold (Fig. 10.5(iv)),

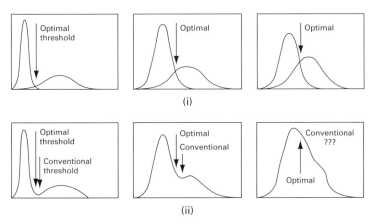

Figure 10.4 (i) Gray-level histograms approximated by two normal distributions, where the intersection represents the optimal threshold. (ii) The resulting optimal and conventional thresholds in the combined histogram. (From SONKA/HLAVAC/BOYLE. *Image Processing, Analysis, and Machine Vision*, 3E. © 2008 Brooks/Cole, a part of Cengage Learning, Inc. Reproduced by permission. www.cengage.com/permissions.)

i.e. one with fewer pixels misclassified, than thresholding at the conventional (bottom of the valley) threshold. Subsequent erosion (Fig. 10.5(v)) and dilation (Fig. 10.5(vi)) can be used to clean up the thresholded image.

Since noise can result in a misclassification of pixels by shifting them to the "wrong" side of a threshold, images are often smoothed using an averaging or median mask prior to thresholding to mitigate this effect. Figure 10.6(i) shows the effect of smoothing the image from Figure 10.5(i) using a median mask. Its resulting histogram (Fig. 10.6(ii)) is much more separable. In this case a threshold can be chosen anywhere on the valley floor to give a segmented image (Fig. 10.6(iii)) with very few misclassified pixels.

There are a number of approaches to implementing optimal thresholding. The general methodology is to consider the pixels, foreground and background, as belonging to two *classes* or *clusters*. The goal is to pick a threshold such that each pixel on each side of the threshold is closer in value to the mean of the pixels on that side of the threshold than the mean of the pixels on the other side of the threshold. The algorithms proceed automatically, without user intervention, and are said to be *unsupervised*.

The Otsu method describes the gray-level histogram of an image as a probability distribution, so that

$$p_i = n_i/N \tag{10.1}$$

where n_i is the number of pixels with gray value i and N is the total number of pixels in the image, so that p_i is the probability of a pixel having gray value i. If we threshold at level k, we can define

$$\omega(k) = \sum_{i=0}^{k} p_i \tag{10.2a}$$

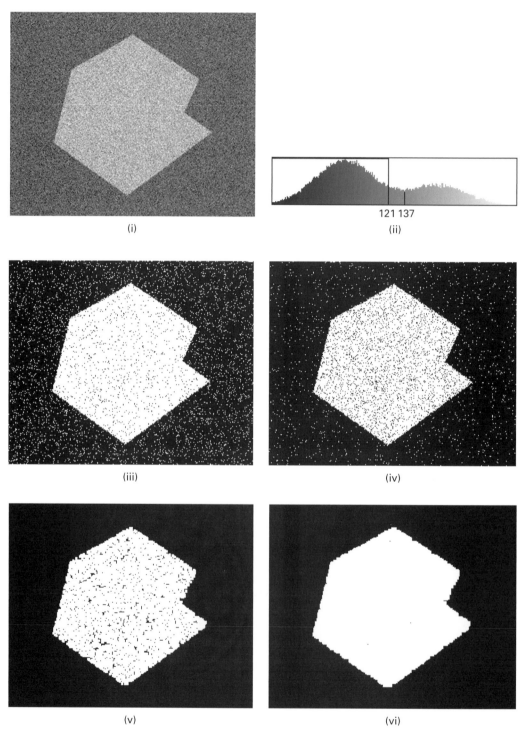

Figure 10.5   (i) An 8-bit image and (ii) its histogram with optimal threshold (121) and conventional threshold (137) marked. (iii) After thresholding using the optimal threshold (121); (iv) after thresholding using the conventional threshold (137); (v) after eroding the image in (iii); (vi) after dilating the image in (v).

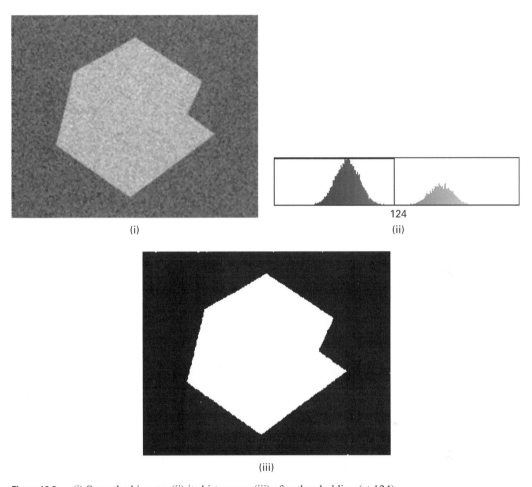

(i)

124

(ii)

(iii)

Figure 10.6   (i) Smoothed image; (ii) its histogram; (iii) after thresholding (at 124).

$$\mu(k) = \sum_{i=k+1}^{L-1} p_i \tag{10.2b}$$

where L is the number of gray levels (e.g. 256, for an 8-bit image). By definition

$$\omega(k) + \mu(k) = \sum_{i=0}^{L-1} p_i = 1 \tag{10.3}$$

We would like to find k to maximize the difference between $\omega(k)$ and $\mu(k)$. This can be done by first defining the image average as

$$\mu_T = \sum_{i=0}^{L-1} i p_i \tag{10.4}$$

and then finding the value of k which maximizes

$$\frac{(\mu_T \omega(k) - \mu(k))^2}{\omega(k)\mu(k)} \tag{10.5}$$

which effectively maximizes the *between-class variance* (or minimizes the *within-class variance*). Thus k is chosen to maximize the separation of two classes ("foreground" and "background"), or alternatively minimize their spread, so that their overlap is minimized. (Appendix B, Section B.4, has further details.) The method is quite general and can be applied to features other than the brightness. The optimal threshold which it finds is stable, based as it is on integration of the gray-level histogram (a global property) rather than its differentiation (a local property such as the valley). The between-class variance is always smooth and unimodal, which makes it easy to find the maximum. When the distributions are constrained to be normal (i.e. Gaussian) the method is equivalent to *mixture modeling*.

Maximum entropy thresholding is very similar to Otsu's method except rather than maximizing the between-class variance, it maximizes the between-class entropy. Entropy is a measure of the uncertainty of an event taking place (Section 5.1.2), and can be derived from the gray-level histogram.

Optimal thresholding can be implemented iteratively by the *isodata* (iterative self-organizing data analysis technique algorithm) method. The steps are as follows:

(i) threshold the image using the mean of the two peaks or the mean pixel value, T_0;
(ii) calculate the mean value of the pixels below this threshold, μ_1, and the mean of the pixels above this threshold, μ_2;
(iii) threshold the image at a new threshold, $T_i = (\mu_1 + \mu_2)/2$;
(iv) repeat steps (ii)–(iii) until $T_i - T_{i-1} \leq \Delta$ (where the change, Δ, can be defined in several different ways, either by measuring the relative change in threshold value or by the percentage of pixels that change sides (foreground to background or vice versa) between iterations).

The isodata algorithm is essentially the *k-means clustering algorithm* used in pattern recognition (Section 11.2.4) applied to two clusters. From a statistical point of view, the cluster means obtained by k-means clustering or by the isodata variant can be interpreted as the Maximum Likelihood Estimates (MLE) if each cluster comes from a normal distribution with different means but identical variance and zero covariance (Section 11.2.2). Indeed the algorithms work well if the spreads of the individual distributions are approximately equal, but they do not perform well where the distributions have differing variances or are far from normal in shape.

Figure 10.7 shows the results of different optimal thresholding algorithms: since the results depend on the individual histograms, the choice of the most appropriate algorithm differs with each particular image. Activity 10.1 illustrates the use of the different thresholding algorithms.

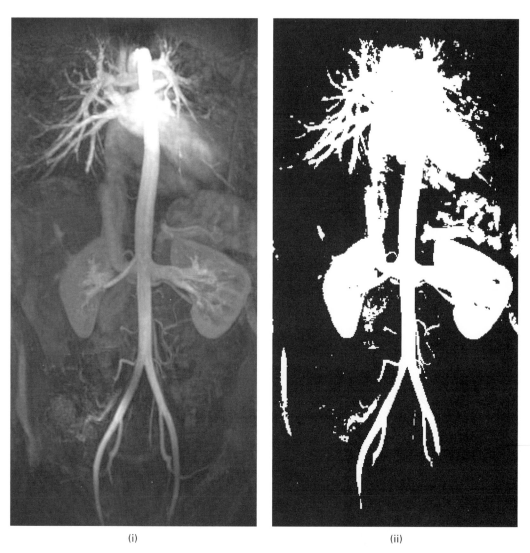

(i) (ii)

Figure 10.7 (i) An MR angiography image showing the aorta and other blood vessels: segmented using (ii) mixture modeling, (iii) Otsu thresholding, (iv) isodata and (v) maximum entropy.

Multi-thresholding or *classification* (Chapter 11) refers to problems where there are more than two classes and several thresholds are required. This is typically used when multiple images of the same scene are available, e.g. T_1-weighted, T_2-weighted and proton-density-weighted MRI images of the same subject. Multiple features (e.g. brightness, texture, gradient) can be measured in each image. Figure 10.8 shows an MRI image of the brain segmented automatically into five different classes, corresponding to known anatomical regions (white matter, gray matter, cerebral spinal fluid, edema (swelling due to excess fluid) and tumor) using multi-channel input. Typically pseudocolor would be added to the multi-thresholded result in order to

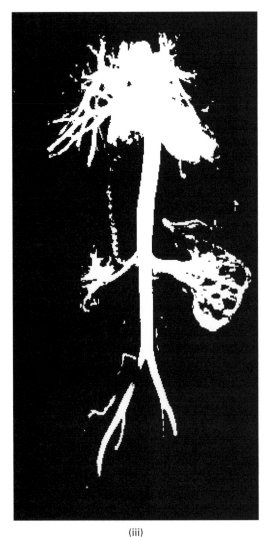
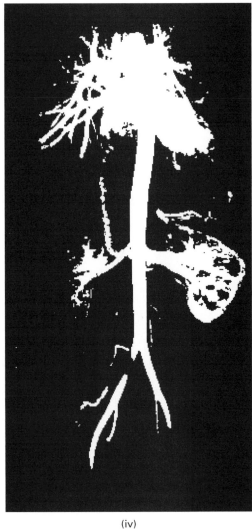

(iii)   (iv)

Figure 10.7   (cont.)

distinguish the regions more readily. The Otsu method can be extended easily to multi-thresholding.

Multi-spectral or *vector images* refers to images in which a number of separate measurements are available for each pixel in the image. Each pixel is thus "vector valued." Examples of vector images are: colored images, for which each pixel has red, green and blue components in an RGB image or hue, saturation and intensity in an HSI image; dual-energy x-ray images, which have two different values for each pixel as a result of different attenuations at the different x-ray energies used; and MRI images, where T_1, T_2 and proton density values at the same pixel can be obtained. Additionally, a CT image and an MRI image which have been registered can be treated as a fused vector

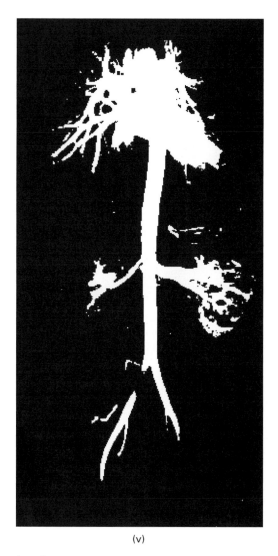

(v)

Figure 10.7 (cont.)

image. Such images are very powerful because multiple features (e.g. brightness, texture, gradient) can be measured in each of the individual channels or *bands*.

10.2.2 Adaptive thresholding

Sometimes it is not possible to segment an image with a single global threshold. This might happen in an image with a varying background, such as the image in Figure 10.9, where the background is darker at the bottom and left-hand side of the image. A profile along the dark central line in Figure 10.9(i) shows that the background varies considerably (Fig. 10.9(ii)). No single threshold (e.g. T_1 or T_2) can successfully separate the

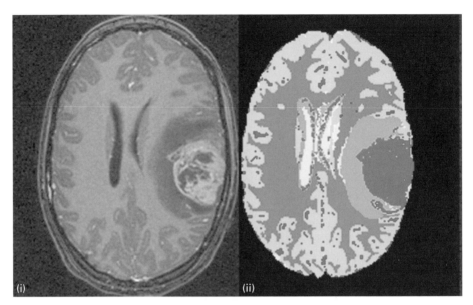

Figure 10.8   (i) Axial slice of MRI brain image and (ii) automatic segmentation into five classes, including a tumor. The segmentation was done in three dimensions. (Courtesy: Professor Guido Gerig, Department of Computer Science, University of North Carolina at Chapel Hill.) See also color plate.

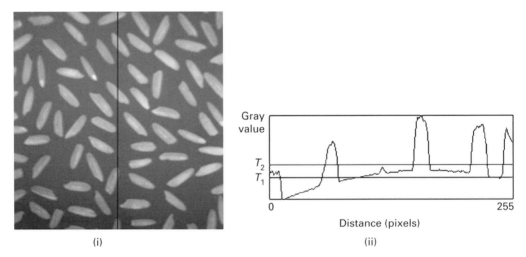

Figure 10.9   (i) An image and (ii) a profile taken along the dark vertical line drawn on the image; global thresholds such as T_1 or T_2 are not able to separate objects (foreground) from background.

objects from the varying background. One way around this problem would be to subtract (or divide) the image by an image of the background alone, either obtained independently or obtained from the image itself by blurring it (Section 6.1.2). Alternatively *adaptive thresholding* could be used.

Instead of applying a single global threshold to all pixels in the image, adaptive thresholding changes the threshold dynamically over the image. In *local adaptive thresholding*, each pixel is considered to have an $n \times n$ neighborhood around it from which a threshold value is calculated (from the mean or median of these values) and the pixel set to black or white, according to whether it is below or above this local threshold, T_L. The size of the neighborhood, n, has to be large enough to cover sufficient foreground and background pixels so that the effect of noise is minimal, but not too large that uneven illumination becomes noticeable within the neighborhood. Often the technique is even more successful when the local threshold, T_L, is chosen as

$$T_L = \{\text{mean or median}\} - C \qquad (10.6)$$

where C is a constant. The method is not unsupervised since values for the parameters n and C must be chosen. Figure 10.10 compares the performance of local adaptive thresholding and Otsu thresholding on an image with a variable background.

Adaptive thresholding is an alternative to subtracting out the background (Activity 6.1) or using morphological thresholding (Activity 9.10). You can practice the method in Activity 10.2.

10.3   Region-based methods

Region-based methods find connected regions based on some similarity of the pixels within them. The objective is to produce connected regions that are as large as possible

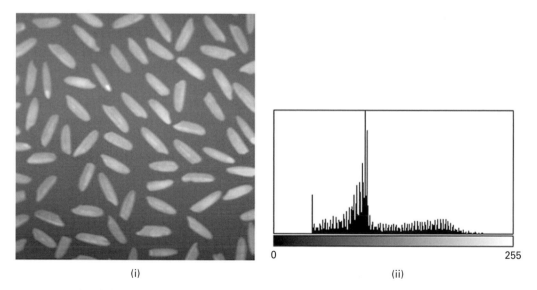

(i)   (ii)

Figure 10.10   (i) Original (256×256) image and (ii) its histogram; (iii) segmented image of (i) using local adaptive thresholding (with $n = 45$, $C = 3$); (iv) segmented image of (i) using Otsu thresholding.

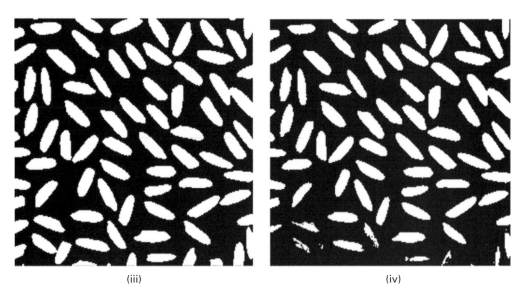

(iii)   (iv)

Figure 10.10   (cont.)

(i.e. produce as few regions as possible), allowing for some flexibility within each region. However, if we require that the pixels in a region be too similar, we may over-segment the image, and if we allow too much flexibility we may merge what should be separate objects. The goal is to find regions that correspond to objects as a person sees them, which is not an easy goal.

Region growing is a *bottom-up* procedure that starts with "seed" pixels, and then grows regions by adding neighboring pixels that have similar properties (e.g. brightness, color, texture, gradient, geometric properties) to the seed. Connectivity (4- or 8-) is used to define which are neighboring pixels. We can specify a variance for the property; region growing stops when a pixel is encountered that is not within this variance. The seeds can be chosen interactively (Activity 10.3), although automatic segmentation is preferable. Figure 10.11 shows a region growing from a single seed point.

Starting with a particular seed pixel and letting this region grow completely before trying other seeds biases the segmentation in favor of the regions which are segmented first. This can have several undesirable effects: the current region dominates the growth process and ambiguities around the edges of adjacent regions may not be resolved correctly, different choices of seeds may give different segmentation results and problems can occur if the (arbitrarily chosen) seed point lies on an edge. One way to counter these problems is to scatter seed points randomly around the image and grow from several seed points simultaneously. It is usually necessary to follow up with a merge process to merge regions with different seed points but similar properties, otherwise the segmentation result is highly dependent on the random location of the seed points.

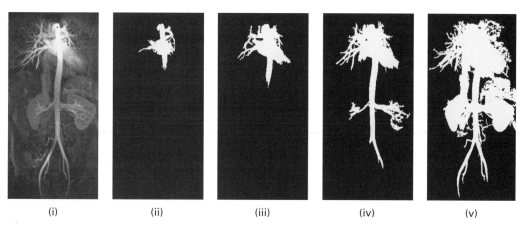

| (i) | (ii) | (iii) | (iv) | (v) |

Figure 10.11   (i) Image with seed point marked within aortic arch at top center of image; (ii)–(v) region growing from seed (to connected pixels with values different by 50, 100, 150 and 200).

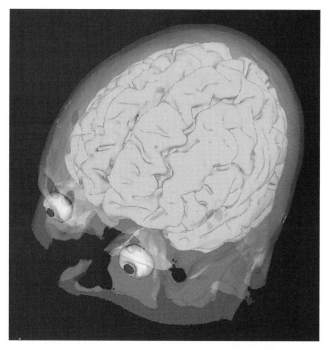

Figure 10.12   Segmentation of a three-dimensional MRI image by region growing. The white and gray matter regions were combined before three-dimensional rendering (Chapter 12). See also color plate.

Figure 10.12 shows the segmentation of a three-dimensional MRI image. The image was segmented using seven seed points placed in different anatomical regions (white matter, gray matter, skull, left eye, left lens, right eye and right lens).

Region growing techniques are generally better in noisy images where edges are extremely difficult to detect. They are particularly useful with images which have *multi-modal* histograms.

10.4   Boundary-based methods

Boundary-based methods are based on finding pixel differences rather than pixel similarities. The goal is to determine a closed boundary such that an inside (the object or foreground) and an outside (the background) can be defined.

10.4.1   Edge detection and linking

Edges in an image are detected by using a gradient operator such as the Sobel operator (Section 6.4.2), and then thresholding the magnitude of the gradient image. The strongest edges are distinct, but some weaker edges appear broken (Fig. 10.13); noisy images compound the problem, resulting in spurious edges (Fig. 10.14). Smoothing the noisy image reduces the spurious edges, but also widens the edges and removes some weak edges completely (Fig. 10.15).

Some *linking* of the edges to form a connected boundary is needed. Adjacent edge pixels could be linked if they have similar properties, e.g. a similar gradient magnitude and orientation based on the Sobel results:

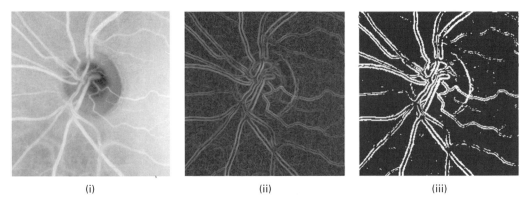

(i)   (ii)   (iii)

Figure 10.13   (i) Original image of retinal vessels; (ii) result of Sobel operator; (iii) after thresholding.

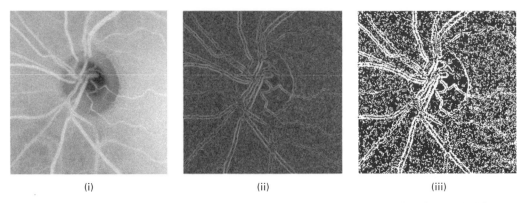

(i)   (ii)   (iii)

Figure 10.14   (i) Original noisy image of retinal vessels; (ii) result of Sobel operator; (iii) after thresholding.

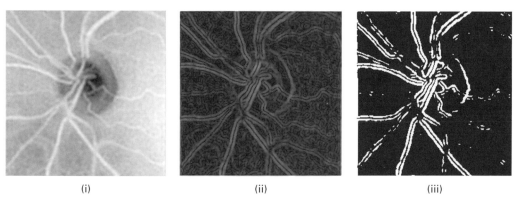

(i)	(ii)	(iii)

Figure 10.15 (i) Noisy image of retinal vessels smoothed with a Butterworth filter; (ii) result of Sobel operator; (iii) after thresholding.

$$| \, \|\nabla f(x,y)\| - \|\nabla(x',y')\| \, | \leq T \qquad \text{for some magnitude threshold } T \qquad (10.7)$$

$$| \, \phi(\nabla f(x,y)) - \phi(\nabla f(x',y')) \, | \, \leq \, A \qquad \text{for some angular threshold } A \qquad (10.8)$$

Once the links are established, the linked edges become the borders. The linked pixels need to be constrained by, for example, scanning along rows or columns, otherwise clusters of linked pixels are formed rather than long single-pixel thick chains. Edge linking is usually followed by post-processing to find sets of linked pixels separated by small gaps, which can then be filled in.

10.4.2 Boundary tracking

Boundary tracking may be applied to a gradient image or any other image containing only boundary information. Once a single point on the boundary has been identified, simply by locating a gray-level maximum, the analysis proceeds by following or tracking the boundary, assuming it to be a closed shape, with the aim of finding all other pixels on that specific boundary, and ultimately returning to the starting point before investigating other possible boundaries. In one implementation, the search for the highest gray-level pixels continues in broadly the same direction as in the previous step, with deviations of one pixel to either side permitted, to accommodate curvature of the boundary (Fig. 10.16).

This simple method is liable to fail under conditions of high noise, when the boundary makes seemingly random and abrupt changes of direction which cannot successfully be tracked in this way. Substantial low-pass filtering is needed beforehand to reduce noise, unless the algorithm used is refined or assisted manually.

Simultaneously tracking both sides of a long, thin object, such as a blood vessel, requires each tracking to continuously check the other border and becomes difficult when the object branches or crosses other objects (Sonka *et al.*, 1999). The extension of boundary tracking to surfaces is complicated.

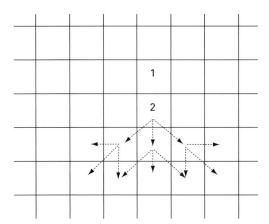

Figure 10.16   Boundary tracking: find boundary pixel (1); search eight neighbors to find next pixel (2); search in same direction allowing deviation of one pixel either side; repeat final step until end of boundary.

10.5   Other methods

10.5.1   Active contours

Segmentation of medical images is a difficult task complicated by noise and sampling artifacts. Often we are looking for an object in an image which is smooth and has a closed boundary. An *active contour* or *snake* is a controlled continuity contour which elastically snaps around and encloses a target object by locking on to its edges. It is possible to control the snake through a function called the *energy* by analogy with physical systems. The snake is *active* because it is continuously evolving so as to reduce its energy. By specifying an appropriate energy function we can make a snake that evolves to have particular properties such as smoothness. The method can easily be extended to dynamic image data and three-dimensional image data.

The energy function for a snake is in two parts, the *internal* and *external* energies. Thus

$$E_{\text{snake}} = E_{\text{internal}} + E_{\text{external}} \tag{10.9}$$

The internal energy depends on the intrinsic properties of the snake, such as its length or curvature. The external energy depends on factors such as image structure and particular constraints the user has imposed.

The physical analogy can be extended, and the motion of the snake can be regarded as being due to simulated forces acting on it to make it reduce its total energy. To design a snake with specified properties it is normal to work out a suitable energy function and then calculate the forces needed to reduce it.

If we want the snake to shrink like an elastic band, we need to define an internal energy that increases with its length. User-defined control points, approximately equally spaced, specify the starting position of the snake, which should be a reasonable approximation to its desired position; the internal energy function can be taken as the sum of the squares of the distances between adjacent control points, to simulate springs which obey

Hooke's Law connecting the control points. The sum is multiplied by an adjustable constant, K, corresponding to the strength of the springs. Thus

$$E_{\text{internal}} = E_{\text{elastic}} = K \sum_{i=1}^{N} (d_{i,i-1})^2 \qquad (10.10)$$

where i is the *index* of the control point with coordinates (x_i, y_i). Because the snake is a loop, control point 0 is the same as control point N. The corresponding forces on the ith control point, obtained by differentiating the energy function, are given by

$$F_i(x) = 2K((x_{i+1} - x_i) - (x_i - x_{i-1})) \qquad (10.11a)$$

$$F_i(y) = 2K((y_{i+1} - y_i) - (y_i - y_{i-1})) \qquad (10.11b)$$

Such forces pull a control point towards its two nearest neighbors. Geometrically, the force is towards the average position of the neighbors. Such forces applied to every control point will pull the snake inwards and will pull the control points into line with one another, smoothing the snake.

Now we know what forces act on each control point, we have to use them to adjust the position of the snake. We can implement the *dynamics* of the snake by moving each control point by an amount proportional to the force acting on it at each time step. Thus, the updating equations are given by

$$x_i + CF_i(x) \rightarrow x_i \qquad (10.12a)$$

$$y_i + CF_i(y) \rightarrow y_i \qquad (10.12b)$$

where C is another user-defined constant, which determines how far the point moves for a given force. In practice, we calculate the new coordinates for all the points before updating any of them, i.e. we use the old value of x_i, not the new one, to find the shift in x_{i+1}. Figure 10.17 shows a snake obeying this equation. The elastic force rapidly pulls the snake into a smooth oval, which keeps contracting. The most outlying points get pulled in fastest. One or two points start moving outwards because they are pulled into line with their neighbors before the overall contraction gets to them. After a few iterations you can also see the trajectories of the control points, which move to be equidistant from

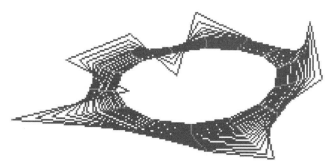

Figure 10.17 Twenty iterations of a snake (red), starting from an outer contour, moving under an internal elastic function. The trajectories of the control points are shown in green. See also color plate.

each other. We have *simulated* a physical system in order to give a computational structure a desired property.

Other terms could be added, for example to favor a particular shape. Alternatively, if we wanted the snake to behave like a thin metal strip rather than like an elastic band, i.e. it should try to be a smooth curve or straight line but should not contract, the energy function should be defined as the sum of the squared *curvatures* of the snake measured at the control points.

Now consider the external energy of the snake, which determines its relationship to the image. Suppose we want a snake to latch on to bright structures in the image. Then the external energy function is minus the sum of the gray levels of the pixels covered by the snake. Reducing this energy function (i.e. making it more negative) will move the snake towards brighter parts of the image. Thus

$$E_{\text{external}} = E_{\text{image}} = -k \sum_{i=1}^{N} P_i \qquad (10.13)$$

where P_i is the pixel value of the ith pixel and the constant k is user-selected. In this implementation, the energy is actually only calculated for the pixels which lie under control points, not under the lines between them. The force that this produces has a rather simple approximation:

$$F_i(x) = \frac{k}{2}(P_{x_{i+1},y_i} + P_{x_{i-1},y_i}) \qquad (10.14a)$$

$$F_i(y) = \frac{k}{2}(P_{x,y_{i+1}} + P_{x,y_{i-1}}) \qquad (10.14b)$$

That is, if the pixel in the direction of increasing x is brighter than the pixel in the direction of decreasing x, then the control point is pulled in the positive x direction, and likewise for y. In short, the force on the control point is in the direction of the gray-level gradient. We can demonstrate the effect of this by placing an initial snake in a ramp image (Fig. 10.18). The snake stays the same shape but wanders in the direction of the brighter part of the image. To avoid the effects of very local structure, more useful snakes use a more sophisticated estimate of the gray-level gradient, which averages over more pixels.

The external energy can have contributions other than the image energy. A *constraint energy*, $E_{\text{constraint}}$, is often included which is determined by constraints applied by the user. For instance the snake might be attracted to lines or edges or pulled to particular points as if by springs, or might be repelled by a particular point.

A snake used for image analysis attempts to minimize its total energy, which is the sum of the internal and external energies. When energies are added their associated forces add too. Snakes start with a closed curve and minimize the total energy function to deform until they reach their optimal state (Activity 10.4). In general, the initial contour should be fairly close to the final contour but does not have to follow its shape in detail: the active contour/snake method is semi-automatic since it requires the user to mark an initial contour. The initial contour in Figure 10.19 was well chosen, so the final contour converged quickly (in about 25 iterations).

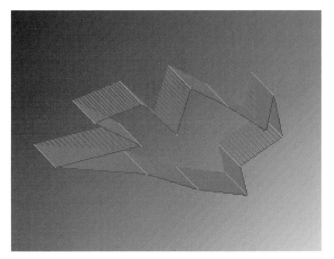

Figure 10.18 Twenty iterations of a snake (red), starting from an outer contour, moving under an external energy function given by Equation (10.13). The trajectories of the control points are shown in green. See also color plate.

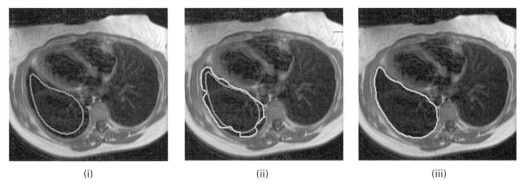

| (i) | (ii) | (iii) |

Figure 10.19 (i) Initial contour; (ii) intermediate contour in yellow (initial contour in green); (iii) final contour. See also color plate.

The main advantage of the active contour method is that it results in closed coherent areas with smooth boundaries, whereas in other methods the edge is not guaranteed to be continuous or closed. However, conventional snake model algorithms suffer from the inability to mold a contour to severe concavities in an object and they often generate unwanted contour loops; more recent loop-free snake algorithms have been developed to prevent these problems.

Level sets can be used to track changes in a contour as we iterate towards a final contour, and lets us track contours within a series of images. It describes a contour, $C(s)$, as an implicit three-dimensional level-set function $\varphi(x, y, t)$, where the third dimension is the "level" of φ. The connection between f and $C(s)$ is defined by the additional requirement that f happens to be identical to $C(s)$ on the 0 level:

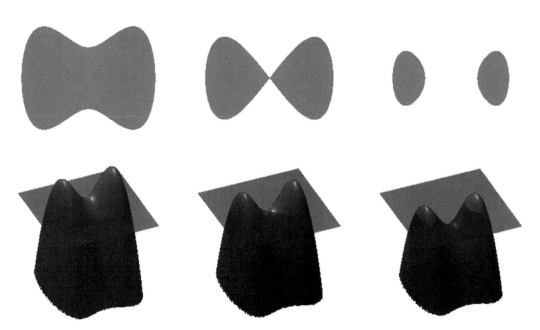

Figure 10.20   Contours (top row) and their relationship to the level set function, φ. See also color plate.

$$\varphi(x, y, 0) = C(s) \qquad (10.15)$$

Figure 10.20 (top left) shows the shape of a well-behaved boundary contour. Below it, the red surface is the graph of a level set function φ determining this shape, and the flat blue region represents the x–y plane. The boundary of the shape is then the zero level set of φ, while the shape itself is the set of points in the plane for which φ is positive or zero.

In the top row of Figure 10.20 we see a shape changing topology by splitting in two. It would be difficult to describe this transformation numerically by parameterizing the contour and following its evolution. On the other hand, if we look at the bottom row, we see that the level set function merely translates downward. If the zero level set moves in the normal direction to itself with a speed v, this movement, φ_t, can be represented by means of a so-called Hamilton–Jacobi equation for the level set function:

$$\varphi_t = v|\nabla \phi| \qquad (10.16)$$

This is a partial differential equation which can be solved numerically. Fast Marching algorithms are used to compute the evolving curve most efficiently.

The level sets model frees us from the need to handle each and every special case of joining and separating contour lines as we iterate through different contours towards the final one. It overcomes all the topological hazards because now all contours are always connected in the third dimension and thus they are continuous functions. Furthermore, using the level set model we can easily take care of breaking and merging of contours within a series of images, such as seen in a time sequence of CT or MRI images (Fig. 10.21).

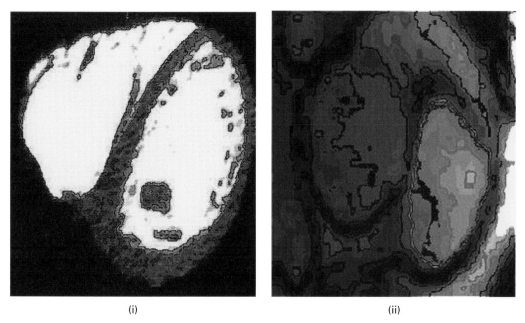

(i)   (ii)

Figure 10.21 Segmentation of (i) CT and (ii) MRI images of the heart using level sets. Each of these images is part of a time series. The snake is shown in red in (i) and in green in (ii). (Courtesy: Dr. Rene Vidal, Biomedical Engineering, Johns Hopkins University.) See also color plate.

10.5.2 Watershed segmentation

Watershed segmentation is a way of automatically separating or cutting apart particles that touch in a segmented (binary) image when, for example, they need to be counted.

The *distance map* (Section 9.2.5) of the initial segmented image containing overlapping objects (Fig. 10.22(i)) is obtained. It is a grayscale image (Fig. 10.22(ii)), which is then thresholded at a value high enough to produce objects which are not touching (Fig. 10.22(iii)) in the final binary output image. The distance transform can be considered as a three-dimensional image with the gray level representing height. Thresholding can be then be thought of as a flooding of the topographic surface to a level that separates the original objects which had become hills in the distance transform. Watershed segmentation works best for smooth convex objects which do not overlap too much (Activity 10.5).

A gray-level image can be considered as a topographic surface by considering the pixel values as heights, and watershed segmentation can be applied directly to it helping to separate objects that are close together. The tomographic surface is often complemented initially so that peaks become valleys. We imagine that this surface is then pierced at the regional minima, and that we immerse the surface slowly in water (Fig. 10.23). Water starts filling the distinct catchment basins, and dams are built to prevent the merging of water from adjacent catchment basins. Once the surface is totally immersed in water, the dams form the *watershed lines*, which mark the boundaries of the catchment basins and segment the image into the desired regions.

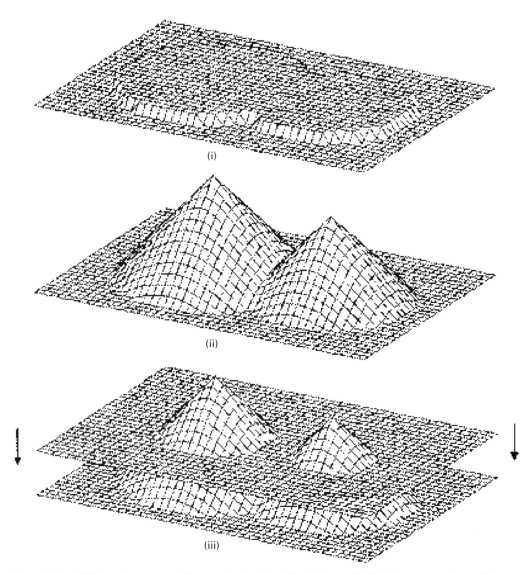

Figure 10.22   (i) Binary image containing overlapping (touching) objects. (ii) The distance transform. (iii) Choosing a threshold to produce objects above the threshold which are not touching. (After Castleman (1996).)

Figure 10.24 demonstrates the process. An image (Fig. 10.24(i)) is segmented by Otsu thresholding to produce an image (Fig. 10.24(ii)) in which several overlapping features appear as single features. This image is then inverted (Fig. 10.24(iii)), and its distance transform taken (Fig. 10.24(iv)). The resulting image, considered as a three-dimensional topology, is then "flooded" to give the watershed lines which are overlaid on the previously segmented image (Fig. 10.24(v)) to separate the overlapped features.

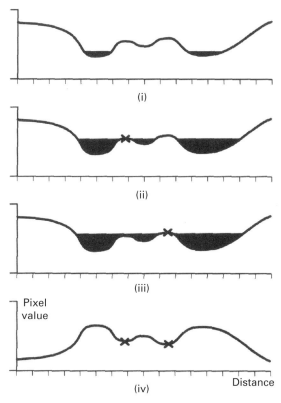

Figure 10.23   (i) Water begins to fill the complemented image profile. (ii) When two catchment basins meet a dam is built to separate them. (iii) As the water level rises further dams are built between catchment basins. (iv) These dams form the watershed lines separating objects from their neighbors. (After Baxes, 1994.)

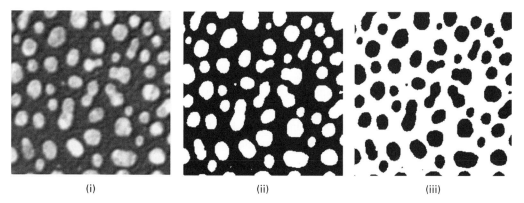

Figure 10.24   (i) Original image; (ii) after Otsu thresholding; (iii) after inversion; (iv) after distance transform; (v) watershed lines overlaid on image (ii).

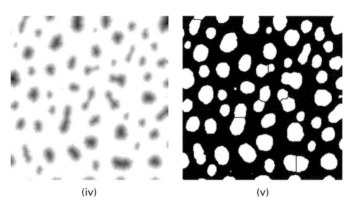

(iv)   (v)

Figure 10.24   (cont.)

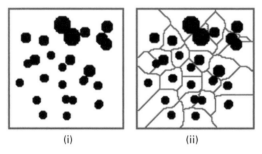

(i)   (ii)

Figure 10.25   (i) Binary image with overlapping features and (ii) watershed lines (in red) overlaid on the original image. See also color plate.

Figure 10.25 shows the result of using the watershed transform on a binary image, which contains some overlapping features. Note that the watershed lines for a binary image correspond to the "skiz" (skeleton of influence zone) (Section 9.2.5).

Often it is preferable to segment the morphological gradient of an image (Section 9.3.1) rather than the image itself. Each object is now a low-level depression bounded by peaks that were the original edges (Fig. 9.39). As water fills the surface, it meets at these peaks, which are then marked as the watershed lines (Fig. 10.26).

In practice, watershed segmentation often produces over-segmentation due to noise or local irregularities in the input image (Fig. 10.27). To reduce this it is common to apply some form of smoothing operation to the input image to reduce the number of local minima. Even so, objects are often segmented into many pieces, which must be merged in a post-processing step based on similarity (e.g. variance of the pixels of both segments together).

A major enhancement of the process consists in flooding the topographic surface from a previously defined set of markers. This prevents over-segmentation (Fig. 10.28).

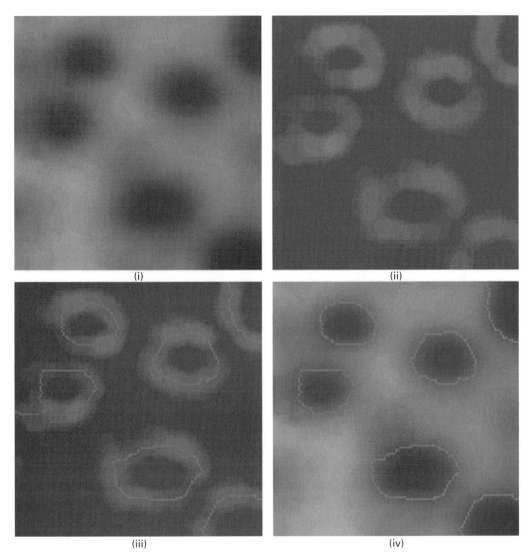

(i)   (ii)

(iii)   (iv)

Figure 10.26   (i) Original image and (ii) gradient image. (iii) Watershed lines overlaid on the gradient image. (iv) Watershed lines overlaid on the original image. See also color plate.

Computer-based activities

Activity 10.1 Thresholding – comparison of optimal methods
Open **angiogram** in ImageJ, and make four duplicate images (**Image/Duplicate...**). Threshold each in turn into two classes using the four different optimal algorithms (**Plugins/Ch.10 Plugins/Multithresholder**). Note the position of the (automatically derived) threshold in each case.

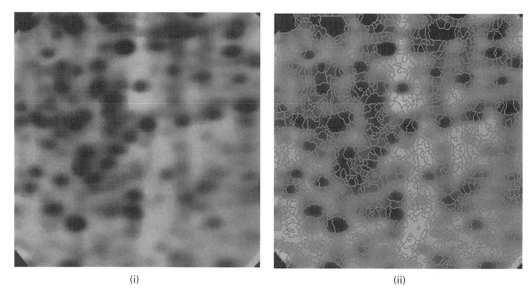

Figure 10.27   (i) Image of electrophoresis gel. (ii) Watershed transform of the gradient image. See also color plate.

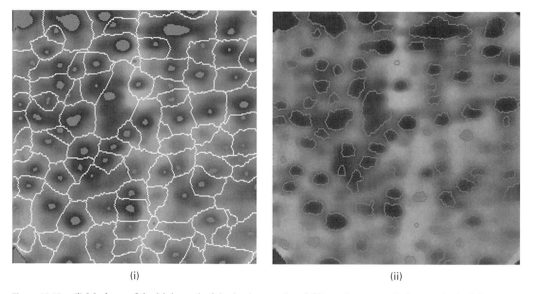

Figure 10.28   (i) Markers of the blobs and of the background and (ii) marker-controlled watershed of the gradient image. See also color plate.

Activity 10.2 Local adaptive thresholding

Open the **rice** image in ImageJ and observe its gray-level histogram (using **Plugins/Ch.10 Plugins/Live Histogram**). The image contains an uneven background. Use adaptive thresholding (**Plugins/Ch.10 Plugins/Adaptive threshold** and choose to display the mean image), trying different values of the neighborhood size, n, and the constant, C, to obtain an image which separates the rice grains from the uneven background. (Note: n needs to be at least the size of a rice grain. Start with $n = 45$ and $C = 3$.) Note the separability of the histogram of the new image, which can be easily segmented with a single global threshold (**Image/ Adjust/ Threshold ...**).

Repeat with the images `uneven` and `sonnet`.

Activity 10.3 Region growing

Open `mra` (which is identical to Fig. 10.5(i)) in ImageJ and invert it (**Edit/Invert**). Move the cursor around inside the aortic arch, the curved portion of the large blood vessel at the top center of the image, and find the (x, y) coordinates of a black pixel (pixel value $= 0$) within it to use as a seed, e.g. $x = 140$, $y = 60$. Open the region growing plugin (**Plugins/3D Toolkit/Connected Threshold Grower ...**), enter the (x, y) coordinates of the chosen seed point, and set the threshold limits as 0 and 50. This allows the region to grow out to connected points having pixel values up to 50. Press "OK" to see the region grown from the seed point under these conditions. Repeat on the original image using an upper threshold of 100, then 150, and then 200. Note the growth of the region.

Activity 10.4 Snakes

Open `mri` in ImageJ, and using the freehand tool draw a closed contour around the brain. Start the snake plugin (**Plugins/Ch.10 Plugins/SnakeD**); accept the default values and click "OK" to start. Watch the red snake adjust during each iteration to close in on the brain, and observe the resulting segmented image. Repeat, adjusting the parameters, to see whether you can achieve a more accurate result. Note that the final segmentation depends to some extent on your initial contour.

Repeat the exercise, drawing your initial contour inside the brain, and watch the snake iterate outwards. Which produces the better segmentation of this image, the outside or inside starting contour?

Activity 10.5 Distance transform and morphological watershed

Open `circular objects` in ImageJ, and threshold it using the Otsu method (**Plugins/Ch.10 Plugins/Multithresholder**, choosing "Otsu"). Note that many of the objects in the image touch each other, which would confound counting them. Make a duplicate of this image.

Find the distance transform (**Process/Binary/Distance Map**) of the thresholded image, and adjust its contrast (**Process/Enhance Contrast**, and check "Normalize"). Show the surface plot (**Analyze/Surface Plot**, check "Shade") to see the surface that fills with water: imagine how the dams are constructed between catchment basins.

Enable debugging in **Edit/Options/Misc ...** Apply watershed segmentation (**Process/Binary/Watershed**) to the thresholded image. The watershed command creates an animation that shows how the watershed algorithm works. Move through the frames of the animation and note how the watershed lines have separated the objects.

Open `cermet`, and threshold it using the Otsu method (**Plugins/Multithresholder**, choosing "Otsu"). Note how several of the objects are elongated as a result of pairs of nearly circular objects overlapping. Apply watershed segmentation (**Process/Binary/Watershed**) to the thresholded image, and note that most of these coalesced objects have been separated.

Exercises

10.1 What is image segmentation and why might one want to segment an image? Describe an image segmentation algorithm and explain its advantages and disadvantages.

10.2 Explain the basis for optimal segmentation using the Otsu method.

10.3 Explain the difference between contextual and non-contextual segmentation methods.

10.4 What segmentation method is particularly useful for segmenting images that contain a variable background? Explain the basis of the method and why it works.

10.5 Distinguish between automatic and semi-automatic methods of segmentation, giving examples of each.

10.6 Design an energy term for a snake to track lines of constant gray value.

10.7 Illustrate the use of the distance transform and morphological watershed for separating objects that touch each other.

10.8 Explain why the watershed lines of a binary image correspond to the "skiz" lines.

11 Feature recognition and classification

Overview

Classification involves sorting objects in an image into separate classes, and is often the final step in a general image analysis process. Automated classification is fundamental to computer-assisted diagnosis in medical imaging and many other applications, such as robotic vision and speech recognition. Often the information available to make a decision is imprecise and frequently the decision procedures are statistical in nature. In such cases statistical approaches are used and the diagnostic accuracy of classification can be measured by receiver-operating characteristic (ROC) curves. However, if the fundamental information is provided by the object structure then structural or syntactic methods are more appropriate. Recent methods, such as neural networks and genetic algorithms, borrow from both approaches.

Learning objectives

After reading this chapter you will be able to:

- distinguish between feature recognition and classification;
- identify the sequence of operations in a general classification system;
- recognize features which are robust, discriminating, reliable and independent;
- discuss the function of a training set of images and the difference between supervised and unsupervised learning;
- outline how the performance of a classifier can be measured;
- explain the concepts of Bayesian classification and the use of discriminant functions;
- describe non-parametric methods in statistical classification;
- illustrate how Principal Components Analysis (PCA) can be used to provide a more informative set of features;
- discuss how maximal separability of classes can be obtained using the Fisher criterion;
- explain how a dendrogram and scree plot are used in hierarchical clustering;
- outline the use of a decision tree in structural classification;
- discuss the applications of classification schemes to diagnostic imaging.

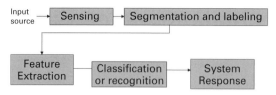

Figure 11.1   A general diagnostic system.

11.1   Object recognition and classification

Classification is often the final step in a general diagnostic process (Fig. 11.1). It involves sorting objects in an image (or images) into separate classes. Typically the image is segmented to isolate different objects from each other and from the background, and the different objects are *labeled*. A *feature extraction* step reduces the data by measuring certain properties or *features* of the labeled objects. These features (or, more precisely, the values of these features) are then passed to a *classifier* that evaluates the evidence presented and makes a decision as to the class each object should be assigned.

The quality of the acquired image depends on the resolution, sensitivity, bandwidth and signal-to-noise ratio of the imaging system. Pre-processing such as low-pass filtering may be required prior to segmentation, which is often a challenging process. The measured features can be transformed or mapped into an alternative feature space, to produce better features, before being sent to the classifier.

Humans are adept at recognizing objects, using size, shape, color and other visual clues. The goal of *recognition* is to recognize or detect an object and make a (yes/no) decision, e.g. does this mammogram show a lesion or not? *Classification* goes a step further by sorting objects into one of several groups or classes, e.g. is this lesion benign or malignant?

Classification techniques can be divided into two broad areas: *statistical* or *structural* (or *syntactic*) techniques, with a third area that borrows from both, sometimes called *cognitive methods*, which include *neural networks* and *genetic algorithms*. The first area deals with objects or patterns that have an underlying and quantifiable statistical basis for their generation and are described by quantitative features such as length, area and texture. The second area deals with objects best described by qualitative features describing structural or syntactic relationships inherent in the object. Statistical classification methods are more popular than structural methods; hybrid, cognitive methods have gained popularity over the last decade or so, but are beyond the scope of this book.

11.2   Connected components labeling

Segmentation provides a simplified, binary image that separates objects of interest (foreground) from the background, while retaining their shape and size for later measurement. The foreground pixels are set to "1," and the background pixels set to "0." Connected components labeling scans the segmented, binary image and groups its pixels into components based on pixel connectivity, i.e. all pixels in a connected component share similar pixel values and are in some way connected with each other. Once all groups have been determined, each pixel is labeled with a number (1, 2, 3, ...), according to the component to which it was assigned, and these numbers can be looked up as gray levels or colors for display (Fig 11.2). The labeling of connected components in an image is central to many automated image analysis applications.

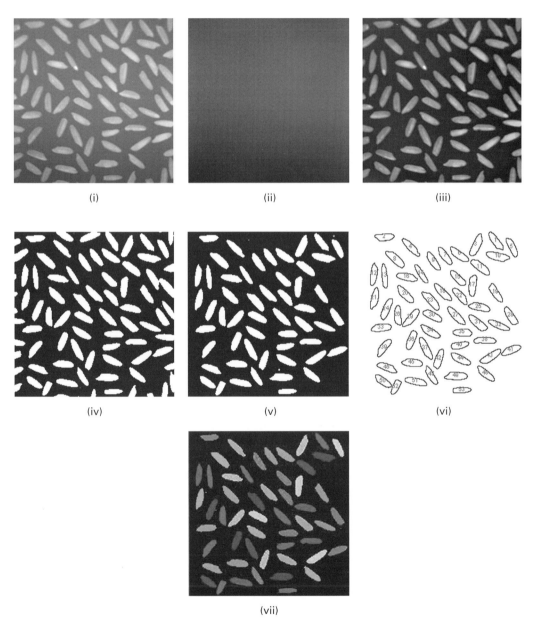

Figure 11.2   (i) Original image; (ii) background (from blurring (i)); (iii) improved image (= (i) − (ii)); (iv) segmented image (Otsu threshold of (iii)); (v) partial objects removed from (iv); (vi) labeled components image; (vii) color-coded labeled components image. See also color plate.

We have noted previously that segmentation is often preceded by pre-processing such as smoothing/blurring of the image to reduce noise, but that was not necessary for the image in Figure 11.2. Post-processing of the segmented image can be used to

- remove partial objects by using a criterion that tests connectivity to the extremities of an image (Fig. 11.2(v)),
- remove objects smaller or larger than certain limits, and
- fill in holes in objects or background by opening or closing.

When a labeled component image comprising a number of components is color-coded, it is often advisable to re-use a palette of colors that are easily distinguishable (Fig. 11.2(vii)) rather than use different colors that are barely distinguishable.

The two-pass algorithm for labeling connected components comprises three distinct phases. The first phase involves scanning the image in a raster pattern. It moves along a row until it comes to a pixel p whose pixel value is "1." It then examines the neighbors of p that have already been encountered in the scan (i.e. generally the neighbors (i) to the left of p, (ii) above it, and (iii) and (iv) the two upper diagonal terms). Based on this information, provisional labeling of p occurs as follows:

- if all four neighbors have pixel values of "0," assign a new provisional label to p, else
- if only one neighbor has a pixel value of "1," assign its provisional label to p, else
- if more than one of the neighbors have pixel values of "1," assign one of the provisional labels to p and make a note of the equivalences.

After completing the scan, the equivalent label pairs are sorted into equivalence classes and a unique label is assigned to each class. In the final phase, a second scan is made through the image, during which each label is replaced by the label assigned to its equivalence classes.

One obvious result of connected components labeling is that the objects in an image can be readily counted. More generally, the labeled binary objects can be used to *mask* the original image to isolate each (grayscale) object but retain its original pixel values so that its properties or features can be measured separately. Masking can be performed in several different ways. The binary mask can be used in an overlay, or alpha channel, in the display hardware to prevent pixels from being displayed. It is also possible to use the mask to modify the stored image. This can be achieved either by multiplying the grayscale image by the binary mask or by bit-wise ANDing the original image with the binary mask. (A binary mask image can be used to combine portions of two (or more) grayscale (or color) images; this is the compositing process used in graphic arts and in the movie industry, where the mask image is known as a digital matte.) Isolating features which can then be measured independently is the basis of *region-of-interest* (RoI) *processing*.

11.3   Features

It is necessary to reduce the dimensionality (an 8-bit deep image of size 256×256 pixels has $256^{65\,536} \approx 10^{157\,826}$ possible realizations!) of the classification task by measuring essential properties or features of the objects. The features are higher-level representations of structure and shape, and should be chosen to preserve the information that is important to the particular task at hand. Examples of features include those describing the contents of the objects and those describing their shape. The first category includes features such as

- features obtainable from the histogram of an object using region-of-interest processing, such as the mean pixel value (grayness or color) and its standard deviation, the contrast, and the entropy; and
- the texture of an object, using statistical moments of the gray-level histogram of the object or its fractal dimension (Appendix C.3).

The second category includes features such as

- the size or area, A, of an object, obtained directly from the number of pixels comprising each object, and its perimeter, P (Appendix C.1);
- the circularity, $4\pi A/P^2$;
- the skeleton or medial axis transform (Section 9.2.5) or points within it such as branch points and end points, which can be obtained by counting the number of neighboring pixels on the skeleton (3 and 1, respectively) (Fig. 11.3);
- the Euler number: the number of connected components (i.e. objects) minus the number of holes in the image (Fig. C.2); and
- statistical moments of the boundary or area (Appendix C.1).

Activity 11.1 illustrates the measurement of some of these features.

The choice of appropriate features depends on the particular image and the application at hand. However, they should be

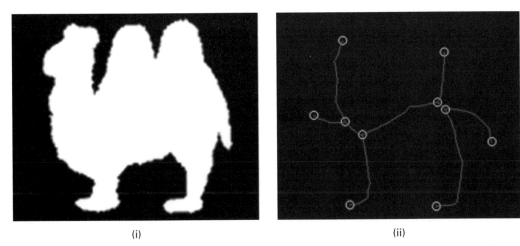

(i)   (ii)

Figure 11.3   (i) Image and (ii) its skeleton (red), with its branch points (white) and end points (green) circled. See also color plate.

- *Robust*; i.e., they should normally be invariant to translation, orientation, scale and illumination, and well-designed features will be at least partially invariant to the presence of noise and artifacts; this may require some pre-processing of the image (e.g. low-pass filtering to reduce noise, and variable background removal and histogram equalization to ensure illumination invariance) before measurement of the features.
- *Discriminating* (i.e. the range of values for objects in different classes should be different and preferably be well separated and non-overlapping).
- *Reliable* (i.e. all objects of the same class should have similar values).
- *Independent* (i.e. uncorrelated; as a counter-example, length and area are correlated and it would be wasteful to consider both as separate features).

It is also helpful if the features incorporate lessons from human perception; in medical imaging, the clinical user's experience with the images will often suggest a qualitative expression of relevant features, which can then be converted into quantitative and repeatable measures. In some cases models of how the patterns are formed can be determined and used to indicate the necessary features, but often this is not the case and features are chosen on a more-or-less ad hoc basis and then tested to find out which are best for the particular task.

For *screening*, i.e. detection of a disease performed on large numbers of patients with the intent of following up suspicious findings, the features should be simple to extract, require minimal user intervention and contribute to the sensitivity (Appendix B.3) of the procedure. Examples of images used in screening include x-ray mammograms for breast cancer, retinal images for eye diseases and visible or x-ray images for childhood scoliosis (curvature of the spine). *Diagnosis* involves classifying features into specific classes, e.g. is a suspicious region in the breast a fibroadenoma, a cyst or a carcinoma? Treatment planning in *radiation therapy* extracts features to identify treatment areas and boundaries. Multi-modality *registration* of images, in the absence of external fiducials (Section 4.3), extracts and compares features from each modality in order to recognize correspondence between equivalent structures.

A *feature vector* or *pattern vector*, x, is a vector containing the measured features, $x_1, x_2, ..., x_n$:

$$x = \begin{matrix} x_1 \\ x_2 \\ \vdots \\ x_n \end{matrix} \tag{11.1}$$

for a particular object or region. The feature vectors can be plotted as points in *feature space* (Fig. 11.4). For n features, the feature space is n-dimensional with each feature constituting a dimension. Objects from the same class should cluster together in feature space (reliability) and be well separated from different classes (discriminating). In classification, our goal is to assign each feature vector to one of a set of classes $\{\omega_i\}$.

The more features that are measured, the higher dimensional will be the feature space and the more parameters will have to be estimated for classification. For a limited number

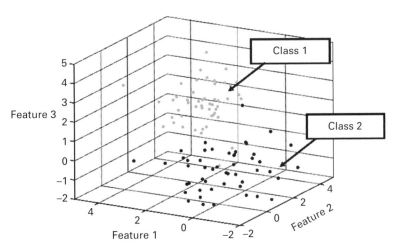

Figure 11.4   Three-dimensional feature space containing two classes of features, class 1 (in gray) and class 2 (in black).

of objects, it is difficult to estimate a large number of parameters well. A solution is to decrease the number of features per object. This involves either (i) *feature selection* – choosing the most informative subset of features, and not using the others, or (ii) *feature extraction* – combining the existing features set into a smaller set of new, more informative features. Ultimately the classifier performance is the criterion for which are the best or most informative features.

A problem in feature selection is that sometimes the *two best* features are not the *best two* features. To find the best two features we can use brute force and try all possible combinations, but this is very expensive computationally: to extract k features from a total set of d features involves $d!/k!(d-k)!$ possibilities, so that exhaustive evaluation is often impossible. What we need is a criterion to evaluate the informativity of a set of features and an efficient search routine which finds the most promising feature sets. When we want to extract just a few features from a large set of features, we can use *forward selection*: this starts with the best individual feature and keeps adding the subsequent best feature until the final number of desired features is reached. When we expect to use most of the features we can use *backward selection*: here we start with the whole set of features, and remove the worst features one by one. Both methods are sub-optimal: it is better to use a hybrid (*branch-and-bound*) feature selection process, where the number of features is increased and decreased several times.

In feature extraction we compute a smaller set of new features which are more informative. The most well known feature extraction method is *Principal Component Analysis* (PCA). This is a mapping where the new features, y, are a linear combination of the original features, x, and are uncorrelated. The new features can be thought of as arising from a rotation of the old features to provide new features which are ranked or ordered in terms of the amount of variation of the original data for which they account. Since they are ranked, it is possible just to retain the first few new features. Figure 11.5 shows how a

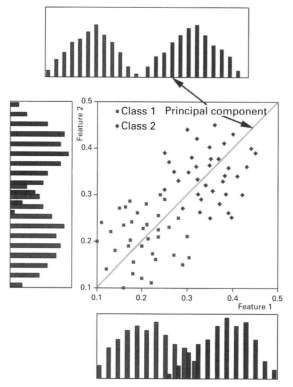

Figure 11.5   The data set is optimally separated (as shown by the histograms) along a line, the first principal component direction, which is a linear combination of the original features. (After Russ 2002 Copyright (2007). From *The Image Processing Handbook*, 5th Edition, by Russ. Reproduced by permission of Taylor and Francis Group, LLC, a division of Informa plc.). See also color plate.

two-dimensional data set can be reduced to a single principal component, which optimally separates the data, by rotation.

The covariance matrix of the feature vector, Σ or **cov(x)**, is a generalization of the concept of variance to higher dimensions. The matrix is symmetric, and its terms are measures of how pairs of features vary together (i.e. co-vary) so that the diagonal terms are in fact variances. For a feature vector x, the covariance matrix is given by

$$\Sigma \text{ (or } \mathbf{cov}(x)) = \begin{bmatrix} \text{var}(x_1) & \ldots & \text{cov}(x_1, x_n) \\ \ldots & \ldots & \ldots \\ \text{cov}(x_n, x_1) & \ldots & \text{var}(x_n) \end{bmatrix} = (x - \mu)^{\text{T}}(x - \mu) \qquad (11.2)$$

The covariance terms can be expressed as

$$\Sigma_{i,j} = \rho_{i,j}\,\sigma_i\sigma_j \qquad (11.3)$$

where $\rho_{i,j}$ is called the *correlation coefficient* between x_i and x_j, and σ_i is the standard deviation of x_i. If x_i and x_j tend to increase together then $\Sigma_{i,j} > 0$; if x_i tends to decrease when x_j increases then $\Sigma_{i,j} < 0$; and if x_i and x_j are uncorrelated then $\Sigma_{i,j} = 0$ (Fig. 11.6).

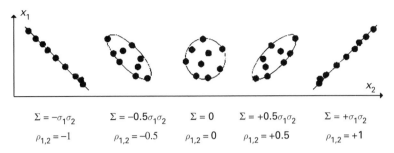

$$\Sigma = -\sigma_1\sigma_2 \qquad \Sigma = -0.5\sigma_1\sigma_2 \qquad \Sigma = 0 \qquad \Sigma = +0.5\sigma_1\sigma_2 \qquad \Sigma = +\sigma_1\sigma_2$$
$$\rho_{1,2} = -1 \qquad \rho_{1,2} = -0.5 \qquad \rho_{1,2} = 0 \qquad \rho_{1,2} = +0.5 \qquad \rho_{1,2} = +1$$

Figure 11.6 The values of covariance and correlation coefficient for various data sets.

Worked example

Consider the following feature vector:

$$x = \begin{bmatrix} 4.0 & 2.0 & 0.60 \\ 4.2 & 2.1 & 0.59 \\ 3.9 & 2.0 & 0.58 \\ 4.3 & 2.1 & 0.62 \\ 4.1 & 2.2 & 0.63 \end{bmatrix}$$

representing a set of five measurements of three features (from left to right – length, width and height of an object). Each row is another measurement of the three features. The mean is given by

$$\mu = [4.10 \quad 2.08 \quad 0.604]$$

and the covariance matrix is given by

$$\Sigma = \begin{bmatrix} 0.025 & 0.0075 & 0.00175 \\ 0.0075 & 0.007 & 0.00135 \\ 0.00175 & 0.00135 & 0.00043 \end{bmatrix}$$

obtained using Equation (11.2).

Thus, 0.025 is the variance of the length, 0.0075 is the covariance between the length and the width, 0.00175 is the covariance between the length and the height, 0.007 is the variance of the width, 0.00135 is the covariance between the width and height and 0.00043 is the variance of the height.

The principal components are actually the eigenvectors of the covariance matrix of the feature vector. *Principal component analysis* is a mapping where the principal components are a linear combination of the original features, and are uncorrelated. The new features can be thought of as arising from a rotation of the old features to provide new features which are ranked or ordered in terms of the amount of variation of the original data for which they account. Since they are ranked, then it is possible just to retain the first few new features. Figure 11.5 shows how an example data set where two features can be reduced by rotation to a single best feature, the principal component, which optimally separates the data. In the two-dimensional case the principal component lies along the *regression line* of the original data.

11.4   Object recognition and classification

Figure 11.7(i) is an image containing both bolts and nuts, some of which lie on their sides and present a different shape. Indeed we can distinguish between them on the basis of their shape. The bolts are long, with an end piece, and the nuts either have a hole in them (the "face-on" nuts) or are short and linear (the "end-on" nuts). Segmentation, in this case by global thresholding, produces a simplified, binary image (Fig. 11.7(ii)). The skeleton of this image shows the essential shape differences between the bolts and the two types of nut (Fig. 11.7(iii)). Branch pixels can be extracted from this image (not shown), on the basis of connectivity. If they are used as a seed image, and *conditionally dilated* under the condition that the seed image is constrained to remain within the bounds of a mask image (the original binary image, Fig. 11.7(ii)), this results in an image of the nuts alone

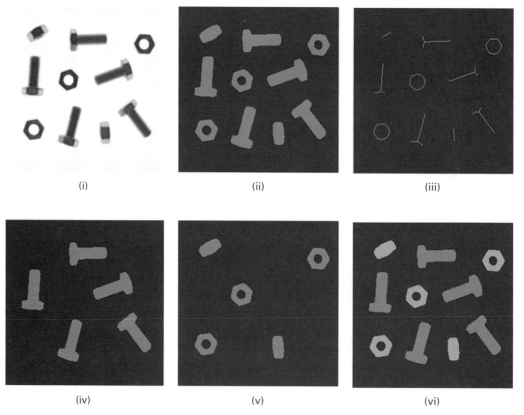

   (i)   (ii)   (iii)

   (iv)   (v)   (vi)

Figure 11.7 (i) Original image; (ii) after thresholding; (iii) after subsequent skeletonization; (iv) after conditionally dilating the branch pixels from (iii); (v) after logically combining (ii) and (iv); (v) color coding the nuts and bolts. See also color plate.

(Fig. 11.7(iv)). The bolts can now be obtained (Fig. 11.7(v)) by logically combining this figure with the original binary figure (using [Fig. 11.7(ii) AND (NOT Fig. 11.7(iv))]). The nuts and bolts can then be joined in a color-coded image (Fig. 11.7(vi)), which illustrates that nuts and bolts have been recognized differently.

An alternative approach to separating the nuts and bolts involves measuring different object (feature) properties, such as the area, perimeter or length. If we measure the area of the labeled objects in the segmented image (Fig. 11.8(i)) by

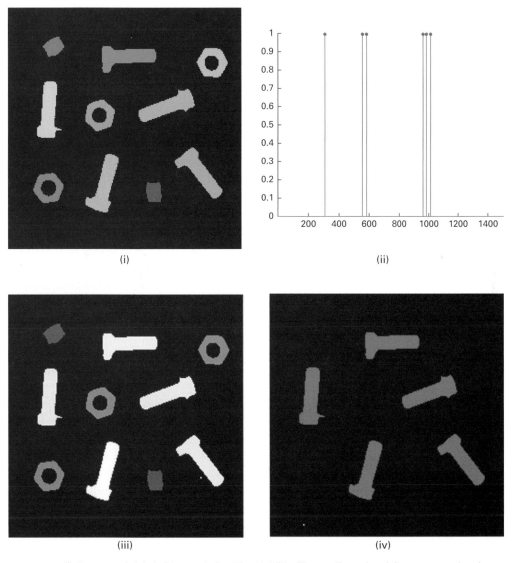

Figure 11.8   (i) Segmented, labeled image (using Fig. 11.5(i)); (ii) one-dimensional feature space showing the areas of the features; (iii) the features "painted" with their measured areas; (iv) after thresholding image (iii) at a value of 800. See also color plate.

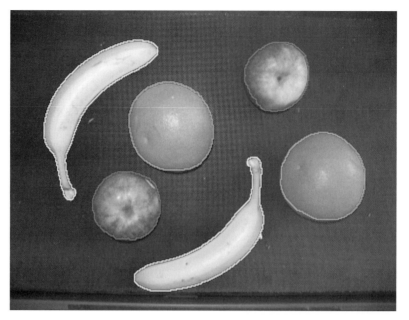

Figure 11.9   Objects have been classified into three classes of fruit, and outlines superimposed on the original image. See also color plate.

counting the pixels belonging to each label and plot these values in one dimension (Fig. 11.8(ii)), we can see that the nuts and bolts are well discriminated on the basis of area, with the bolts having larger areas. There are three *clusters*, comprising the nuts with the highest areas, followed by the face-on bolts with intermediate areas, and the edge-on bolts with the lowest areas. If the objects are then re-labeled with their area values (Fig. 11.8(iii)), that image can be thresholded at a value of 800 (i.e. an area of 800 pixels) to show just the bolts. The nuts can then be found by logically combining this image with the segmented nuts-and-bolts image as before. Only one feature (area) is required to discriminate the two classes, so that feature space (Fig. 11.8(ii)) is one-dimensional.

Similar techniques have been used to classify the fruit in Figure 11.9 into three different classes. Think about the features that would be most discriminating in this case (circularity, size, perhaps texture?). The single-pixel outlines of the fruit can be obtained from subtracting the segmented image from a dilated version of itself. (See Activity 11.2.)

A typical classification problem comprises the following task: given example images typical of a number of classes (the *training set*), classify another image into one of these classes. The training set images should cover a variety of objects belonging to each class. Features need to be identified such that the in-class variabilities are less than the between-class variabilties. For the example shown in Figure 11.10, color and texture are probably good candidates, even though textured materials often have very different appearances with variations in illumination and camera position.

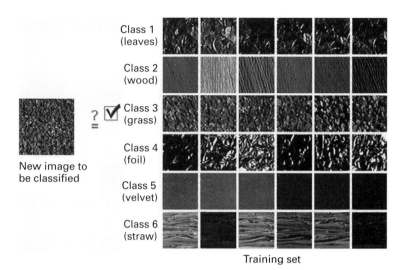

Class 1
(leaves)

Class 2
(wood)

? ☑ Class 3
(grass)

Class 4
(foil)

New image to
be classified

Class 5
(velvet)

Class 6
(straw)

Training set

Figure 11.10   The image at left has to be classified into one of the classes defined by the training set images.
A good classifier will assign it to class 3. See also color plate.

11.4.1   Classification

In any effort at designing a classifier it is essential to have a *training set* of images. Either
the classes to which the images belong are known (*supervised* learning) or they are
unknown (*unsupervised* learning), in which case the most appropriate classes must be
found.

The process of using data to determine the best set of features for a classifier is known
as *training* the classifier. The most effective methods for training classifiers involve
learning from examples. A performance metric for a set of features, based on the
classification errors it produces, should be calculated in order to evaluate the usefulness
of the features. Learning refers to some form of algorithm for reducing the classification
error on a set of training data.

11.5   Statistical classification

There are two general approaches to statistical classification, *parametric* and *non-
parametric* methods. Parametric methods require probability distributions and estimate
parameters derived from them such as the mean and standard deviation to provide
a compact representation of the classes. Examples include *discriminant analysis*
(Fig. 11.11(i)), a parametric method based on functions which separate the classes, and
clustering (Fig. 11.11(ii)), a non-parametric method which finds natural groups of samples
in unlabeled data. Parametric methods tend to be slow at training, but once trained are fast
at classifying test data. Non-parametric methods, on the other hand, either estimate the
probability distributions (non-parametric estimation) or bypass the probabilities and go
directly to decision functions (non-parametric classification).

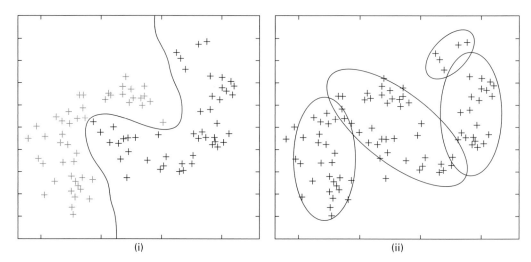

Figure 11.11 Outline of (i) discriminant analysis and (ii) clustering, in two-dimensional feature space.

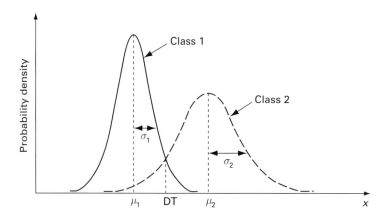

Figure 11.12 Probability density functions for two classes, 1 and 2; often they will be Gaussian in shape.

11.5.1   Parametric methods

Probability theory (Appendix B.3) is a solid basis for classifier design. Consider the case where there are just two classes – class 1 (ω_1) and class 2 (ω_2), and a single feature, x. We have a training set, i.e. representative examples from both classes, so that we can measure the feature for both classes and construct probability distributions for each (Fig. 11.12). These are formally known as the probability density functions or *class-conditional probabilities* (Appendix B.3), $p(x|\omega_1)$ and $p(x|\omega_2)$, i.e. the probabilities of measuring the value x, given that the feature is in class 1 or class 2, respectively. If we have a large number of examples in each class, then the probability density functions will be Gaussian in shape (the Central Limit Theorem).

The classification problem is: given another feature measurement, x, to which class does this feature belong? If the two distribution functions overlap, then this cannot be answered definitively, only statistically. The probability is known as the posterior probability, $P(\omega_i|x)$, i.e. the probability that given a feature value of x, the feature belongs to class ω_i. Probability theory, and specifically Bayes' Rule, relates the posterior probabilities to the class-conditional probabilities or *likelihoods* (the derivation is given in Appendix B.3):

$$P(\omega_i|x) = p(x|\omega_1) \cdot P(\omega_i)/p(x) \qquad (11.4)$$

where $P(\omega_i)$ is the *a priori* or *prior probability* (i.e. the probability of being in class ω_1 or ω_2 based on the relative numbers of those classes in the population, prior to taking the test) and $p(x)$ is often considered a mere scaling factor (the *evidence*) that guarantees that the posterior probabilities sum to unity. (Uppercase P is used to denote a probability mass function, and lowercase p to denote a probability density function.) In words, Bayes' rule is often paraphrased as

$$\text{posterior (probability)} = \frac{\text{likelihood} \times \text{prior (probability)}}{\text{evidence}} \qquad (11.5)$$

This enables us to find the posterior probability in terms of the measured probability density functions of the training set (*training*) and the measured or estimated prior probability (*prior knowledge*). We want to maximize the posterior probability, $P(\omega_i|x)$ (which is the same as maximizing $p(x|\omega_1) \cdot P(\omega_i)$).

Bayes' decision rule is:

$$\text{decide } \omega_1 \text{ if } P(\omega_1|x) > P(\omega_2|x); \text{ otherwise decide } \omega_2. \qquad (11.6)$$

Worked example

Suppose that the class-conditional probability functions for ω_1 and ω_2 are Gaussians with (μ_i, σ_i) of (4, 2) and (10, 2), and that they have equal prior probabilities ($P_1 = P_2 = 1/2$). What is the optimal decision threshold?

The problem can be solved by finding the intersection of the two (scaled) Gaussians. This is equivalent to finding the value of x which makes the posterior probabilities equal. Thus

$$\exp\left(-\frac{1}{2}(x-4)^2\right)/\exp\left(-\frac{1}{2}(x-10)^2\right) = 1$$

Taking natural logs and simplifying,

$$(x-4)^2 - (x-10)^2 = 1$$

from which $x = 7$, which is intuitively obvious.

If the priors are changed to $P_1 = 2/3$ and $P_2 = 1/3$ (i.e. before a feature is measured, there is twice the probability of being in class 1 than class 2), the decision threshold can be found by scaling the Gaussian for ω_2 so that it has half the area as the Gaussian for ω_1. This is equivalent to solving

$$\exp\left(-\frac{1}{2}(x-4)^2\right)\Big/\exp\left(-\frac{1}{2}(x-10)^2\right)=\frac{1}{2}$$

which gives

$$(x-4)^2-(x-10)^2=2\ln 2=1.40$$

from which $x = 7.12$, larger than the earlier value, which agrees with intuition.

If there is more than one feature, $x = \{x_1, x_2,...\}$, the classification is performed in multi-dimensional feature space, where each class is characterized by a multi-dimensional (Gaussian) probability distribution function (Fig. 11.13).

It can be shown that instead of considering the full expression for the posterior probability, it is sufficient to consider the "distance" (Fig. 11.14) from the feature x to

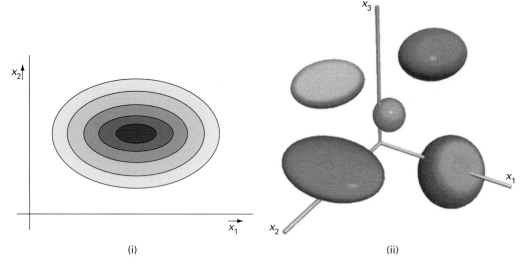

(i)   (ii)

Figure 11.13   Multi-variate normal distributions for (i) two features and (ii) three features. (Note that in these examples, the principal axes are parallel to the feature axes.)

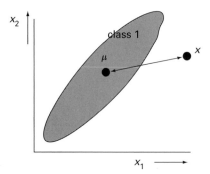

Figure 11.14   The Mahalanobis distance between a feature and the mean of a class; the features x_1 and x_2 have been standardized prior to plotting.

the mean of the class, μ, and assign (classify) it to the class with the minimal "distance" (Appendix B.3). (The appropriate "distance" is the *Mahalanobis distance*, which is a generalization of the usual Euclidean distance that uses standardized features to take into account the different dimensions and variances of the original features.)

A feature could be a numerical score on a test for a particular disease, and might be based on the size or number of objects (lesions?) within an image. Class 1 (ω_1) might be patients free of the disease and class 2 (ω_1) patients who have the disease. We want to know the probability of that having scored x a patient has the disease or is disease-free.

In medical diagnosis the consequences of missing a true case of disease (false negatives) are different from those of falsely indicating the disease (false positives). These costs can be factored into the classification task by introducing a *loss function*, λ, which indicates the cost of each possible decision (α_i), and allows us to convert from a probability into a decision (Appendix B.3). The loss function acts as a multiplier on the posterior probabilities, so that Bayes' decision rule for deciding on ω_1 becomes

$$\text{decide } \omega_1 \text{ if } \lambda_{21}P(\omega_1|x) > \lambda_{12}\ P(\omega_2|x); \text{ otherwise decide } \omega_2 \qquad (11.7)$$

where λ_{ij} is used as shorthand for $\lambda(\alpha_i | \omega_j)$, the loss incurred for deciding ω_i when the true class is ω_j (relative to $\lambda_{ij} = \lambda_{ji} = 1$). The effect of the loss function is illustrated in Activity 11.3.

Discriminant analysis is a type of classification that partitions feature space by specifying *decision boundaries* between classes. These boundaries, described by *discriminant functions*, are obtained from the classifier (e.g. the Bayes' classifier). A classic example of discriminant analysis uses Fisher's iris data (Fisher, 1936), comprising fifty samples from each of three species (*setosa, virginica* and *versicolor*) of iris flowers (Fig. 11.15): four features (the length and width of the sepal and petal, in centimeters) were measured from each sample. The task is to classify the flowers into three classes, which should correspond with the three different species, on the basis of these features.

Although the features were measured manually from physical flowers, they could be measured from suitable RGB images. Petals and sepals would need to be visible, and it would be easier if the flowers were pressed into two dimensions before image acquisition. It may be possible to distinguish the brightly colored petals from the green sepals by looking at the red, green and blue channels separately; the sepals should predominate in

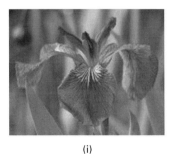 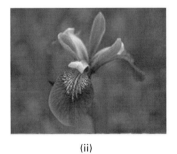 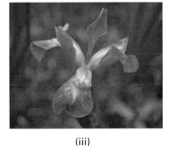

(i) (ii) (iii)

Figure 11.15 (i) *Iris setosa*, (ii) *Iris versicolor* and (iii) *Iris virginica*. See also color plate.

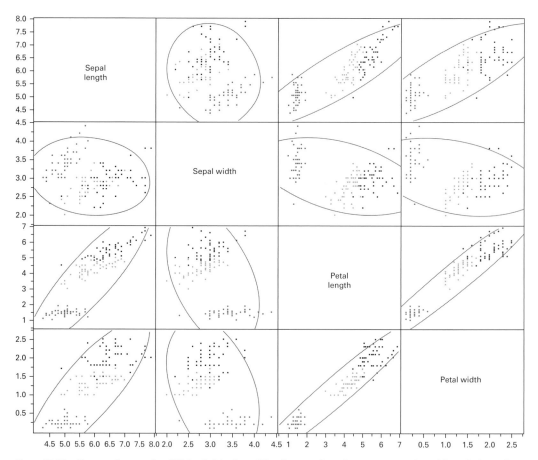

Figure 11.16 Scatter plot matrix of Fisher's iris data. (The features from *Iris setosa* are plotted in red, those from *Iris versicolor* are plotted in green, and those from *Iris virginica* are plotted in blue; the elliptical contours enclose 95% of the features in each plot.) See also color plate.

the green channel. Background removal and smoothing would be performed on the appropriate channels before automated segmentation. Segmentation will deliver the shapes, which can be used to mask the appropriate channels so that the features can be measured conveniently.

A *scatter plot matrix* of the features is useful to see whether any of the features are correlated, i.e. whether they are connected to some degree within the data set (Fig. 11.16). The correlation coefficients from the scatter plot matrix form a correlation matrix (Table 11.1).

The petal length is highly correlated with the petal width, and somewhat less correlated with the sepal length and the sepal width. Because of the high correlation, the petal width is not providing much information that is not already provided by the petal length, and we could consider dropping it as a discriminant feature in order to reduce the task to three-dimensional feature space. The data can then be presented as a three-dimensional

Table 11.1 Correlation matrix, showing the correlation coefficients corresponding to the scatter plot matrix of Figure 11.16.

	Sepal length	Sepal width	Petal length	Petal width
Sepal length	1	−0.118	0.872	0.818
Sepal width	−0.118	1	−0.428	−0.366
Petal length	0.872	−0.428	1	0.963
Petal width	0.818	−0.366	0.963	1

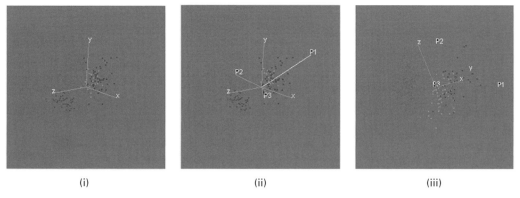

(i) (ii) (iii)

Figure 11.17 Spinning plots: (i) x, y and z are petal length, sepal length and sepal width, respectively; (ii) the principal components, P_1, P_2 and P_3, are shown overlaid; (iii) a projection in the plane of P_1 and P_2. (The features from *Iris setosa* are plotted in red, those from *Iris versicolor* are plotted in green, and those from *Iris virginica* are plotted in blue.) See also color plate.

spinning plot (Fig. 11.17), which can be rotated to show the most prominent directions of the data.

As the spinning plot is rotated, some directions will show more variation in the data than others. The direction in which the features have the most variance is known as the *first principal component*, P_1, and is a linear combination of the *standardized* (i.e. values divided by their standard deviations) original features. Each subsequent principal component (P_2, then P_3) is the linear combination of the standardized original features that has the greatest possible variance and is uncorrelated with all previously defined principal components (and is therefore orthogonal to them). The set of principal components has the same total variation and structure as the original features. The restriction that each successive component be uncorrelated (orthogonal) with the previous components ensures that each new component will have a lower variance than its predecessor. It follows that the first few principal components often capture most of the sample variation.

Formally, the principal components are eigenvectors of the diagonalized covariance matrix, which describes the variance of all the features (Appendix B.3). The eigenvalues show how much variance of the data is explained by each principal component (Table 11.2), so that *principal components analysis* can be used to determine the relative importance of

Table 11.2 The eigenvalues show how much of the total variance is explained by each principal component; the eigenvectors are a linear combination of the original features, with the coefficients above.

The coefficients do not add to unity for each principal component because the features need to be standardized.

	P_1	P_2	P_3
Eigenvalue	2.021	0.907	0.071
percent	67.38	30.24	2.37
Eigenvectors			
Petal length	0.688	0.075	0.721
Sepal length	0.629	0.433	−0.645
Sepal width	−0.361	0.898	0.251

the components in explaining the variance and may prompt a reduction in the dimensionality of a classification problem. In this case P_1 and P_2 between them account for about 97.6% of the total variance in the data.

Therefore, for this data set, the (two-dimensional) projection of the spinning plot (Fig. 11.17(iii)) contains almost all the variance in the data set, and a set of discriminant functions (not shown) could be superimposed on it to show the decision boundaries. In general these decision boundaries will be quadratic, i.e. second-order, and give rise to ellipses, hyperbolas or parabolas in two-dimensional feature space. If the covariance matrices for both classes, ω_1 and ω_2, are equal, then the decision boundary reduces to a linear boundary and the classifier is called a *linear classifier*.

While the principal components transformation identifies the directions of maximal variance, it does not guarantee maximal separability. Another transformation, the Fisher transformation, specifically optimizes class separability. The basis vectors of this transformation, known as canonicals (which are also linear combinations of the original features), are found by maximizing the Fisher criterion, F, which for two-class problems is given by

$$F = \frac{(\mu_1 - \mu_2)^2}{\sigma_1^2 + \sigma_2^2} \tag{11.8}$$

That is, the mean classifier outputs for the two classes should be as well separated as possible and their variances should be as small as possible. This is equivalent to the *Otsu method* of segmentation (Appendix B.4), which finds the threshold that makes each distribution of gray values as tight as possible, which in turn minimizes their overlap.

For multi-class data the canonical plot is normally presented for only the two most significant canonicals, and shows the data in the directions that best separate the classes. Figure 11.18 is the canonical plot for the Fisher data. For this data the first canonical explains 99.1% of the variance in the data, and the second canonical explains the remaining 0.9%. Each multi-variate mean is surrounded by confidence ellipses which are circular in canonical space, and the discriminant functions (not shown) are linear. *Iris setosa* is well separated from the other two species.

Table 11.3 Confusion matrix showing the results of discriminant analysis
used to distinguish three species of iris flower.

| | Actual | | |
Predicted	*setosa*	*versicolor*	*virginica*
Class 1 (*setosa*)	50	0	0
Class 2 (*versicolor*)	0	48	1
Class 3 (*virginica*)	0	2	49

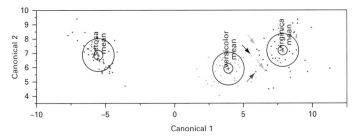

Figure 11.18 Canonical plot for the Fisher data. The three features that are misclassified (see Table 11.3) using this classifier are marked with colored arrows; the black arrow shows an additional feature that is misclassified if cross-validation is used. (The small colored circles are 95% confidence limits for the positions of the means; and the larger colored circles contain 50% of the features for that class.) See also color plate.

Features are assigned to the class whose multi-variate mean is closest. (Since different features have different scales, and likely have different dimensions, the appropriate distances to calculate are the Mahalanobis distances rather than Euclidean distances.) For this data, the three features marked in Figure 11.18 will be misclassified, i.e. assigned to the wrong classes. Two features from *Iris versicolor* will be misclassified as class 3 (which we were hoping to identify as *Iris virginica*), because they are closer to the mean of class 3, and one feature from an *Iris virginica* will be assigned to class 2 (which we were hoping to identify as *Iris versicolor*) because it is closer to the mean of class 2. The final classifications can be tallied in a *confusion matrix* (Table 11.3), which is a contingency table in which the actual and the predicted classes of the data (or vice versa in some implementations) are presented. Entries on the diagonal of the matrix are the correct classifications; and entries off the diagonal are the misclassifications. The confusion matrix shows the performance of the classifier. In this case, three features were misclassified and appear as off-diagonal entries, representing a total misclassification rate of 2% (i.e. 3 out of 150).

Cross-validation shows the prediction for a given observation if it is left out of the estimation sample (a re-sampling technique known as *jack-knifing* (or *leave-one-out*)). In this case an additional feature is misclassified (Fig. 11.18). The cross-validation matrix is displayed in Table 11.4.

The performance of a classifier can also be specified in terms of its *receiver-operating characteristic* (ROC) curve (Appendix B.3). It represents a plot of the classifier's true

Table 11.4 Cross-validation matrix.

Predicted	Actual		
	setosa	versicolor	virginica
Class 1 (setosa)	50	0	0
Class 2 (versicolor)	0	47	1
Class 3 (virginica)	0	3	49

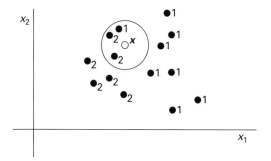

Figure 11.19 3-NN classifier; in this case, the new feature is assigned to class 2.

positive detection rate (correctly classifying a target object as belonging to the target class) versus its false positive rate (incorrectly classifying a non-target object as belonging to the target class). In discriminant analysis, moving the decision values either side of their optimal values (i.e. the values giving the minimum total misclassifications, given by the intersections of the multi-variate Gaussian distributions) changes the *sensitivity* (true positive fraction) and *specificity* (true negative fraction) of the classifier and generates data for the ROC plot. The area under the ROC curve (AUC) is an indicator of classifier performance; a value of 0.5 indicates performance at the level of guessing, and a value of 1.0 indicates perfect performance.

11.5.2 Non-parametric techniques

A common approach is the *k-nearest-neighbor* (k-NN) classifier. The number of nearest neighbors, k, is chosen by the user, and is generally between 0 and 5. In the 1-NN classifier the distances from a new feature to all the features in the training set are computed, and the new feature is assigned the label of the nearest feature in the training set. (In three-dimensional feature space, using Euclidean distances will result in spheres and using Mahalanobis distances will result in ellipsoids.) For the k-NN classifier the nearest k features are considered, and the new feature is assigned the label of the most frequently occurring label in the k nearest neighbors (Fig. 11.19). The value of k should be odd to avoid a tie. The method can be computationally expensive for larger values of k in a high-dimensional feature space.

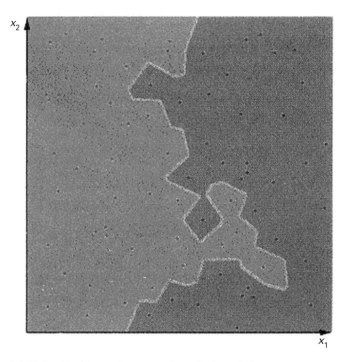

Figure 11.20 1-NN classification produces very irregular boundaries.

For new features close to a decision boundary, 1-NN classification produces irregular boundaries that are not robust (Fig. 11.20).

When distinguishing normal and abnormal classes in, for example, tumor detection, it is more useful to modify the criterion to assign a new vector to a particular class if at least l of the k nearest neighbors are in that particular class. This is useful when (i) the penalty for misclassifying one class (e.g. abnormal as normal – *false negatives*) is much greater than the penalty for misclassifying the other class (e.g. normal as abnormal – *false positives*) and (ii) when there is an unbalanced training set, with many more samples in one class than the other.

11.5.3 Unsupervised methods

With unsupervised classification, the class labels are unknown, and the data are plotted to see whether they cluster naturally. The clusters may or may not correspond with human perception of similarity.

k-means clustering

In *k-means clustering* each cluster is represented by one prototype object, and a new data sample is assigned to the nearest prototype and therefore to that cluster. The training consists of a very simple iterative scheme to adjust the placing of the prototypes:

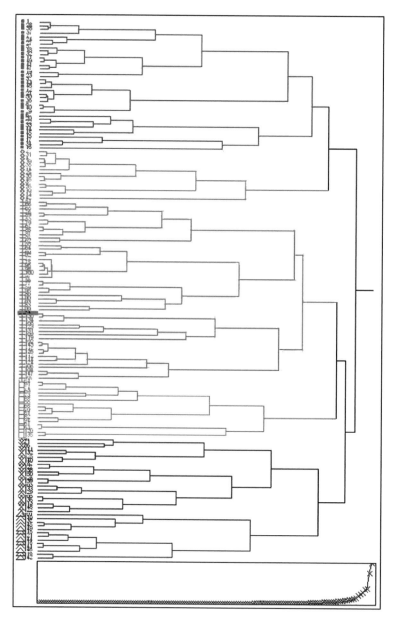

Figure 11.21 Dendrogram and scree plot obtained by hierarchical of the canonical data from the Fisher iris database. The number of classes can be chosen by drawing a vertical line down the dendrogram at a particular position. The scree plot helps determine this position: as shown it is placed to identify six clusters (shown colorized), although the scree plot suggests just three clusters. See also color plate.

(i) randomly choose k objects from the training set, which become the prototypes;
(ii) assign all the other objects to the nearest prototype;
(iii) calculate the new prototype of the class as the mean of all objects having the same label;
(iv) if the prototypes have changed significantly, return to step (ii).

The *k-means* approach is a special case of a general approach called the *Expectation Maximization* (EM) *algorithm*. It is intended for use with larger data tables, from approximately 200 to 100 000 observations. With smaller data tables, the results can be highly sensitive to the order of the observations in the data table.

Hierarchical clustering

In *hierarchical clustering* each feature starts off as its own cluster, and is subsequently joined to the "nearest" feature to form a new cluster. At each step of the clustering, larger clusters are obtained. The algorithm is

(i) find the two features that are "closest" in multi-variate space;
(ii) replace them with a single feature at their mean;
(iii) repeat with the next two closest features, and continue until all the features are subsumed into one cluster.

The result is a *dendrogram* (Fig. 11.21), a visual tree-like representation of the clustering process. Branches that merge on the left were joined earlier in the iterative algorithm. A vertical line drawn through the dendrogram determines the number of clusters in the model. Although there is no standard criterion for the optimal number of clusters, the *scree plot* offers some guidance. It gets its name from the rubble that accumulates at the bottom of steep cliffs. The place where the scree plot changes from a sharp downward slope to a more level slope, not always obvious, is an indication of the optimal number of clusters.

Figure 11.22 shows how the classification changes as the number of clusters is changed. Three clusters (Fig. 11.22(iii)) is a satisfyingly simple classification, and corresponds to the leveling off of the scree plot. (It is also desirable to have three classes, corresponding closely (one hopes!) to the three species of iris.)

There are a number of data points in the bottom right side of the plot which originate from *Iris virginica* and are mistakenly classified as *Iris versicolor*, and several other points which originate from *Iris versicolor* and are mistakenly classified as *Iris virginica*. These points are enclosed within the black lines overlaid on Fig. 11.22(iii). The resulting

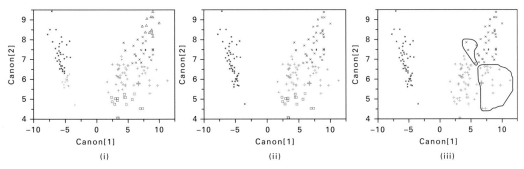

Figure 11.22 Scatter plots of Fisher's canonicals with data colorized according to the number of clusters chosen in the dendrogram obtained by hierarchical clustering: (i) 6 clusters (ii) 4 clusters and (iii) 3 clusters. See also color plate.

Table 11.5 Confusion matrix showing the results of hierarchical clustering used to distinguish three species of iris flower.

Predicted	Actual		
	setosa	*versicolor*	*virginica*
Class 1 (*setosa*)	50	0	0
Class 2 (*versicolor*)	0	46	18
Class 3 (*virginica*)	0	4	32

confusion matrix is given in Table 11.5. The misclassification rate of 14.7% is significantly worse than the 2% achieved using discriminant analysis on the same data set.

11.6   Structural/syntactic classification

In some applications the relevant information is not available in the form of *continuous* data (i.e. measured numerical values), but rather as *categorical* data (i.e. labels or attributes) which may be ordered (*ordinal* data) or unordered (*nominal* data). Nominal data, for example, might comprise a list of attributes describing the structure or shape of objects (Fig. 11.23(i)).

It is natural and intuitive to classify a pattern through a sequence of questions, in which the next question depends on the answer to the current question. Such an approach is particularly useful for non-metric classification, and leads to a *decision tree* (Fig. 11.23(ii)). Such a system is referred to as an *expert system* or *rule-based system*, since it relies on questions based on rules for the class boundaries that have been drawn up with prior knowledge from human experts. The order in which the questions are asked is important for an efficient implementation. An advantage of such a scheme is that the categories are easily interpretable; a disadvantage is that if another category (class) is added the rules may have to be completely re-shuffled or even changed. Training can help discover the most efficient paths.

Syntactic methods are used when the patterns can be represented as ordered sequences or *strings* of discrete symbols (e.g. the bases in a deoxyribonucleic acid (DNA) sequence such as "ATCGGAACTA"), and the strings are generated from certain rules which can be described by an underlying *grammar*. *Parsing* is the task of determining whether the string is a member of the language generated by this grammar.

11.7   Applications in medical image analysis

Classification techniques play an important role in medical imaging, especially in the detection and classification of tumors. After segmenting a suspicious region, a feature

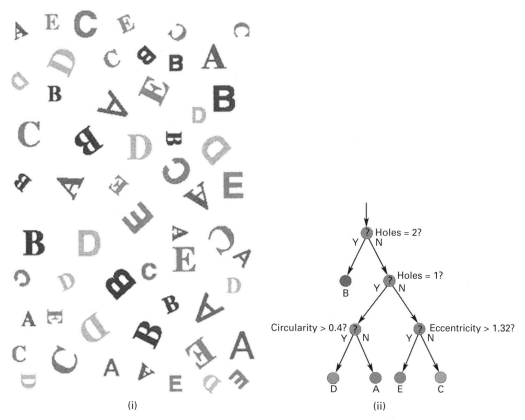

Figure 11.23 Expert system to classify (i) the letters A to E, using (ii) rules based on shape factors that are invariant to size, orientation, position and font. (After Russ, 2002.)

extraction and selection scheme is performed in order to extract the relevant information from the region; and a classification technique is chosen so that the best results are achieved, based on the available features and the tumor classes.

A very important application is the detection of breast cancer. Among the most frequent and distinctive signs indicative of cancer are clustered microcalcifications and spiculated lesions. Microcalcifications are tiny calcium deposits, whose size ranges from smaller than 0.1 mm to 5 mm in diameter. A cluster is typically defined as including three to five microcalcifications within a 1 cm^2 region. Spiculated lesions have a star-shaped appearance with blurred boundaries, and are far more difficult to detect. Their distinct shape (Fig. 11.24) is the result of radially oriented spicules extending from the tumor center into the surrounding breast tissue; they are always malignant. Their gray-level gradient provides a contour, whose shape and orientation can be important features for classifying such lesions.

Typically many features, such as size, brightness, contrast, shape and texture as features (Karssemeijer, 1993), are extracted from microcalcification clusters and spicula-tions in an attempt to match the radiologist's technique, and these are used as input to a

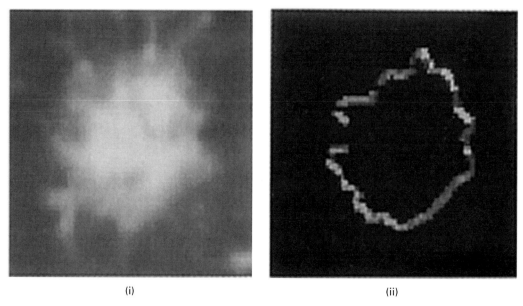

(i)   (ii)

Figure 11.24   (i) A spiculated lesion and (ii) its gray-level gradient.

k-NN or Bayes' classifier (Kegelmeyer, Pruned and Bourland 1994; Karssemeijer and te Brake, 1996). Texture features based on artificial neural networks (Sahiner *et al.*, 1996; Li *et al.*, 2001), designed to emulate the processing abilities of biological neural systems, have been used in the continuing quest for automatic classification and computer-aided diagnosis (CAD).

The extraction of tumor boundaries in 3-D images poses a challenging problem. Several attempts have been made to apply neural network architecture to MRI brain images (e.g., Zhu and Yan, 1997). Fuzzy cluster analysis and principal component analysis have both been applied to functional MRI images (Baumgartner *et al.*, 2000).

Acoustic neuromas are benign tumors which generally grow near the acoustic nerve and can be detected in MRI images. Features such as the mean and standard deviation (representing texture) of the gray level, shape (especially circularity), position relative to the acoustic nerve and the symmetry in position of clusters of neuromas are typical features for characterization.

Structural/syntactic classification has been used in diagnosing heart disease from the stenoses (narrowings) of images of the coronary artery (Ogiela and Tadeusiewicz, 2002). After segmentation and skeletonization of the artery, the external contour was straightened by a straightening transformation. All the potential shape elements characterizing both concentric and eccentric stenoses were defined and an attributed grammar proposed. A recognition rate of 93% was obtained in determining the correct location of a stenosis and its type.

Discriminant analysis of tortuosity features is being used to classify the skeletons of retinal blood vessels, in an attempt to distinguish between normal and pathological vessels (Section 13.5).

Computer-based activities

Activity 11.1 Shape measurements and particle analysis

Open **mri** in ImageJ, and outline the brain using the Freehand Selections tool.

Under **Analyze/Set Measurements ...**, check Area, Mean Gray Value, Standard Deviation, Centroid, Skewness and Kurtosis. Choose **Analyze/Measure** to obtain a Results box with the measurements.

Open **cermet** and threshold using **Plugins/Ch.10 Plugins/Multithreshold**, and choose the isodata algorithm. Under **Analyze/Set Measurements ...**, check Area and Centroid. Choose **Analyze/Analyze Particles ...**; change pixel size to "50 – Infinity" and choose Show Outlines. Study the resulting drawing and data.

Activity 11.2 Object recognition and classification

Open **fruit**, and classify the objects into three classes (bananas, oranges and apples), using features of your choosing. Superimpose outlines of the objects onto the original image.

Activity 11.3 Loss function

Open **discriminant.xls** and look at formulation I, which assumes that both distributions are Gaussian. Enter the healthy, non-diseased distribution as mean $\mu = 4$ and standard deviation $\sigma = 2$, and the diseased distribution as $\mu = 10$, $\sigma = 2$ (with the priors each equal to 0.5, and the loss factors both equal to 1). The program finds the optimal decision threshold by finding the intersection of the two Gaussians, suitably scaled by the priors and the loss factors. The four mutually exclusive events can be found, from which the sensitivity (true positive fraction – the proportion of target objects that are correctly classified as belonging to the target class) and specificity (true negative fraction – the proportion of non-target objects incorrectly classified as belonging to the target class) can be calculated and the contingency tables and the posterior probabilities calculated.

The performance of a classifier can also be specified in terms of the area under its *receiver-operating characteristic* (ROC) curve, known as the area-under-the-curve, AUC (Appendix B.3), which can take a value between 0.5 (the performance is equivalent to guessing) and 1.0 (perfect performance). Scroll down to see the ROC curve, and note the value of the AUC. The second page of the Excel file shows the distributions drawn to scale, and you can verify the intersection.

Now change the loss factors to 2 and 10, and check how this affects the decision threshold and the posterior probabilities, and the value of the AUC.

Exercises

11.1 Discuss the invariance of shape features to translation, rotation, scaling, noise and illumination. Illustrate your answer with specific examples of features.

11.2 Explain the following terms: (i) pattern, (ii) class, (iii) classifier, (iv) feature space, (v) decision rule, (vi) discriminant function.

11.3 What is a training set? How is it chosen? What influences its desired size?

11.4 Consider the following feature vector:

$$x = \begin{bmatrix} 7 & 4 & 3 \\ 4 & 1 & 8 \\ 6 & 3 & 5 \\ 8 & 6 & 1 \\ 8 & 5 & 7 \\ 7 & 2 & 9 \\ 8 & 2 & 2 \\ 7 & 4 & 5 \\ 9 & 5 & 8 \\ 5 & 3 & 3 \end{bmatrix}$$

representing a set of ten observations of three features of an object. Calculate the covariance matrix.

11.5 Suppose that the class-conditional probability functions for ω_1 and ω_2 are Gaussians with (μ_i, σ_i) of (4, 2) and (10, 1), and that they have equal prior probabilities $(P_1 = P_2 = 1/2)$. What is the optimal decision threshold?

11.6 Describe the conceptual differences between supervised and unsupervised learning.

11.7 You are given the following labeled samples, (x_1, x_2):

Class 1: (2.491, 2.176), (0.550, 4.202), (1.063, 0.766), (5.793, 3.452), (2.054, −1.476)

Class 2: (−2.138, −2.474), (4.219, −2.076), (−1.795, −2.838), (−1.165, −2.992), (−1.795, −2.838)

Class 3: (−3.711, 4.3630, (−4.476, 2.298), (−2.521, 0.483), (−1.165, 3.162), (−13.438, 2.414)

Classify each of the following feature vectors, using (i) 1-NN and (ii) 3-NN classification: (−7.427, 2.328), (−4.797, −1.408), (1.079, −1.754), (4.821, 2.435), (2.545, 0.065).

11.8 Consider the recognition of the character 'E' in different sizes, orientations and both handwritten and in various printed fonts. What features would you extract to achieve recognition invariance under these conditions?

11.9 Describe an application of structural classification in medical diagnosis.

12 Three-dimensional visualization

Overview

The advent of multi-modality three-dimensional and four-dimensional imaging has fueled developments in multi-dimensional visualization. There are numerous techniques for viewing such data sets on two-dimensional monitors, but the three main classes are multi-planar viewing, surface rendering and volume rendering. The rendering technique can play a dominant role in determining which information is displayed to the user. The optimal choice of rendering technique is generally determined by the clinical application.

Learning objectives

After reading this chapter you will be able to:

- explain the importance of three-dimensional visualization in medical imaging;
- discuss the different techniques used in three-dimensional visualization;
- outline the differences between surface and volume rendering;
- choose an appropriate rendering technique for a specific application;
- describe the applications of virtual reality systems.

12.1   Image visualization

Medical images have a number of different dimensionalities: (i) two-dimensional, such as a digital radiograph, a fluoroscopic image or a tomographic (US/CT/MRI/PET/SPECT) slice; (ii) three-dimensional, either a stack of tomographic (2-D) slices or direct three-dimensional volumetric data (e.g. from spiral CT or MRI); and (iii) four-dimensional, a time sequence of three-dimensional images. The focus of this chapter is on three-dimensional visualization. The three-dimensional data can be considered as an image stack, either from a single modality or a mix of modalities, where the two-dimensional slices have been registered (Sections 4.3.1 and 6.3) and may have been pre-processed, e.g. to remove noise or enhance contrast. The visualizations are displayed on a two-dimensional computer monitor, although three-dimensional holographic displays and head-mounted displays, as used in virtual reality systems, are being developed.

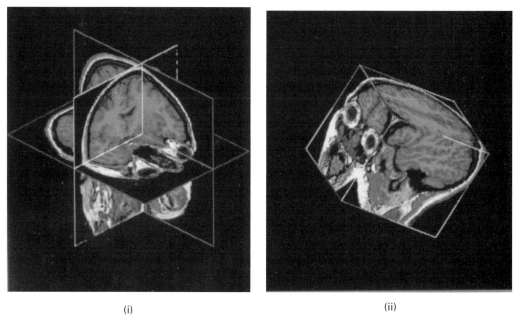

(i)   (ii)

Figure 12.1   Orthogonal sections of a three-dimensional volume image as (i) intersecting orthogonal planes and (ii) a cubic volume. (After Robb, 2000.)

A typical stack might comprise up to about 50 parallel slices, each with a resolution of $512 \times 512 \times 12$ bits. Each slice is a reconstruction of a plane with a slice thickness of about 1 mm, which avoids the superpositioning of objects in the z direction that occurs in planar imaging. The slices are usually contiguous or separated by a few millimeters, but may be overlapping. An immediate advantage is that the data can be viewed from any view point. Reformatting of the data to show orthogonal orientations is particularly simple, although with appropriate interpolation oblique sections can also be chosen. This is known as *multi-planar viewing* (see Activity 4.3). The operator selects single or multiple planes, and can often view them singly or simultaneously, either as intersecting planes or as cubic volumes, and maneuver them interactively (Fig. 12.1).

Visualization of three-dimensional biomedical images is typically performed by either *surface rendering* or *volume rendering* techniques. Each has its own advantages and disadvantages, and the choice between them depends on the nature of the images and the desired result.

12.2   Surface rendering

With surface rendering techniques the surfaces of structures or organs are first extracted. This requires a segmentation and classification step, in which each voxel is classified according to the structure to which it belongs. The classification step searches for voxels that lie on edges and are connected. Once the structures have been classified and their

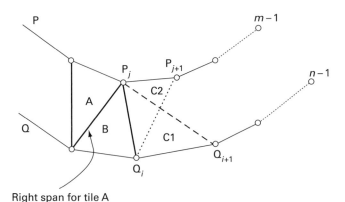

Right span for tile A
(left span for tile B)

Figure 12.2 Tiling parallel contours.

boundaries identified, the boundaries can be represented by a wire-frame or *triangular mesh*. The *tiling problem*, i.e. how to join the triangles (tiles) to form a surface, can be solved by using Delaunay triangulation or more heuristically. For example, in Figure 12.2, tile C2 would be chosen rather than C1 either because it has the smaller area or because it has the smaller span. Figure 12.3 shows a tiled face.

Surfaces with the same value of a property, such as brightness, gradient or texture, so-called *iso-surfaces*, can also be generated directly from the voxel data by an algorithm such as the *marching cube* algorithm (Lorensen and Cline, 1987). The basic idea is that we can define a cube (voxel) by the pixel values at its vertices. If one or more of these values is less than the user-specified iso-value, and one or more have values greater than this value, then the voxel must contribute some component of the iso-surface. By determining which edges of the cube are intersected by the iso-surface, we can create triangular patches which divide the cube between regions within the iso-surface and regions outside. By connecting the patches from all cubes on the iso-surface boundary, we get a surface representation.

Once the surface is obtained, by whichever algorithm, a viewing direction and projection is chosen. Perspective is a strong cue for depth (Fig. 12.4): closer items appear larger than more distant items. However, in some situations, it is helpful to have perspective-free images: it is computationally simpler and allows a region to remain a constant size in different views. Perspective-free viewing is generally chosen for view-points outside a structure, and perspective viewing when inside a structure.

The surface is rendered visible with *shading* and using *hidden surface removal* so that both topography and three-dimensional geometry are more easily understood (Fig. 12.5). The shading value depends on the angle between the viewing direction and the normal to the tile or patch, and the distance to the viewer. There are a variety of algorithms used to perform hidden surface removal. When viewing a three-dimensional object, we only observe surfaces facing the viewer: a simple way to remove hidden surfaces is *backface culling*. For convex bodies all back-facing polygons are removed: a polygon is

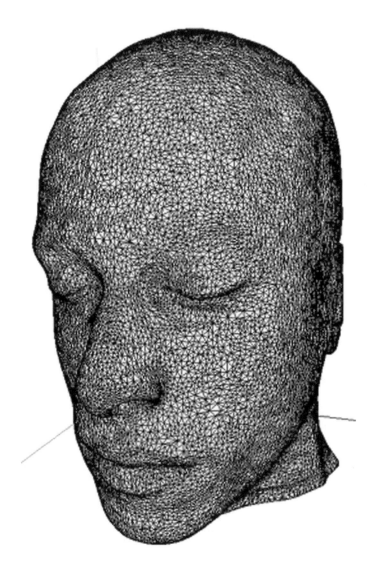

Figure 12.3   Human face tiled with a triangular mesh.

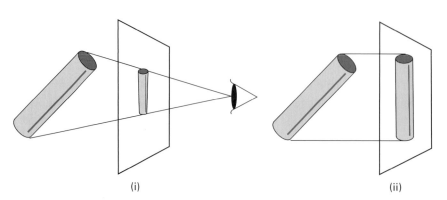

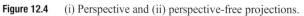

(i)   (ii)

Figure 12.4   (i) Perspective and (ii) perspective-free projections.

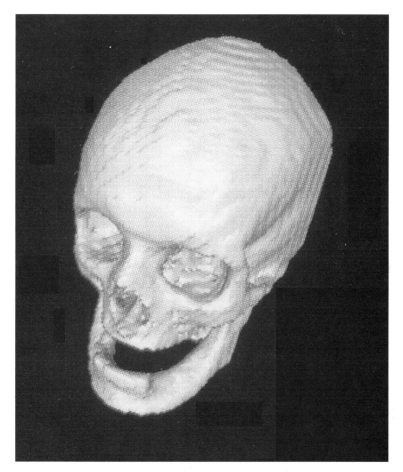

Figure 12.5   Surface-rendered image of a skull.

backfacing if its normal N is facing away from the viewing direction V, i.e. if $N \cdot V = \cos(\alpha) > 0$ (Fig. 12.6). For the perspective-free projection we can direct V along the z axis. The value of $\cos(\alpha)$ is used to determine the shading. The backface culling algorithm has a huge speed advantage since the test is cheap and we expect that at least half the polygons will be discarded. If objects are not convex, the algorithm is more complex. Usually it is performed in conjunction with a more complete hidden surface algorithm. Additional three-dimensional cues can be provided by techniques such as stereoscopic display, rotation and shadowing.

The benefit of surface rendering is that it is generally very fast, since only the points on the surface need to be re-computed following, for example, a rotation rather than every single voxel in the image if volume rendering is used. The contour-based surface descriptors can be used with computer-aided manufacturing (CAM) to control milling machines that can create exact models of the structure. Surface rendering has several disadvantages. The surface brightness does not depend on underlying tissue, and to

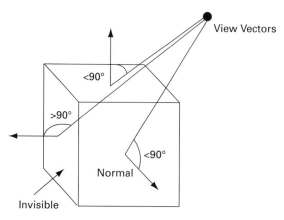

Figure 12.6   Backface culling: if the dot product of view vector and normal is positive then the polygon is visible; otherwise it is not visible.

obtain sharp edges soft tissue is typically eroded. Since the decision on which surface will be visualized has been made during contour extraction, there can be no interactive, dynamic determination of which surface to render. Another disadvantage is that the technique is prone to sampling and aliasing errors, due to the discrete nature of the placement of the triangular mesh. Activity 12.1 shows a surface rendered display.

12.3   Volume rendering

Volume rendering presents a display of the entire three-dimensional image after it has been projected on to a two-dimensional plane. The most common approach is based on *ray casting* techniques, which are a generalization of ray tracing, in which a two-dimensional array of rays is projected through the three-dimensional image. Each ray intersects the three-dimensional image along a series of voxels, and these voxels are weighted to achieve the desired rendering. If the structures in the three-dimensional image have been segmented and classified, the voxels can be weighted accordingly to achieve a translucent representation (Fig. 12.7(i)). An alternative approach is to display only the voxels with the maximum intensity along each ray, the so-called *maximum intensity projection*, MIP (Fig. 12.7(ii)), which does not require any segmentation. The result is a flat looking image that looks like a planar image. This technique is typically a poor choice for most three-dimensional data sets. The exception is some three-dimensional CT scans and angiograms, where the MIP is able to identify bright objects embedded inside another object.

The voxels along each ray are weighted according to

$$C_{out} = C_{in}(1 - \alpha(i)) + c(i)\alpha(i) \tag{12.1}$$

where C_{out} is the value of the ray as it exits the ith voxel, and C_{in} is the value as it enters the ith voxel. There are two values associated with each voxel: $c(i)$, a shading or

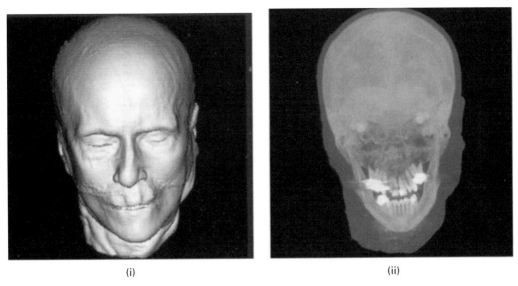

(i)   (ii)

Figure 12.7   (i) Volume-rendered image using the voxel gradient and (ii) maximum intensity projection image.

luminance value, which can be based on the voxel value or calculated from a reflection model using the local gradient, and $\alpha(i)$, an opacity derived from the tissue type. For example, if $\alpha(i) = 0$, then the ray passes through the ith voxel as if it were transparent; if $\alpha(i) = 1$, then the voxel is opaque or luminescent depending on the value of $c(i)$. The values of $\alpha(i)$ are added along each ray and C_{out} is displayed when the sum reaches 1. It is possible to interpolate from the vertex values of the voxel which the ray passes through, but it is better to consider the neighboring voxels (8 or 26) and trilinearly interpolate. This yields values that lie exactly along the ray.

The values of α and c can be changed during the projection process to produce effects "on-the-fly," such as changing the degrees of transparency/opacity or selecting different segmented surfaces. Depth shading can also be incorporated by adding a function of distance from the viewer into the display value. Hidden surface removal is implemented by having any ray stop at the first voxel encountered along its path that satisfies a threshold criterion.

Splatting is an alternative to ray casting. Every voxel is thrown or splatted, like a snowball, on to the image plane, leaving footprints on the image which are then rendered. The technique trades quality for speed.

Volume rendering is computer-intensive, requiring a large number of rays to be used to generate satisfactory results, although modern computers are sufficiently rapid to allow real-time exploration, editing and measurement. Figure 12.8 shows two examples of volume-rendered CT images. The approach is best suited to simple scenes with little clutter: it allows the user to section and mask pixels interactively to reveal underlying voxels from the raw data and manipulate them as in *virtual surgery*.

Activity 12.2 involves rendering a stack of MRI images.

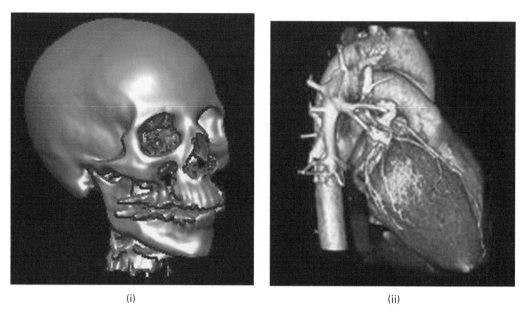

(i) (ii)

Figure 12.8 Volume-rendered CT images of (i) the skull and (ii) the heart.

12.4   Virtual reality

Medicine is starting to use virtual reality (VR) systems, which use very fast, usually stereoscopic, three-dimensional visualization and specialized, intuitive input devices. They are being used in training and education, therapy planning and surgery assistance (Activity 12.3). They range from (i) desktop VR systems with fast rendering capabilities through (ii) immersive systems, where the user typically wears a head-mounted display, and feels immersed in a synthetic three-dimensional environment that includes visual and auditory stimuli and sometimes tactile and force sensations, to (iii) augmented or enhanced reality systems where the user sees the real world, with virtual objects super-imposed on it. Head-tracking and eye-tracking information can be used to navigate through a three-dimensional scene.

In virtual endoscopy, the three-dimensional environment is constructed from data obtained from helical CT scanning (Section 3.2.5). Virtual colonoscopy, examination of the colon, is an important clinical application since cancer of the colon is one of the biggest causes of death from cancer. Virtual colonoscopy is faster than conventional colonoscopy, is minimally invasive and does not involve sedation. The radiation exposure incurred during a virtual colonoscopy examination is currently equivalent to that of two plain abdominal films and will probably decrease with continued software and hardware developments.

Virtual reality systems can also be used to improve the way surgeons plan procedures using simulations. And augmented reality surgery can be used for minimally invasive surgery, with the overlay of pre-calculated images on to the patient.

Computer-based activities

Activity 12.1 Surface-rendered display

Open the mpg file **cfairway.mpg**, the surface display of the airways of a patient with mild cystic fibrosis (courtesy of Division of Physiologic Imaging, Department of Radiology, University of Iowa). Note the bronchiectasis (ballooning) of the upper lobe airways. This is characteristic of patients with cystic fibrosis.

Activity 12.2 Volume rendering

Open the sample stack of MRI images of the head (**File/Open Samples** and choose **MRI Stack**). Open the plugin **VolumeJ**, and accept all the default parameters except those in bold following: Rotate **100**, **20**, 0; Scale 1.0; Aspect 1, 1, **5**; Classifier: Gradient no index (this makes the voxels more opaque the closer their intensity is to the threshold (128.0) and the higher their surface gradient (set by the deviation, 2.0)); Interpolation: trilinear; Light 1,1,**10**. Choose the "raytrace rendering algorithm," and click "Render" to view the rendered result.

Activity 12.3 Visualizations

Run the mpg files **ventricles.mpg** and **brain.mpg**. Which is three-dimensional visualization and which is a simulated file?

Exercises

12.1 Explain the importance of three-dimensional visualization in medical imaging.

12.2 Discuss the maximum intensity projection (MIP) technique used in three-dimensional visualization. What are its advantages and disadvantages?

12.3 Explain the differences between surface and volume rendering. Which approach is preferable for brain imaging?

Part IV

Medical applications and ongoing developments

13 Medical applications of imaging

Overview

Imaging science visualizes an object and quantitatively characterizes its structure and/or function. Biomedical imaging applies imaging science to the presentation of and interaction with multi-modality biomedical images with a view to using them productively to examine and diagnose disease in human patients. This chapter discusses a number of specific applications in medicine that illustrate many of the concepts introduced in this book. The examples have been chosen to demonstrate a wide range of algorithms and approaches; none represent complete solutions, but are rather examples of continuing research.

Learning objectives

After reading this chapter you will be able to:

- appreciate the complexity and problems associated with imaging tasks;
- recognize broad schemes for approaching image analysis;
- analyze the component parts in an imaging problem;
- select potential strategies for analyzing images from a variety of applications.

13.1   Computer-aided diagnosis in mammography

Mammography (Section 3.2.3) is the single most important technique in the investigation of breast cancer, the most common malignancy in women. It can detect disease at an early stage when therapy or surgery is most effective. However the interpretation of screening mammograms is a repetitive task involving subtle signs, and suffers from a high rate of *false negatives* (10–30% of women with breast cancer are falsely told that they are free of the disease on the basis of their mammograms (Martin, Moskowitz and Milbrath, 1979)), and *false positives* (only 10–20% of masses referred for surgical biopsy are actually malignant (Kopans, 1992)). Computer-aided diagnosis (CAD) aims to increase the predictive value of the technique by pre-reading mammograms to indicate the locations of suspicious abnormalities, and analyze their characteristics, as an aid to the radiologist.

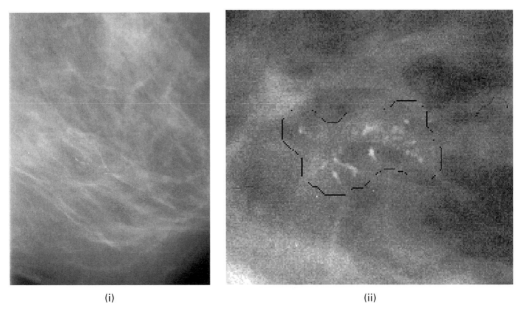

(i)   (ii)

Figure 13.1   (i) A mammogram showing a cluster of microcalcifications and (ii) computer-estimated margin
around a cluster of microcalcifications.

About 90% of breast cancers arise in the cells lining the milk ducts of the breast, and
are known as *ductal carcinoma in situ* (DCIS). Once the tumor extends beyond the lining
of the ducts it is termed invasive, and can spread (*metastasize*) to other sites in the body.
Radiographic indications fall mainly into two categories, microcalcifications and lesions
(Section 3.2.3). Microcalcifications are the primary means of detecting *in situ* carcinomas; they are typically on the order of several hundred microns or smaller in diameter,
comprise calcified dead cells, and tend to occur in clusters (Fig. 13.1). Most lesions are
invasive cancers; they are ill-defined in shape, often with tissue strands or spiculations
radiating out from them, and similar in radio-opacity to the surrounding normal tissue
(Fig. 13.2). The imaging requirements in mammography are stringent, both in terms of
spatial and contrast resolution.

Computer-assisted diagnosis of mammograms involves image processing, segmentation and feature extraction. Segmentation of the breast region serves to limit the search
area for lesions and microcalcifications. Background subtraction may be necessary to
compensate for a varying background optical density in the anode–cathode direction of
the mammography system, known as the heel effect: simple subtraction of the low-pass
filtered image from the original image can be effective (Dougherty, 1998). It is useful to
adjust the gray values of the image to compensate for varying tissue thickness: one way
to do this is to add gray values according to the *Euclidian distance map* (Section 9.2.5),
mapping distances to the skin line in a smoothed version of the mammogram (Bick
et al., 1996). Noise in the image can be reduced by median filtering, although this
can disturb the shape and/or contrast of small structures. An improved technique

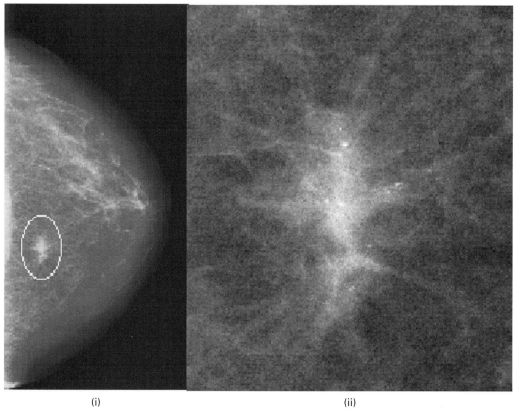

(i)   (ii)

Figure 13.2   (i) A mammogram showing a stellate lesion and (ii) a magnified image of the lesion.

(Nishikawa *et al.*, 1993a) combines the result of morphological erosion and dilation using multiple structuring elements.

Lesions can be extracted using a region-growing technique (Section 10.3.1) with a stopping criterion based on size or circularity (Huo *et al.*, 1995). Features which are useful for characterizing mass lesions include their degree of spiculation, shape and texture. Spiculation features commonly involve the calculation of image gradient using, for example, the Sobel masks (Section 6.4.2). The cumulative edge gradient (Appendix C.3.1), from the Sobel magnitude-of-edges image, can be plotted as a histogram of the radial angle, from the Sobel phase-of-edges image, to determine the degree of spiculation (Giger *et al.*, 1990; Huo *et al.*, 1998). The FWHM (full width at half maximum) of the gradient is able to distinguish spiculated masses from smooth masses. Others have used multi-scale oriented line detectors to detect and measure spiculated masses (Karssemeijer, 1994; Goto *et al.*, 1998; Parr *et al.*, 1998.) The centers of mass lesions tend to be circular so that specific filters can be used (Kobatake and Murakami, 1996). The boundary of the lesion can be unwrapped, and its difference from a smoothed version used to characterize the degree of spiculation (Giger *et al.*, 1994). Other relevant features include asymmetry, which would include automatic registration of left and right breast

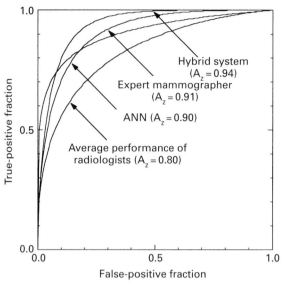

Figure 13.3   Receiver operating characteristic (ROC) curves illustrating the performances of a computer classification method and radiologists in the task of distinguishing between malignant and benign lesions. ANN indicates an artificial neural network using cumulative edge gradient features, and the hybrid system used several features. (Reprinted from Huo *et al.*, 1998, with permission from Elsevier.)

images (Yin *et al.*, 1994), and changes with time (Sallam and Bowyer, 1996). Most researchers extract several features and use principal component analysis (Section 11.3) to identify the most successful combinations. Different methods can be evaluated by receiver operating characteristic (ROC) analysis (Fig. 13.3), but cannot be compared with each other unless the same image databases were used (Appendix B.3).

Microcalcifications can be described by the morphology (shape, area, brightness, etc.) of individual calcifications and the spatial distribution and heterogeneity of individual calcifications within a cluster. They can be enhanced by spatially filtering the mammogram twice, once to enhance the signal-to-noise ratio and a second time to suppress it, and taking the difference of both images (Nishikawa *et al.*, 1990). An alternative is to threshold the image, and morphologically open it using a structuring element to eliminate very small objects while preserving the size and shape of the calcifications (Dougherty, 1998). Isolated calcifications have little clinical significance, so that many investigators have incorporated a clustering algorithm into the classification system, in which only clusters that contain more than a selected number of microcalcifications within a region of chosen size are retained (Nishikawa *et al.*, 1993b). Such schemes are easily implemented using the *k*-nearest-neighbor (*k*-NN) algorithm (Section 11.5.2). Both spatial distribution and heterogeneity of the features within a cluster can be used qualitatively to correlate with a radiologist's criterion, and a classifier such as a neural network used to estimate the likelihood of malignancy (Jiang *et al.*, 1999). Bayesian methods (Bankman *et al.*, 1993), discriminant analysis (Swets *et al.*, 1991), rule-based methods (Chang *et al.*, 1998) and genetic algorithms (Zheng *et al.*, 1999) have also been used in classification.

Computer-aided diagnosis (CAD) systems do not have to be perfect since they are used with a radiologist and not alone. Since the cost of a missed cancer is much greater than the misclassification of benign findings, they should be developed to reduce false negatives (i.e. have a high sensitivity) even at the cost of some acceptable number of false positives (i.e. reasonable specificity).

13.2   Tumor imaging and treatment

Multi-modality imaging is essential in the diagnosis and treatment of cancer (Fig. 4.28). In diagnosis it is used to detect, localize and characterize the "tumor burden" (Dougherty, 1995). Once a tumor is characterized, imaging is used in guiding surgical resection and radiation treatment planning (RTP) and assessment of treatment. Each imaging modality – radiography, CT, SPECT, MRI, PET and others – provides complementary information to understand better the structure and function of the tumor and adjacent organs. Progress in imaging systems has enabled the acquisition of volumetric data sets from which the tumor can be visualized with appropriate rendering (Sections 12.2 and 12.3).

Dynamic imaging uses a tracer material injected into the circulatory system, the kinetics of the tracer distribution providing functional information. The tracer or contrast material is administered as a *bolus* that propagates through the circulatory system and is detectable by the imaging modality. Different tracer materials have been developed for specific imaging modalities. The functional nuclear medicine modalities rely on the uptake and/or metabolism of a radioactive tracer to identify and characterize high-grade recurrent tumors: the poor spatial resolution of these modalities precludes their use for detecting small (<0.5 cm diameter) tumors.

It is important to be able to distinguish benign from malignant tumors, and this can be achieved by studying the microcirculation and/or oxygenation status. High tumor perfusion is indicative of a high blood and oxygen supply to the tumor, which are key elements in its growth. Perfusion imaging is done using contrast-enhanced computed tomography or magnetic resonance imaging, as well as with nuclear medicine methods and ultrasonography. Perfusion, the flow rate per unit volume, is computed pixel-by-pixel using a series of dynamic images (Miles, 1999). Often multi-modalities, PET with CT or MRI, can be used to study the same tumor (Schaefer *et al.*, 1997), and image registration techniques can be used to register images from existing CT and MR systems. Combination CT/PET scanners are now available commercially: the PET scan picks up the metabolic signal of actively growing cancer cells in the body, and the CT scan provides a detailed picture of the internal anatomy that reveals the size and shape of abnormal cancerous growths. When the two images are fused together they provide accurate information on both tumor location and metabolism.

The goal of three-dimensional radiation therapy planning is to deliver a lethal dose to cancer cells without damaging surrounding healthy tissue, some of which (e.g. the brain stem and optic nerve) may be extremely sensitive to ionizing radiation, in order to minimize side effects. Figure 13.4 shows a fused CT/PET image of a slice through the head of a patient with a tumor in the nasal cavity in front of the brain. The lines represent incremental

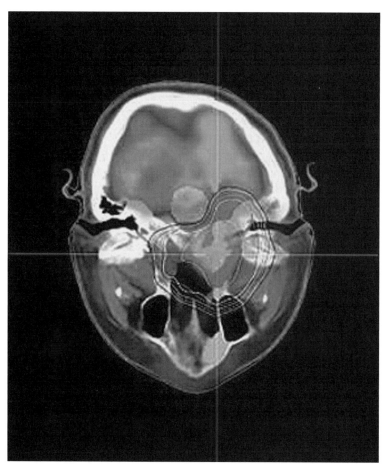

Figure 13.4   Fused CT/PET image showing radiation iso-dose lines around a nasal tumor. (Photo courtesy of Varian Medical Systems of Palo Alto, California. Copyright © Varian Medical Systems. All rights reserved.)

levels of radiation dose, encircling the tumor, computed by a three-dimensional conformal treatment plan. The brain, eyes and lenses receive only minimal doses of radiation, about 10% of the tumor dose.

13.3   Angiography

Coronary artery disease is the leading cause of death worldwide. It occurs when the coronary arteries that supply blood to the heart muscle become hardened and narrowed due to the build-up of *plaque* (fat deposits) on their inner walls, termed *atherosclerosis*. As the plaque increases in size, the interior of the arteries, the lumen, gets narrower (stenoses) and less blood can flow through them. Eventually, blood flow is reduced and the heart muscle does not receive sufficient oxygen. This can result in a *myocardial infarction* (heart attack) when a blood clot develops at the site of the plaque and suddenly cuts off most or all of the blood supply causing permanent damage to the heart muscle.

Once the lumen becomes impaired it can be studied by x-ray arteriography using a radio-opaque contrast agent injected into each artery with a small tube-like device, a catheter, under fluoroscopic guidance. X-ray arteriography is a two-dimensional projection technique, with *biplane* (preferably orthogonal) measurements often taken to characterize the stenosis under the assumption of an elliptic cross-section (Morton *et al.*, 1995). The percentage area stenosis, S, is given by

$$S = \frac{A_1 - A_2}{A_1} \times 100 \qquad (13.1)$$

where A_1 and A_2 are the reference (normal) and stenosed cross-sectional areas, respectively. However, the densitometric (gray) values within a single arteriogram can be used to estimate the thickness in the perpendicular direction (Dougherty and Kawaf, 2001); this is preferable for the very irregular lumens obtained following balloon angioplasty, a therapeutic procedure to remove the obstructions in the arteries. Densitometry can be inaccurate in the presence of significant beam hardening (Section 3.2.5) if the vessel is not oriented close to perpendicular to the x-ray beam and if branches from other vessels lie close-by and interfere with the background correction. Helical CT angiography (CTA) delivers a three-dimensional image of the arteries directly, from which the area stenosis and the degree of calcification of the lesion (Breen *et al.*, 1992; Dougherty, 1997) can be readily calculated, but it is not used routinely.

Commercial packages for assessing morphology and stenosis, quantitative coronary arteriography (QCA), use a minimum cost analysis (MCA) algorithm to detect the outline of the vessels and calculate the stenosis assuming circular cross-sections. The user defines the start and end point of an arterial segment interactively, and the software finds the medial axis (Section 9.2.5) automatically. The contours of the vessel are found in two iterations. First, scanlines are drawn perpendicular to the medial axis along the length of the segment. The edge strength of each pixel along the scanlines is computed, and these are stored in a rectangular "cost" matrix after geometric warping and interpolation. The minimum cost algorithm iteratively searches for optimal contour paths in the cost matrices, using information in the position of each border to help identify the position of the other (Sonka *et al.*, 1995). Geometric corrections for pincushion distortion can be attempted if necessary (Hoffman *et al.*, 1996). Enhancement of vessel edges for better visualization can be easily realized in real time using unsharp masking (Section 6.4.2), but it increases the errors in the measured diameters in quantitative coronary arteriography and is not recommended (Van der Zwet and Reiber, 1995). The reconstruction of three-dimensional space from two-dimensional projections is ambiguous. However, on-line three-dimensional reconstruction of the coronary arterial tree, based on two views acquired from routine angiograms at arbitrary orientation and using gantry angulations, has been used to give multiple projection images, from which a set of views with minimal vessel overlap are chosen (Chen and Carroll, 1998).

Intravascular ultrasound imaging (IVUS), a catheter-based technique which provides real-time high-resolution tomographic images of both the lumen and the arterial wall, is complementary to x-ray angiography. An array of miniaturized solid-state transducers in

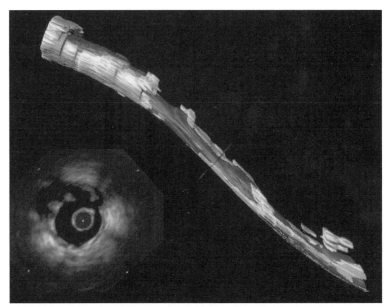

Figure 13.5   Three-dimensional visualization of coronary artery (top) reconstructed from sequence of intravascular ultrasound images (see example at bottom left). The lumen is shown as dark gray and the plaque as lighter gray. (From Robb, 2000. Reprinted with permission of John Wiley and sons, Inc.)

a cylindrical pattern acquire cross-sectional images. The catheter is navigated using the three-dimensional path from the biplane images, and the local coronary artery cross-section reconstructed from the IVUS data. Segmentation of these images to show lumen and plaque is made easier by using multi-frequency transducers. The lumen can then be reconstructed and rendered in three dimensions, with each cross-section registered to it for visualizing the extent of the plaque and precise measurement of the stenosis (Fig. 13.5). Such an image-guided system can be used to diagnose the disease, deliver radiation of topical chemicals to the plaque, or position a rigid support tube, a *stent*.

Magnetic resonance angiography (MRA) has a similar spatial resolution to computed tomography angiography. It also potentially allows the assessment of myocardial function, perfusion and metabolism in the same acquisition session, making it a very attractive and powerful technique. However it offers a bewildering array of data acquisition protocols, each providing somewhat different angiographic information: its greatest challenge is in selecting the optimal protocol for producing the most diagnostic images in the shortest scan time.

13.4   Bone strength and osteoporosis

Osteoporosis is a prevalent bone disease characterized by a loss of bone strength and consequent fracture risk. Because it tends to be asymptomatic until fractures occur, diagnosis is often retrospective and relatively few people are diagnosed in time for

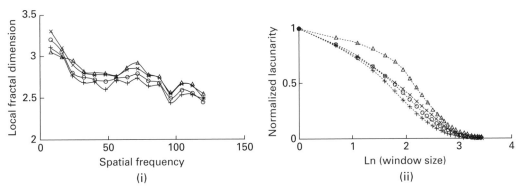

Figure 13.6   (i) Fractal signatures and (ii) normalized lacunarity plots of a typical series of CT images (slice thicknesses: × 1 mm, ○ 3 mm, + 5 mm) and the corresponding projection image (△).

effective therapy to be administered. Clinically, bone mineral density, BMD, is widely used to diagnose and assess osteoporosis, and changes in bone mass are commonly used as a surrogate for fracture risk. Although bone mineral density is correlated with bone strength, it has been increasingly realized that internal bone architecture is also an important determinant of the mechanical strength of bone and can lead to an earlier and more accurate diagnosis of osteoporosis (Goldstein, Goulet and McCubbrey, 1993). The relative contributions of trabecular and cortical bone to overall bone strength are unclear, but most studies have concentrated on trabecular bone since it is the metabolically more active. The limited resolution of commercial CT scanners precludes proper resolution of the trabecular structure; however, CT images retain some of this architectural information (Dougherty, 2001), albeit degraded by the inadequate modulation transfer function (MTF) of the imaging system, and this is referred to as *texture* (Appendix C.2). Fractal analysis (Appendix C.3) of trabecular bone in such images enables the characterization of the microarchitecture (Fazzalari and Parkinson, 1996) and hence bone strength (Millard *et al.*, 1998).

For natural texture images fractalness is limited to a range of scales, and the fractal dimension as a function of spatial frequency within the image presents as a fractal signature (Fig. 13.6(i)) which can distinguish different architectures (Dougherty and Henebry, 2001). Lacunarity measures the distribution of gap sizes in data and contains significant information on the spatial structure of the trabeculae (channels) in the trabecular bone (Fig 13.6(ii)). Both metrics are sufficiently sensitive to distinguish a range of bone conditions (Dougherty and Henebry, 2002) and are potentially useful in monitoring bone strength and predicting future fracture risk using CT or MRI images (Dougherty, 2001).

13.5   Tortuosity

The clinical recognition of elevated *tortuosity* or integrated curvature is important in the diagnosis of many diseases. Increased vascular tortuosity, for example, affects the flow hemodynamics and can lead to *aneurysm* (rupture of the blood vessels), and the tortuosity of retinal blood vessels can be an early indicator of systemic diseases.

Several possible metrics of tortuosity have been proposed, but none has gained universal acceptance. Vessel tortuosity does not have a formal clinical definition but there are clearly some intuitive properties which a reasonable index must satisfy in order for it to correlate with the qualitative assessment of an expert observer. The measure should be invariant to affine transformations of a vessel: translation, rotation and scaling. Most clinicians consider that an ideal tortuosity measure should be additive, i.e. the tortuosity of a composite vessel, comprising several portions, should equal the sum of the tortuosities of those portions. Some of the line integral measures (Hart *et al.*, 1999) and the second difference index (Dougherty and Varro, 2000) satisfy these conditions. However, in their implementations, they are highly sensitive to noise, both from artifacts introduced during vessel extraction to obtain the vessel mid-line, and to digitization errors due to limited image resolution. The latter are compounded because of the use of small groups of consecutive, closely separated, discretely sampled data points to compute local curvatures. Various low-pass filters have been applied to vessel mid-lines to mitigate digitization errors (Smedby *et al.*, 1993; Hart *et al.*, 1999; Dougherty and Varro, 2000), but these are ultimately arbitrary and affect the value of tortuosity obtained: the more severe the filtering, the smoother the mid-line and the lower the measured tortuosity. The use of cubic smoothing splines to filter noisy data (Grisan, Forrachia and Ruggeri, 2003) relies on an arbitrary weighting parameter and does not address the length of data sub-segment required.

A recent paper proposes the use of tortuosity metrics related to the curvature of a unit speed curve, obtained by approximating polynomial spline fitting to the discrete data points representing the mid-line of the vessel (Johnson and Dougherty, 2006). The fitted curve is not required to pass through each mid-line data point, but rather to approach it to within a distance related to the radius of the local blood vessel, and it is not restricted to the discrete pixel grid so that it can more closely correspond to the actual blood vessel. Approximating polynomial spline fitting captures the essential tortuosity of the vessels without having to place undue reliance on the accuracy of each extracted mid-line point, or employ arbitrary smoothing methods. The analysis is construed directly in three dimensions (3-D) so that it can be applied to three-dimensional data sets, which are becoming increasingly available due to the thin, contiguous images now obtainable with helical computed tomography and magnetic resonance angiography.

For real (i.e. noisy) data there exists a unique shortest path which passes through "data balls" of radius r_i, centered on the points x_i, defining the mid-line; this shortest path is a unit speed piece-wise linear function, f. The radii of the data balls can be specified in terms of the local radius of the vessel, R_i. This "shortest path," f_1, between the data balls is used to define the mean curvature, $M(f)$. Once this is obtained, an algorithm is used to find the "smoothest path," f_2, connecting these data balls (Fig. 13.7) and hence to calculate the root-mean-square curvature, $K(f)$. The putative tortuosity metrics were tested on a simulated two-dimensional blood vessel and synthesized three-dimensional helices, and were shown to be scale invariant and additive, insensitive to digitization errors and largely independent of the resolution of the imaging system.

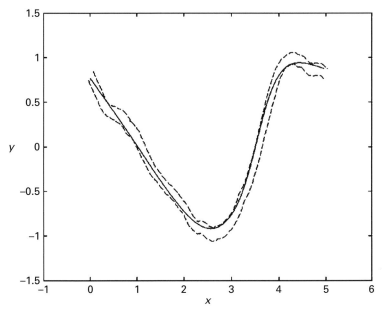

Figure 13.7 The smoothest path (solid line) through a synthesized blood vessel (dashed lines) using a data ball size equal to the local radius of the vessel.

The clinical validity of the metrics has been established (Dougherty and Johnson, 2008a) by applying them to a number of clinical vascular systems, including both two-dimensional (standard angiograms) and three-dimensional data sets (from computed tomography angiography, CTA (Fig. 13.8) and magnetic resonance angiography, MRA). Accurate tortuosity values greatly benefit the treatment and successful outcome of vascular surgery, for example in the endovascular repair of occlusions and aneurysms by endovascular stent insertion (Wolf *et al.*, 2001).

The appearance of the retinal blood vessels is an important diagnostic indicator for many systemic pathologies, including diabetes mellitus, hypertension and atherosclerosis (Hoover, Kouznetsova and Goldbaum, 2000). Normal retinal blood vessels are straight or gently curved, but they became dilated and tortuous in a number of disease conditions (Fig. 13.9), including high blood flow, angiogenesis and blood vessel congestion (Hart *et al.*, 1999). In addition, disease associated with retinopathy of prematurity (ROP), for example, is known to be defined both by increased diameter and tortuosity of retinal blood vessels in the posterior pole, with tortuosity tracking the disease better than dilation (Capowski, Kylstra and Freedman 1995). Tortuosity metrics based on the approximating polynomial spline fits are able to distinguish between normal vessels and some retinal pathologies in retinal fundus images (Dougherty and Johnson, 2008b).

Discriminant analysis allows us to investigate the utility of using both tortuosity metrics to test for the three chosen pathologies (retinitis pigmentosa, diabetic retinopathy and vasculitis) simultaneously. The canonical plot in Figure 13.10 shows the linear combinations of the tortuosity features (M and K) in the two dimensions that best separate the

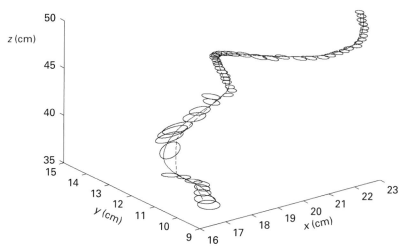

Figure 13.8 The shortest (dashed) and smoothest (solid) paths through computed tomography angiography (CTA) data of the right iliac artery showing the ellipses that were fitted to the outline of the vessel in each slice.

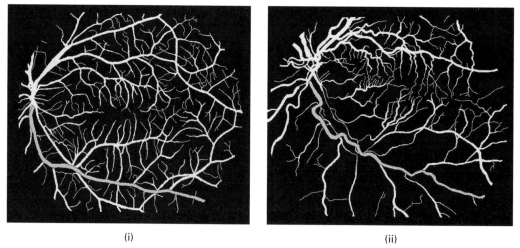

(i)   (ii)

Figure 13.9 Selected blood vessel (in gray) in an image of (i) normal blood vessel and (ii) blood vessel in a patient with retinitis pigmentosa.

groups. Ideally the directions of M and K would be orthogonal to each other in canonical space, indicating that they are independent. Clearly they are not orthogonal and are therefore dependent to some extent, as would be expected based on their definitions. However, they are not collinear, indicating that they are not measuring exactly the same properties. The prevalences (i.e. likelihoods) of the abnormal conditions are very low in the general population (retinitis, 0.025%; diabetic retinopathy, 2.8%; vasculitis, 0.002%), and their values affect the classification. Taking these into account results in 14 of the 35 vessels (40%) being misclassified. In addition, 3 (out of 8) of the retinitis results are misclassified

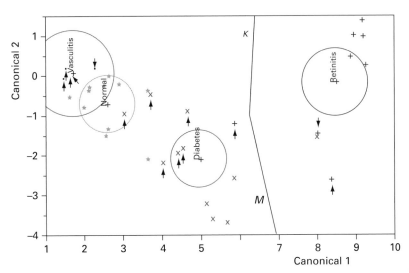

Figure 13.10 Canonical plot of data from retinal vessels. Data from the ground truth conditions are indicated by separate symbols (▪ vasculitis; * normal; × diabetes; + retinitis). The directions of the features, M and K, are shown in the canonical space by the labeled rays. The size of each circle corresponds to a 95% confidence limit for the mean (marked with +) of that group; groups with significantly different values of tortuosity have non-intersecting circles. The small arrows indicate misclassified data points. See also color plate.

as diabetes; 6 (out of 11) of the diabetic results are misclassified as normals; and all the vasculitis results are misclassified as normals.

Such a high misclassification rate precludes the use of this method for screening for all of these conditions simultaneously in the general population. However, a more likely application would be as a test for a single condition, most likely a diagnostic test in referred patients already suspected of being at risk. In the case of retinitis, assuming that the prevalence of the condition in the referred patients is 50%, all cases would be classified correctly. (Even if the prevalence of the general population was used, all the normals would be classified correctly as would 7 out of the 8 retinitis cases – a total misclassification of 5.2%.) These groups are easy to distinguish because the tortuosity in retinitis is significantly larger than normal. In the case of diabetes, again assuming a 50% prevalence in the referred patients, 1 (out of 11) of the normal patients would be misclassified as diabetic (a false positive), and 2 (out of 11) diabetic retinopathy cases would be misclassified as normals 9 (a false negative). This corresponds to a total misclassification rate of 13.6%. In the case of vasculitis, assuming a 50% prevalence in the referred patients, 2 (out of 11) of the normals would be misclassified as vasculitis (false positives), but all (5) vasculitis cases would be correctly classified; a total misclassification rate of 12.5%. False positives are not considered as serious as false negatives, since further testing should identify them correctly; false negatives are unlikely to be tested further.

Clearly tortuosity is a valuable feature in distinguishing any of these three conditions from normal vessels. However, classification would be even more successful if other independent and discriminating features could be identified. In diabetic retinopathy, it would be useful to add features that would quantify the presence of hemorrhaging and microaneurysms.

Scoliosis is a complicated condition characterized by a lateral curvature of the spine and accompanied by rotation of the vertebrae about its axis. Despite the risks associated with repeated exposure to ionizing radiation (Nash *et al.*, 1979), radiography remains the most accurate method of assessing the scoliotic curvature. A scoliotic angle, quantifying the extent of lateral curvature within the affected region of the spine, is routinely used to clinically characterize the curvature (Diab *et al.*, 1995). However, since the curvature occurs in three dimensions it may be characterized more accurately by a tortuosity index if three-dimensional images of the spine are available (Dougherty and Johnson, 2008c).

14 Frontiers of image processing in medicine

Overview

The recent rapid advances in medical imaging and automated image analysis will continue and allow us to make significant advances in our understanding of life and disease processes, and our ability to deliver quality healthcare. A few of the synergistic developments involving a number of disciplines are highlighted.

Learning objectives

After reading this chapter you will be able to:

- recognize the limitations of current imaging technology;
- appreciate the trends and ongoing developments in medical imaging.

14.1 Trends

"A picture is worth a thousand words."

The rapid advances of the last two or three decades in medical imaging technology, which have delivered high-resolution, three-dimensional anatomical and physiological images, is continuing apace, enabling ever more powerful advances in diagnosis and intervention. Improved, miniature detectors are pushing spatial resolution below 1 mm, which will require large computer memories and storage capacities and improved software capabilities to visualize the larger data sets interactively. Advances in post-processing, especially in automated registration, segmentation, classification and rendering, will be required (Van Leemput *et al.*, 1999; Huber and Hebert, 2003; Way *et al.*, 2006). The availability of *multi-modality imaging*, such as combined CT/PET scanners, is increasing, along with the means to share such images around the clinical setting and remotely, fueling improvements in PACS and telemedicine systems (Section 4.3).

14.1.1 The inverse problem

A basic aspect of most imaging modalities is to reconstruct an image based on minimally invasive measurements from a number of sensors. The *inverse problem* determines the properties of the unknown system from the observed measurements. The goal of the reconstruction can be either structural information, such as the anatomy that comes from CT or MRI imaging, or functional information from nuclear medicine imaging or electrical impedance tomography (EIT). An important key feature of inverse problems is their *ill-posedness*, i.e. they do not fulfil classical requirements of existence, uniqueness and stability under data perturbations. The last aspect is especially important since in the real world measurements always contain noise; approximation methods for solving inverse problems with minimal sensitivity to noise, so-called *regularization methods*, are being studied. Electrical impedance tomography is an example of a severely ill-posed inverse problem because very small noise content is typically translated into unpredictable and huge variations in the image, unless proper care is taken during the reconstruction process. Powerful numerical methods, such as *finite element methods* for approximating partial differential equations and the *level set method* for handling topological changes are being developed.

14.1.2   Functional magnetic resonance imaging (fMRI)

Functional MRI (fMRI) provides functional (i.e. physiological) as well as anatomical information by following changes in the flow of fluid, essentially water (or blood) in the body. A major topic of recent interest in the area of model-based image analysis is *functional neuroimaging*, which involves the use of functional MRI to map the activity of the brain to millimeter spatial resolution when it is challenged with sensory stimulation or mental processing tasks. Changes in blood flow and blood oxygenation in the brain are closely linked to neural activity. When nerve cells are active they consume oxygen carried by the hemoglobin in red blood cells circulating in local capillaries. The local response to this oxygen utilization is an increase in blood flow to regions of increased neural activity (occurring after a delay of 1–5 s), leading to local changes in the relative concentration of oxyhemoglobin and deoxyhemoglobin. Hemoglobin is diamagnetic when oxygenated but paramagnetic when deoxygenated; the magnetic resonance signal of blood is therefore slightly different depending on the level of oxygenation. These differential signals can be detected using an appropriate MRI pulse sequence such as blood-oxygen-level-contrast (BOLD) contrast. Higher BOLD signal intensities arise from decreases in the concentration of deoxygenated hemoglobin since the blood magnetic susceptibility now more closely matches the tissue magnetic susceptibility.

However, the slow response time limits its usefulness to characterizing where, rather than how, the brain performs its tasks. Neuron activity can elevate electromagnetic signal changes as well as the hemodynamic and metabolic changes observed with functional MRI. These rapid changes can be measured by electroencephalography (EEG) and magneto-encephalography (MEG) using sensors placed around the head. (EEG has a much higher temporal resolution but rather poor spatial resolution, whereas MEG has a much higher temporal resolution and similar spatial resolution.) The integration of fMRI and EEG/MEG provides high-resolution spatiotemporal multi-modal neuroimaging (Liu, Ding and He, 2006).

Diffusion tensor imaging (DTI) is a related use of magnetic resonance to measure the diffusion of molecules, typically water molecules, in tissue. Two aspects of diffusion tensor imaging render the modality very powerful. First, the microscopic length scale of water diffusion in tissue gives it microscopic spatial sensitivity. Second, in fibrous tissues, the anisotropic nature of the diffusion reflects the gross arrangement of the fiber bundles themselves. The method has been used to probe illnesses such as multiple sclerosis that disrupt the normal organization or integrity of cerebral white matter (Ciccarelli *et al.*, 2003), and the underlying changes in cartilage structure during osteoarthritis (Meder *et al.*, 2006).

Functional imaging methods are also being used to evaluate the appropriateness and efficacy of therapies in, for example, disorders such as Parkinson's disease, depression, schizophrenia, and Alzheimer's disease and for controlling metabolic disorders such as osteoporosis and atherosclerosis.

14.1.3   Molecular imaging

Molecular imaging is the *in vivo*, non-invasive investigation of molecular cellular events involved in normal and pathological processes. It combines molecular agents with powerful new imaging tools, such as PET, to capture pictures of specific molecular pathways in the body, particularly those that are key targets in disease processes. Molecular imaging has the unique ability simultaneously to find, diagnose and treat disease inside the body, as well as to assess the impact of particular therapies. In the future, molecular imaging is expected to aid in identifying the presence of drug-resistant genes that will enable clinicians to pre-determine which treatment regimens will be most effective. Researchers are working to integrate molecular imaging with *nanotechnologies* (using molecular-size (≤ 100nm) structures or sensors) to detect the precise location of disease and deliver drug therapies directly to diseased cells. *Quantum dots* (qdots) are fluorescent nanoparticles of semiconductor material that can be designed to detect the biochemical markers of cancer (Carts-Powell, 2006).

Nanotechnologies are being designed to self-assemble at the appropriate time and to implant themselves to repair bones or tears and even grow new blood vessels or tissue such as heart muscle. During all of these processes, imaging technologies will monitor the process and monitor the results.

14.1.4   Other imaging modalities

There are a number of other emerging imaging modalities with the potential to contribute significantly to diagnostic imaging (Dhawan, 2003). They include: *multispectral optical imaging*, which has been used to study skin lesions and image the breast; *electrical impedance tomography*, based on the naturally varying conductivity of the body; and *microwave imaging*, based on differences in the dielectric properties at microwave frequencies of, for example, breast carcinomas and normal breast tissue.

14.1.5   Surgical interventions

Medical images are used not only for diagnosis, but also in surgical interventions. In robotic surgery a surgeon uses a joystick to control a robot, which is armed with surgical tools and a camera. It is used for minimally invasive procedures, such as repairing blockages between the kidney and the ureter or to remove the prostate. The surgeon also receives haptic (tactile) feedback through small servo motors in the robotic arms. Visual input is stereoscopic and three-dimensional (3-D), with the surgeon wearing optically treated 3-D glasses. Gross movements are scaled to control much finer movements at the remote instrument tip so that they can be manipulated to tolerances far beyond the physiologic capability of unaided human hand-eye kinetics.

Telemedicine currently offers a wide range of remote medical diagnostics and consultations. Increasingly telesurgery will expand to offer robotic surgical operations over a telemedicine network. Sufficient bandwidth will be required to avoid lag time in the audio-visual and haptic data which can lead to "simulator sickness" involving dizziness, nausea or headaches. Virtual reality surgical simulators will doubtless become more common in educational and training environments, to study anatomy from a new three-dimensional perspective or practice surgical procedures with a scalpel and clamps (Robb, 2000; Suetens, 2002).

14.2   The last word

Physics, mathematics, computer sciences, engineering and the life sciences are all contributing to a remarkable synergy of efforts to achieve dynamic, quantitative imaging of the body using minimally invasive, non-invasive or even virtual methods. The structural and functional relationships between the cells, tissues, organs and organ systems of the body are being advanced by molecular imaging, and laboratory imaging techniques such as confocal microscopy for cellular imaging and micro-array genomic imaging to probe gene function. With continuing evolutionary progress in biomedical imaging, visualization and analysis, we can fully expect to benefit from new knowledge about life and disease processes, and from new methods of diagnosis and therapy.

Imagination is more important than knowledge. For knowledge is limited, whereas imagination embraces the entire world, stimulating progress, giving birth to evolution.

Albert Einstein, 1879–1955

Appendix A The Fourier series and Fourier transform

Any periodic function, $f(x)$, can be expressed in terms of an infinite, weighted sum of sines and cosines, namely its Fourier series:

$$f(x) = \frac{1}{2}a_0 + \sum_{n=1}^{\infty} a_n \cos(nx) + \sum_{n=1}^{\infty} b_n \sin(nx) \tag{A.1}$$

where n is an integer, x is an angle that runs from 0 to 2π, and a_n and b_n are the weights or *Fourier coefficients*. Cosines are *even* functions ($\cos(-nx) = \cos(nx)$) and sines are *odd* functions ($\sin(-nx) = -\sin(nx)$).

The computation of the Fourier series is known as *Fourier analysis*, and it is extremely useful as a way to break down an arbitrary periodic function into a linear combination of elementary functions. In the Fourier series, sinusoids (i.e. sines and cosines) are taken as these elementary or *basis functions*: they are naturally occurring waveforms related to uniform circular motion (Fig. A.1). Sinusoids are traced out by rotating phasors (see **phasor1** and **phasor2**). The reverse process, *Fourier synthesis*, allows a periodic function to be built up from a set of elementary functions.

The Fourier series has widespread applications. For example, since the superposition principle holds for solutions of a linear homogeneous ordinary differential equation, if such an equation can be solved in the case of a single sinusoid, the solution for an arbitrary function is immediately available by expressing the original function as a Fourier series.

It is more useful in imaging to let x traverse a distance, say $-L/2$ to $+L/2$, rather than an angle, in which case the Fourier series can be written as

$$f(x) = \frac{1}{2}a_0 + \sum_{n=1}^{\infty} a_n \cos(2\pi nx/L) + \sum_{n=1}^{\infty} b_n \sin(2\pi nx/L) \tag{A.2}$$

where the Fourier coefficients are given by

$$a_n = \frac{2}{L} \int_{-L/2}^{L/2} f(x)\cos(2\pi nx/L)\mathrm{d}x \tag{A.3a}$$

$$b_n = \frac{2}{L} \int_{-L/2}^{L/2} f(x)\sin(2\pi nx/L)\mathrm{d}x \tag{A.3b}$$

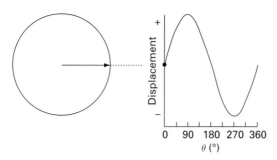

Figure A.1   The projection of a phasor, a vector rotating counter-clockwise at uniform speed, on to a line gives a sinusoid with time: a sine when the projection is on to the vertical, a cosine when the projection is on to the horizontal.

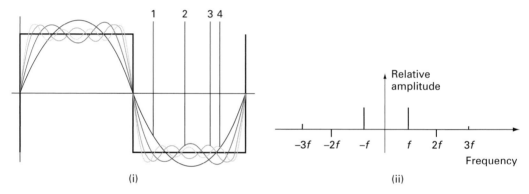

Figure A.2   (i) Harmonic analysis of a periodic square waveform and (ii) its Fourier spectrum.

The Fourier coefficients can be conveniently obtained because the various sine and cosine functions are mutually independent or *orthonormal*, so that the coefficients can be calculated separately.

Figure A.2(i) shows how a periodic square wave can be built up from sinusoids. Near points of discontinuity, an overshoot or "ringing," known as the Gibbs phenomenon, occurs. The Fourier coefficients for this shape, comprising its Fourier spectrum, are shown in Figure A.2(ii): they occur at multiples of a fundamental frequency, f. Note that the negative frequency coefficients are redundant.

The notion of a Fourier series can be extended to a sum of complex exponential functions, with $j = \sqrt{(-1)}$, and complex coefficients, C_n,

$$f(x) = \sum_{n=-\infty}^{n=\infty} C_n \exp(j \cdot 2\pi nx/L) \qquad (A.4)$$

since sines and cosines can be expressed as complex exponentials using Euler's formula,

$$e^{j\theta} = \cos\theta + j\sin\theta \qquad (A.5)$$

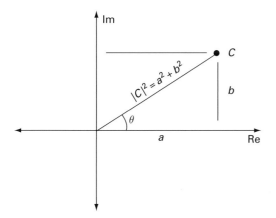

Figure A.3 A complex number, C, has both real (Re) and imaginary (Im) components. Its length is its magnitude, $|C|$, and the angle, θ, it makes with the positive real axis is its phase.

from which we obtain

$$\sin|\theta| = (e^{j\theta} - e^{-j\theta})/2j \qquad (A.6a)$$

$$\cos|\theta| = (e^{j\theta} + e^{-j\theta})/2 \qquad (A.6b)$$

The complex Fourier coefficients, C_n, are given by

$$C_n = \frac{1}{L} \int_{-\infty}^{\infty} f(x)\exp(-j\cdot2\pi nx/L)dx \qquad (A.7)$$

and have both a magnitude (or amplitude) and a phase (Fig. A.3).

The analysis can be extended to non-periodic shapes by considering that the period continues to infinity. In this case the coefficients become continuous rather than discrete, and the summation becomes an integral:

$$f(x) = \int_{-\infty}^{\infty} F(k)\exp(j\cdot2\pi kx)dk \qquad (A.8a)$$

where

$$F(k) = \int_{-\infty}^{\infty} f(x)\exp(-j\cdot2\pi kx)dx \qquad (A.8b)$$

and where k is introduced as the spatial frequency: just as a waveform that varies with time has a frequency, which is inversely proportional to the repeat time, so a waveform which varies with distance has a spatial frequency, which is inversely proportional to the repeat distance.

$F(k)$ is identified as the Fourier transform of $f(x)$ (Equation (A.8b)) and, for a non-periodic shape, it replaces the Fourier coefficients of the periodic shape. It is a

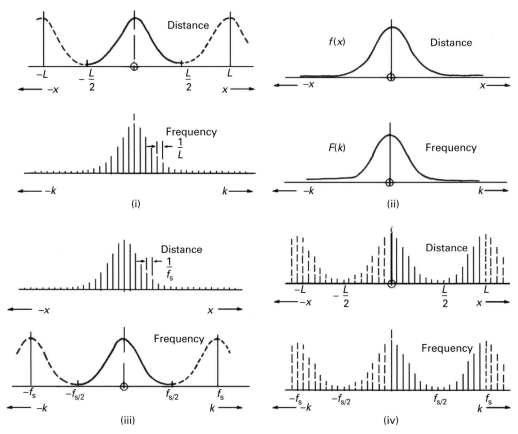

Figure A.4 Various forms of the Fourier transform. (i) The Fourier series: the waveform is continuous and periodic over a distance L in the spatial domain and discrete (i.e. harmonics only) in the spatial frequency domain. (ii) The Fourier transform: the waveform is continuous and non-periodic in the spatial domain and in the frequency domain. (iii) The Fourier transform of a sampled waveform is discrete in the spatial domain and continuous and periodic in the frequency domain: f_s is the sampling frequency. (iv) The discrete Fourier transform, where the waveform in both the spatial and frequency domains is discrete and periodic. (After Randall, 1987, Fig. 2.6.)

continuous function, i.e. all frequencies are present for a non-periodic shape (Fig. A.4(ii)), not just the discrete harmonics that are present in a periodic shape (Fig. A.4(i)). Equation (A.8b) is known as the Fourier transform, and Equation (A.8a) as the inverse Fourier transform; together they form the Fourier transform pair. They are essentially the same, apart from the sign of the exponent.

The Fourier transform is a complex quantity, with real and imaginary parts, $\mathrm{Re}(F(k))$ and $\mathrm{Im}(F(k))$. It is often more useful to consider its magnitude and phase given by

$$|F(k)| = \left[\mathrm{Re}^2(F(k)) + \mathrm{Im}^2(F(k))\right]^{1/2} \tag{A.9a}$$

$$\phi = \tan^{-1}\left[\mathrm{Im}(F(k))/\mathrm{Re}(F(k))\right] \tag{A.9b}$$

The equations can be generalized into two, or more, dimensions, where u and v are the components of the spatial frequency in the x and y directions, with $k = (u^2 + v^2)^{1/2}$.

The Fourier transform of $f(x, y)$ always exists if it is a physical quantity, such as image brightness. The Fourier magnitude and phase images provide a picture of the frequency composition of the image and the relative shifts between the components, respectively. The Fourier intensity image, $|F(k)|^2 = \mathrm{Re}^2(F(k)) + \mathrm{Im}^2(F(k))$, known as the *power spectrum* or power spectral density image, does not contain phase information. Although we often concentrate on the intensity image, there is very significant information in the phase image.

The transform can also be applied to a sampled or digital image comprising $M \times N$ pixels, in which case it is known as the discrete Fourier transform, DFT:

$$F(u, v) = \frac{1}{MN} \sum_{x=0}^{M-1} \sum_{y=0}^{N-1} f(x, y) \exp(-\mathrm{j} \cdot 2\pi((ux/M) + (vy/N))) \qquad \text{(A.10a)}$$

with

$$f(x, y) = \int_{-\infty}^{\infty} \int_{-\infty}^{\infty} F(u, v) \exp(\mathrm{j} \cdot 2\pi((ux/M) + (vy/N))) \mathrm{d}u \, \mathrm{d}v \qquad \text{(A.10b)}$$

This situation is illustrated in Figure A.4(iii), and is the reverse of the Fourier series case shown in Figure A.4(i). Because of the symmetry of the Fourier transform pair, a continuous periodic waveform in one domain becomes discrete with equally spaced components in the other domain. In the Fourier series, a periodic and continuous spatial waveform gives rise to a discrete frequency spectrum of equally spaced harmonics; in the case of a non-periodic waveform, sampled at a fixed rate, the frequency spectrum is continuous and periodic.

In practice the frequency domain will also be sampled (Fig. A.4(iv)), and thus the spatial waveform will be rendered periodic. That is, the discrete Fourier transform (DFT) of an image will implicitly assume that the image is repetitive beyond its boundaries. The DFT transform pair is given by

$$F(u, v) = \frac{1}{MN} \sum_{x=0}^{M-1} \sum_{y=0}^{N-1} f(x, y) \exp(-\mathrm{j} \cdot 2\pi((ux/M) + (vy/N))) \qquad \text{(A.11a)}$$

and

$$f(x, y) = \sum_{u=0}^{M-1} \sum_{v=0}^{N-1} F(u, v) \exp(\mathrm{j} \cdot 2\pi((ux/M) + (vy/N))) \qquad \text{(A.11b)}$$

Because the integrals have been replaced by finite sums, the discrete Fourier transform is computationally tractable. Even so, to obtain N frequency components from N spatial samples requires N^2 complex multiplications. Fast Fourier transform (FFT) algorithms are able to obtain the same result with a reduced number, typically $N \log_2 N$, of complex multiplications.

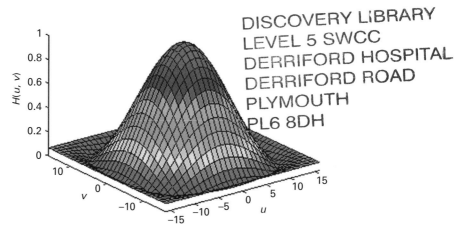

Figure A.5 $|H(u, v)|$ for a 3×3 smoothing mask, with $N = M = 33$.

There are a number of symmetry combinations for Fourier transform pairs. For example, in the case of a real image in the spatial domain, the real part of its complex Fourier transform will have even symmetry (and so will its amplitude) while the imaginary part will have odd symmetry (as will the phase). Such a function is known as a *Hermitian*. Any real image is a combination of components with real and odd symmetries; it is the even symmetries in the real image that give rise to the real, even part of the transform, and the odd symmetries that give rise to the imaginary, odd part of the transform.

The Fourier transform of the point spread function (PSF), $h(x, y)$, of an imaging system is its optical transfer function (OTF), $H(u, v)$. By examining the magnitude of the optical transform function, $|H(u, v)|$ – known as the modulation transfer function (MTF) – it can quickly be determined which spatial frequency components are passed or attenuated by the imaging system.

As an example, consider an imaging system whose point spread function can be modeled by a 3×3 weighted-average mask which describes small amounts of blurring:

$$\frac{1}{15} \begin{bmatrix} 1 & 2 & 1 \\ 2 & 3 & 2 \\ 1 & 2 & 1 \end{bmatrix} \tag{A.12}$$

Figure A.5 shows a plot of the magnitude of its discrete Fourier transform, which is the modulation transfer function, $|H(u, v)|$, of the imaging system. Near $(u, v) \approx (0, 0)$, the modulation transfer function has a value close to 1, indicating that low-frequency components are passed without being changed. Near the perimeter of the plot, the modulation transfer function is close to zero, indicating that high-frequency components are completely blocked, which accounts for the blurring effect.

Appendix B Set theory and probability

B.1 Concepts from set theory

Set theory is used to indicate membership of elements in a set, and is used in probability theory. If set A contains the elements $a_1, a_2, \ldots, a_n$, then

$$A = \{a_1, a_2, \ldots, a_n\} \tag{B.1}$$

Note that a_1 is an element of A, thus

$$a_1 \in A \tag{B.2}$$

but b_1 is not an element of A, thus

$$b_1 \notin A \tag{B.3}$$

An empty or null set is denoted by

$$\phi = \{\} \tag{B.4}$$

If set A is a subset of a larger set D, then

$$A \subseteq D \tag{B.5}$$

Sets can be represented in a Venn diagram, where everything is traditionally placed inside a large rectangle that represents the universal set U. Subsets of U appear inside the rectangle as quasi-circles. The complement of a set A is given by that portion of the rectangle outside of A and is denoted A^C. The notation

$$A^C = \{w \mid w \notin A\} \tag{B.6}$$

reads as "A^C is a set of elements, w, such that w's elements are not elements of A."

The *union* of two sets A and B is the set of all elements belonging to either A or B, or both, and is denoted by

$$C = A \cup B \tag{B.7}$$

and is shown in Figure B.1(i). The *intersection* of two sets A and B is the set of all elements belonging to both A and B, and is denoted by

$$D = A \cap B \tag{B.8}$$

and is shown in Figure B.1(ii).

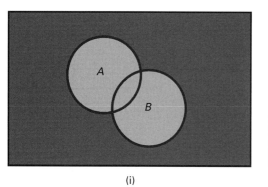 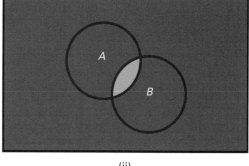

(i)   (ii)

Figure B.1   (i) Union and (ii) intersection of sets A and B, shown as light gray regions.

Morphological operators such as *dilate* and *erode* can be defined in terms of set theory (Gonzalez and Woods, 2008), where A is an image and B is a structuring element. For example, the dilation of A by B can be written as

$$A \oplus B = \{z \mid [(\hat{B})_z \cap A] \subseteq A\} \tag{B.9}$$

where $\hat{B}$ is the reflection of B, defined as

$$\hat{B} = \{w \mid w = -b, \text{ for } b \in B\} \tag{B.10}$$

and $(B)_z$ indicates a translation by z, such that

$$(B)_z = \{w \mid w = b + z, \text{ for } b \in B\} \tag{B.11}$$

Equation (B.9) is based on reflecting the structuring element B and shifting it by z, and then finding the set of all displacements, z, such that $\hat{B}$ and A overlap by at least one element. This is analogous to convolution except that we are using logic operations in place of arithmetic operations. In practice, however, we will use a more intuitive definition of dilation and the other morphological operators (Chapter 9).

B.2   Boolean algebra/logic operations

Boolean algebra captures the essential properties of both set and logic operations. Specifically, it deals with the set operations of intersection, union and complement and the logic operations of AND, OR and NOT. Logic operations are very useful when dealing with binary images, and provides a powerful tool when implementing morphological operations (Chapter 9). They are used in the design of integrated circuits (ICs) in electronics, where an output voltage depends on one or more input voltages. The two states 0 and 1 represent low and high voltage, although more generally in logic they represent "false" and "true." Logic operations are described by *logic gates* and their corresponding *truth tables*.

The output of the logical AND operation is "true" (1) only when both inputs are "true" (1); i.e., the output is true if input A and input B are true (Fig. B.2). The AND operation is written as A AND B (or as $A{\cdot}B$). The output of the OR operation is "true" (1) when either input A or input B, or both, is "true" (1) (Fig. B.2); it is denoted by A OR B (or as

Name	Graphic Symbol	Algebraic Function	Truth Table
AND	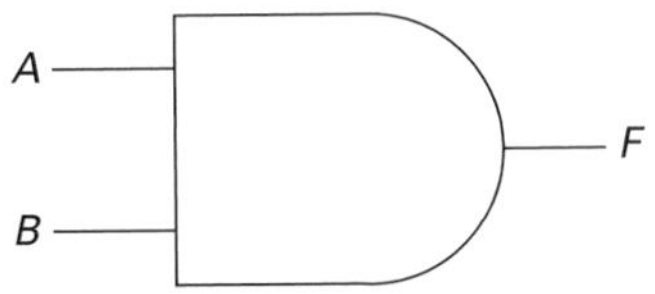 A ——⟩ F B ——	$F = AB$	A B | F 0 0 | 0 0 1 | 0 1 0 | 0 1 1 | 1
OR	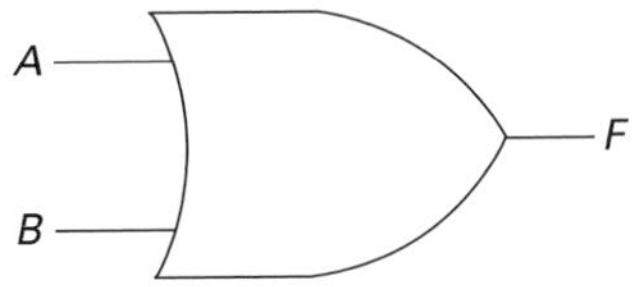 A ——⟩ F B ——	$F = A + B$	A B | F 0 0 | 0 0 1 | 1 1 0 | 1 1 1 | 1
NOT	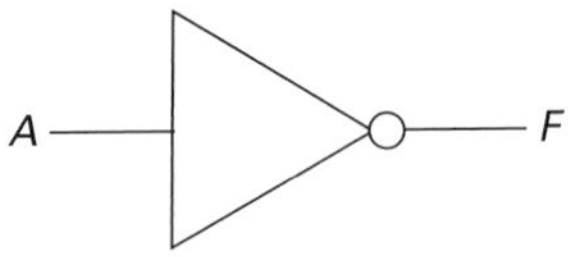 A ——▷o—— F	$F = \bar{A}$	A | F 0 | 1 1 | 0
NAND	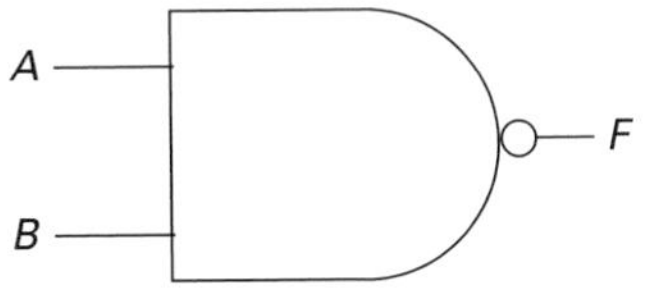 A ——⟩o— F B ——	$F = (\overline{AB})$	A B | F 0 0 | 1 0 1 | 1 1 0 | 1 1 1 | 0
NOR	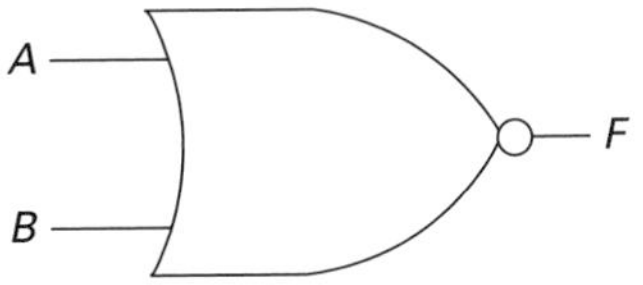 A ——⟩o— F B ——	$F = (\overline{A + B})$	A B | F 0 0 | 1 0 1 | 0 1 0 | 0 1 1 | 0

Figure B.2 Logic operators and truth tables.

$A+B$). An exclusive OR operator (XOR) exists, whose output is "true" (1) when either input A or input B, but not both, is "true" (1). The NOT operation produces the complement of the (single) input, and can be incorporated into other gates to produce the NAND and NOR operations (Fig. B.2). In fact it can be shown that all operations can be built from NAND operations, or alternatively from NOR operations. When used with binary images these operations operate on the images on a pixel-by-pixel basis, taking a pixel from an image A with a correspondingly positioned pixel from image B to produce a pixel in an output image.

The logic operations have a one-to-one correspondence with set operations, except that the former operate only on binary variables. For example, the intersection operation

($\cap$) in set theory reduces to the AND operation for binary variables and the union ($\cup$) reduces to the OR operation for binary variables.

B.3   Probability

In probability a *random experiment* is the process of observing the outcome of a chance event. The *elementary outcomes* are all the possible results of the experiment, and they comprise the *sample space, S.* As examples, the sample space for the single toss of a coin is
    $S = \{H, T\}$, where H is heads and T is tails;
for two tosses of a coin it is
    $S = \{(H, H), (H, T), (T, H), (T, T)\}$;
for the throw of a single die it is
    $S = \{1, 2, 3, 4, 5, 6\}$.
An *event* consists of one or more possible outcomes of the experiment: the *probability* or likelihood of an event occurring is the proportion of its occurrence in a large number of experiments. For example, if there is a finite number of outcomes, N, and each is equally likely, then the probability of each outcome, P, is $1/N$; and the probability of an event consisting of M outcomes is M/N. A probability of 0 indicates that an event is impossible; and a probability of 1 indicates that it is certain.
    Thus for an event A

$$0 \leq P(A) \leq 1 \tag{B.12}$$

$$P(S) = 1 \tag{B.13}$$

$$P(A^C) = 1 - P(A) \tag{B.14}$$

Worked example Throwing two dice
Throw two dice, a white die and a black die. What is the probability of event A, that the black die shows a 6? What is the probability of event B, that the numbers on the dice add to 4?
    The sample space, S, is shown in Fig. B.3. Event A comprises the six elements with the black die showing 6, so that the probability of event A is 6/36, i.e. 1/6. Event B comprises the three outcomes where the numbers on the two dice add to 4, so that its probability is 3/36, i.e. 1/12.

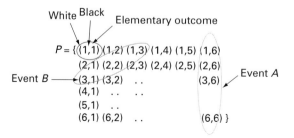

Figure B.3   Throwing two dice. See also color plate.

Events A and B are *independent* if

$$P(A \text{ AND } B) = P(A) \cdot P(B) \tag{B.15}$$

This would be true, for example, in the throwing of two dice; the score on the second is independent of the throw on the first.

Worked example

What is the probability of event E, getting at least one 6 in four rolls of a single die?

This type of problem is best solved by finding the probability of not getting any 6s, and then taking the complement. The probability of not getting any 6s on four rolls is $(5/6 \times 5/6 \times 5/6 \times 5/6)$, i.e. 0.432. The complement of this, the probability of getting at least one 6, is 0.518.

The sample space, S, for throwing three dice comprises outcomes such as $(1, 1, 1)$, $(1, 2, 1)$, etc., and can be considered as a three-dimensional sample space, comprising six slices. The first slice sets die #3 to show 1, and comprises the 36 outcomes of die #1 and die #2; the second slice sets die #3 to show 2, and comprises the 36 outcomes of die #1 and die #2; and so on.

The general *addition rule* is illustrated in Figure B.4:

$$P(A \text{ OR } B) = P(A) + P(B) - P(A \text{ AND } B) \tag{B.16a}$$

or, equivalently,

$$P(A \cup B) = P(A) + P(B) - P(A \cap B) \tag{B.16b}$$

where the third term on the right-hand side has to be subtracted because it has already been included twice (Fig. B.4).

Mutually exclusive events are those that cannot occur in the same experiment, e.g. throw a die and get A = number is even and B = number is 5. If events A, B, C,... are mutually exclusive, they do not overlap (Fig. B.5) and the addition rule reduces to

$$P(A \text{ OR } B \text{ OR } C) = P(A) + P(B) + P(C) \tag{B.17}$$

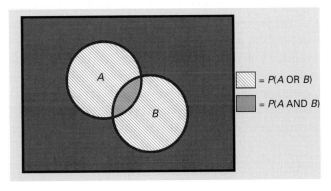

Figure B.4   The general addition rule.

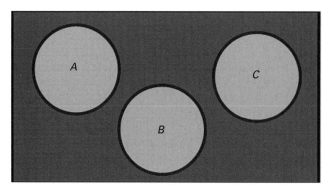

Figure B.5   Mutually exclusive events.

Sex	Age (years)			Total
	<30 (*U*)	30–45 (*B*)	>45 (*O*)	
Male (M)	60	20	40	120
Female (F)	40	30	10	80
Total	100	50	50	200

Figure B.6   A contingency table.

A contingency table (Fig. B.6) is used to record and analyze the relationship between two or more variables, usually *nominal* or *categorical* variables, i.e. variables which are classifying labels, such as sex, race, birthplace, etc. The numbers in the right-hand column and the bottom row are called *marginal* totals and the figure in the bottom right-hand corner (200) is the grand total.

Provided the entries in the table represent a random sample from the population, probabilities of various events can be read from it or calculated. For example, the probability of selecting a male, $P(M)$, is 120/200, i.e. 0.6; the probability of selecting a person under 30 years old, $P(U)$, is 100/200, i.e. 0.5; and the probability of selecting a person who is female *and* under 30 years old, $P(F$ AND $U)$ or $P(F \cap U)$, is 40/200, i.e. 0.2: this is often called the *joint probability*. (Note that the events F and U are independent of each other, so that the joint probability is equal to the product of the individual probabilities, 0.4×0.5.) The probability of selecting a person who is male *or* under 30 years old, $P(M$ OR $U)$ or $P(M \cup U)$, is 160/20, i.e. 0.8.

Conditional probability is the probability of some event A, given the occurrence of some other event B. Conditional probability is written $P(A|B)$, and is read as "the probability of A, given that B is true." Conditional probability can be explained using the Venn diagram shown in Figure B.7. The probability that B is true is $P(B)$, and the area within B where A is true is $P(A$ AND $B)$, so that the conditional probability of A given that B is true is

$$P(A|B) = P(A \text{ AND } B)/P(B) \tag{B.18a}$$

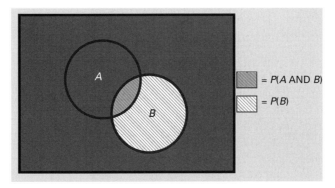

Figure B.7 Conditional probability.

Note that the conditional probability of event B, given A, is

$$P(B|A) = P(A \text{ AND } B)/P(A) \tag{B.18b}$$

(If the events A and B are independent, Equation (B.18a) would reduce to

$$P(A|B) = P(A) \tag{B.19a}$$

and

$$P(B|A) = P(B) \tag{B.19b}$$

which can be used as an alternative to Equation (B.15) as a test for independence.)

The general conditional probability definition, Equation (B.18), can be cross-multiplied to give the so-called *multiplicative rule*

$$\begin{aligned} P(A \text{ AND } B) &= P(A|B) \cdot P(B) \\ &= P(B|A) \cdot P(A) \end{aligned} \tag{B.20}$$

Manipulating this further, equating the equivalent two terms on the right and re-arranging gives *Bayes' Rule*:

$$P(A|B) = \frac{P(B|A) \cdot P(A)}{P(B)} \tag{B.21}$$

where $P(A|B)$ is known as the posterior probability.

Bayes' theorem has many applications, one of which is in diagnostic testing. Diagnostic testing of a person for a disease typically delivers a score, e.g. a red blood cell count, which is compared with the range of scores that random samples from normal and abnormal (diseased) populations obtain on the test. The situation is shown in Figure B.8, where the ranges of scores for the normal and abnormal population samples are shown as Gaussian distributions: we would like to have a decision threshold, below which a person tested would be diagnosed disease-free and above which the person would be diagnosed as having the disease. The complication is that the two ranges of scores overlap, and the degree of overlap will affect the goodness of our diagnosis of the tested patient; i.e., the more the overlap, the less likely that our diagnosis will be definitive.

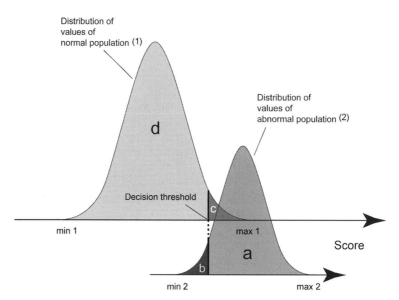

Figure B.8   Diagnostic test score distributions for normal (1) and abnormal (2) population samples.

	A	
	yes	no
B yes	a (TP)	c (FP)
no	b (FN)	d (TN)

Figure B.9   Contingency table for a diagnostic test. The regions a, b, c and d are shown in Figure B.8.

The decision threshold should be in the region of overlap, i.e. between max 1 and min 2. It distinguishes between those who will receive a negative diagnosis (test negative) from those who will receive a positive diagnosis (test positive). The distribution of the scores from the normal population (1) is split into two regions, "d" (below the threshold) and "c" (above the threshold), and the distribution of the scores from the abnormal or diseased population (2) is split into "b" (below the threshold) and "a" (above the threshold).

The sample space thus can be arranged in a contingency table (Fig. B.9), showing event *A* (actually having the disease) and event *B* (having a positive result that indicates having the disease). Thus a person may or may not have the disease, and the test may or may not indicate that he/she has the disease: there are four mutually exclusive events. A person from region "a" tests positive and actually has the disease, and is known as a true positive (TP). A person from region "b" tests negative although he/she actually has the disease, and is known as a false negative (FN). A person from region "c" tests positive but does not have the disease, and is known as a false positive (FP). And a person from region "d" tests negative and does not have the disease, and is known as a true negative (TN). A good test would have a large TP and TN, and a small FP and FN, i.e. little overlap of the two distributions.

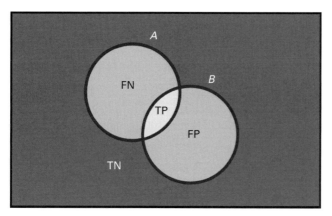

Figure B.10 Venn diagram for diagnostic testing.

The corresponding Venn diagram is shown in Figure B.10, although the areas are not drawn to scale.

The traditional measures of the diagnostic value of a test are its *sensitivity* (the (conditional) probability of the test identifying those with the disease given that they have the disease) and its *specificity* (the (conditional) probability of the test identifying those free of the disease given that they do not have the disease). With reference to Figures B.8 and B.9

$$\text{sensitivity,} \ \ P(B|A) = \text{TP}/(\text{TP} + \text{FN}) = a/(a+b) \tag{B.22}$$

$$\text{specificity,} \ \ P(\bar{B}|\bar{A}) = \text{TN}/(\text{TN} + \text{FP}) = d/(d+c) \tag{B.23}$$

where a, b, c and d are the areas of the labeled regions in Figure B.8. However, sensitivity and specificity do not answer the more clinically relevant questions: If the test is positive, how likely is it that an individual has the disease? Or, if the test is negative, how likely is it that an individual does not have the disease? The answers to these questions require the posterior probabilities from Bayes' rule (Equation (B.21)), which can be paraphrased as:

$$\text{posterior probability} = \frac{\text{likelihood} \times \text{prior probability}}{\text{evidence}} \tag{B.24}$$

where the posterior probability is the probability of having the disease, after having tested positive, i.e. the predictive value of a positive test (P_+), $P(A|B)$; the likelihood is the probability of testing positive, given that you have the disease, i.e. the sensitivity, $P(B|A)$; the prior probability is the occurrence of the disease in the population, $P(A)$; and the evidence is the probability of testing positive, i.e. $P(B)$.

The posterior probabilities are sometimes referred to as the predictive values of a test:

$$\text{predictive value of a positive test } (P_+), P(A|B) = \text{TP}/(\text{TP} + \text{FP}) = a/(a+c) \tag{B.25}$$

$$\text{predictive value of a negative test } (P_-), P(\bar{A}|\bar{B}) = \text{TN}/(\text{TN} + \text{FN}) = d/(d+b) \tag{B.26}$$

The sensitivity and specificity do not take into account the prevalence of the disease in the general population, the so-called *prior probability* (which is the probability of an individual having the disease prior to being tested), while the posterior probabilities (or predictive values) do incorporate the prior probability (see Activity B.1).

Worked example

Suppose a rare disease affects 1 out of every 1000 people in a population, i.e. the prior probability is 1/1000. And suppose that there is a good, but not perfect, test for the disease: for a person who has the disease, the test comes back positive 99% of the time (sensitivity = 0.99) and for a person who does not have the disease the test is negative 98% of the time (specificity = 0.98). You have just tested positive: what are your chances of having the disease?

You may expect it to be rather high, but you need to take into account the rarity of the disease. In this example, the prior, $P(A)$, is 0.001 and the sensitivity, $P(B|A)$, is 0.99. The specificity, $P(\bar{B}|\bar{A})$, is 0.98; and therefore $P(B|\bar{A}) = 1 - 0.98 = 0.02$. The prior, $P(A)$, gives the marginal total for the left-hand column of the contingency table (Fig. B.11), and since the grand total is 1.0, the marginal total of the right-hand column must be 0.999. The top-left event within the contingency table has a probability $P(A \text{ AND } B)$, equal to $P(A|B) \cdot P(B)$ from Equation (B.18b), and is therefore 0.99×0.001, i.e. 0.00099. This gives the term below, $P(A \text{ AND } \bar{B})$, by subtraction. The top-right event has probability $P(\bar{A} \text{ AND } B)$, which is equal to $P(B|\bar{A}) \cdot P(\bar{A})$, and is therefore 0.02×0.999, i.e. 0.01998; subtraction gives the term below, and addition horizontally gives the marginal totals for the rows. With this information, the positive predictive value of the test, $P(A|B)$, the probability of having the disease given that you have tested positive, is 0.472 (using either Equation (B.18a) or Equation (B.21)). This is not as bad as you may have thought given the large values of sensitivity and specificity of the test. Since the probability of having the disease after having tested positive is low, 4.72% in this example, this is sometimes known as the *False Positive Paradox*. The reason for this low probability is because the disease is so rare. Although your probability of having the disease is small despite having tested positive, the test has been useful: by testing positive, your probability of having this disease has increased from the prior probability of 0.001 to the posterior probability of 0.472. It is now time for further testing! The posterior probability, or positive predictive value, $P(A|B)$, is seen to be a more useful parameter than the sensitivity of the test.

	A	$\bar{A}$	
B	0.00099	0.01998	0.02097
$\bar{B}$	0.00001	0.97902	0.97903
	0.001	0.999	1.0

Figure B.11   Contingency table for a particular diagnostic test.

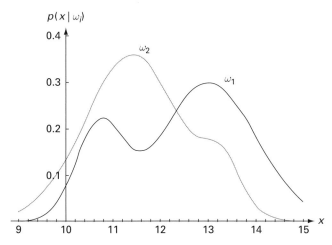

Figure B.12   Hypothetical class-conditional probabilities of measuring x for two classes ω_1 and ω_2. (From Duda *et al.* (2001) with permission.)

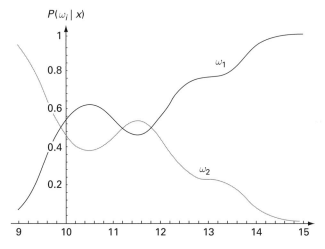

Figure B.13   Posterior probabilities for the classes shown in Figure B.12, for prior probabilities of $P(\omega_1)=2/3$ and $P(\omega_2)=1/3$. Normalization by the "evidence" term keeps the sum of the posteriors equal to unity. (From Duda *et al.* (2001) with permission.)

Bayes' Rule can be formulated in terms of the posterior probability of a score x indicating whether that patient belongs to class 1 (normals) or class 2 (diseased). If the class-conditional probability density functions, $p(x|\omega_i)$, and the prior probabilities, $P(\omega_i)$, for the normal ($i=1$) and diseased ($i=2$) classes are known (Fig. B.12), then the posterior probabilities can be calculated (Fig. B.13). We will conclude that x belongs to class 1 if the posterior probability $P(\omega_1|x)$ is greater than $P(\omega_2|x)$, otherwise we will conclude that it belongs to class 2. To justify this decision, we note that whenever we observe a particular value of x, the probability of making an error in our classification is given by

$$P(\text{error}|x) = P(\omega_1|x) \qquad \text{if we decide } \omega_2$$
$$= P(\omega_2|x) \qquad \text{if we decide } \omega_1 \qquad \text{(B.27)}$$

The average probability of error is

$$P(\text{error}) = \int_{-\infty}^{\infty} p(\text{error}, x)\mathrm{d}x = \int_{-\infty}^{\infty} p(\text{error}, x)p(x)\mathrm{d}x \qquad \text{(B.28)}$$

If for every x we ensure that $P(\text{error}|x)$ is as small as possible, then the integral will be as small as possible, and we have justified *Bayes decision rule*, i.e.

$$\text{decide } \omega_1 \text{ if } P(\omega_1|x) > P(\omega_2|x); \qquad \text{otherwise decide } \omega_2 \qquad \text{(B.29)}$$

This results in minimizing the average probability of error,

$$P(\text{error}|x) = \min[p(\omega_1|x), P(\omega_2|x)] \qquad \text{(B.30)}$$

The four mutually exclusive events (TP, FP, TN and FN) can be found, from which the sensitivity and specificity can be calculated and the contingency tables and predictive values found. If the "cost" involved in false positives is greater than that involved in false negatives, it may be preferable to shift the decision threshold upwards from the optimal value so as to minimize the FPs, although this will involve increasing the number of FNs: this can be incorporated into the scheme by using a *cost factor*, sometimes called a *loss factor*, λ, by which the distributions can be scaled. Re-scaling them relative to each other will result in a different intersection and hence a different decision threshold, which will give rise to different sensitivities and specificities: a re-scaling which shifts the decision threshold upwards will decrease the sensitivity (and P_+) and increase the specificity (and P_-).

One problem with threshold-dependent measures is their failure to use all of the information provided by a classifier. Some tests may not be as straightforward as reading numbers. They could, for example, involve several observers reading features from a noisy image. The different observers may use different criteria or decision thresholds to decide whether or not a feature is present: some may tend to over-read, others to under-read. Moving the decision threshold changes the classification. For example, moving the threshold from low to high reduces the number of false positives, but unfortunately it also reduces the number of true positives (Fig. B.14). Taking the decision threshold at the intercept of the distributions minimizes the total errors (FPF + FNF), and is considered the *optimal threshold* (in the absence of a loss function).

It is useful to measure the performance of a test over a range of decision thresholds, using so-called *Receiver Operating Characteristic* (ROC) *plots*. The term refers to the performance (the "operating characteristic") of a human or mechanical observer (the "receiver") engaged in assigning cases into two classes. An ROC plot is obtained by plotting all sensitivity values (true positive fraction) against their corresponding (1 − specificity) values (false positive fraction) for a range of decision thresholds (Fig. B.14).

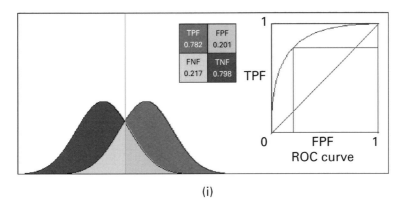

(i)

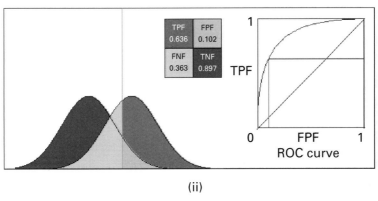

(ii)

Figure B.14 Overlapping distributions. Decision threshold at (i) intercept of distributions and (ii) higher value than (i). The corresponding points on the ROC plot are shown. See also color plate.

The optimal threshold, using the intersection of the distributions, corresponds to a point on the corresponding ROC curve closest to (0, 1). If the threshold is very high, then there will be almost no false positives (but few true positives also). Both TPF and FPF will be close to zero, corresponding to a point at the bottom left of the ROC curve. As the threshold is moved lower, the number of true positives increases (rather dramatically at first, so the ROC curve moves steeply up). At threshold values much lower than the optimal threshold, there is a sharp increase in false positives and the ROC curve levels off. An interesting property of the ROC plot is that the threshold used to obtain a point on the curve is equal to the slope of the curve at that point. ROC plots do not take into account the prior probability.

The area under the ROC curve, denoted AUC or A_Z, indicates the overall performance of the test/system, since it is independent of any particular threshold. The greater the overlap of the two curves, the smaller the area under the ROC curve (Fig. B.15). Values of AUC span the range 0.5 and 1.0. A value of 0.5, corresponding to the forward diagonal, indicates complete overlap of the distributions; no classification is possible. Higher values indicate less overlapping distributions and a better test. When the distributions

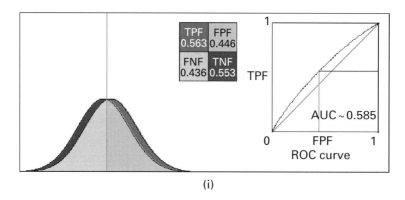

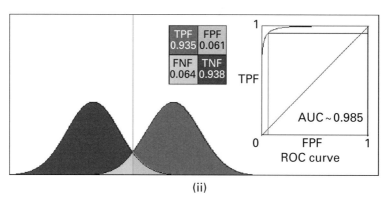

Figure B.15 Distributions with (i) a large and (ii) a small overlap. The corresponding values of AUC are shown with the ROC plots. (The AUC value for the distributions shown in Figure B.14 is 0.859.) See also color plate.

are completely separate, the classification test is perfect and the value of AUC reaches 1.0. A value of 0.8 for AUC means that for 80% of the cases a random selection from the positive group will have a score greater than a random selection from the negative class.

For each decision threshold a point on the ROC curve is plotted using values in the corresponding contingency table, which only depend on whether samples are above or below the threshold and not by how much they are above or below. As a consequence the area under the ROC curve is not significantly affected by the shapes of the underlying distributions, which is a welcome simplification.

The AUC for training data is usually higher than that for test data (Fig. B.16), since most classifiers will perform best on the data used to generate the classification rule (the training data), and less well on new (test) data. Each curve corresponds to a particular value of the discriminability, d', where

$$d' = |\mu_2 - \mu_1|/\sigma \qquad (B.31)$$

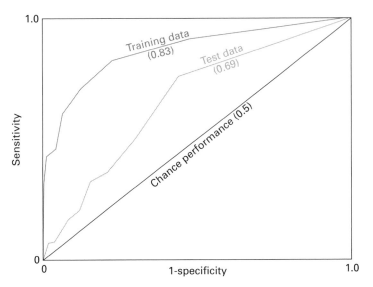

Figure B.16 Typical receiver-operating characteristic (ROC) curves.

B.4 Image segmentation

Segmentation of an image into two classes or clusters (Section 10.2.1), using its gray-level histogram, is similar to finding the optimal decision threshold in diagnostic testing. In this case, we are searching for the optimal threshold to partition the pixels into foreground and background.

If the range of pixels is $[0, L-1]$, and the histogram is bimodal, there are two classes of pixels, class 0 (the background) with values $[0, k]$ and class 1 (the foreground) with values $[k+1, L-1]$, where k is the value of the threshold.

The class probabilities are

$$P(C_0) = \sum_{i=0}^{k} P(i) = \omega_0(k) = \omega(k) \tag{B.32}$$

$$P(C_1) = \sum_{i=k+1}^{L-1} P(i) = \omega_1(k) = 1 - \omega(k) \tag{B.33}$$

the class means are

$$\mu_0(k) = \sum_{i=0}^{k} iP(i|C_0) = \frac{1}{\omega_0(k)} \sum_{i=0}^{k} iP(i) \tag{B.34}$$

$$\mu_1(k) = \sum_{i=k+1}^{L-1} iP(i|C_1) = \frac{1}{\omega_1(k)} \sum_{i=k+1}^{L-1} iP(i) \tag{B.35}$$

and the individual class variances are

$$\sigma_0{}^2(k) = \frac{1}{\omega_0(k)} \sum_{i=0}^{k} [i - \mu_0(k)]^2 P(i) \tag{B.36}$$

$$\sigma_1{}^2(k) = \frac{1}{\omega_1(k)} \sum_{i=k+1}^{L-1} [i - \mu_1(k)]^2 P(i) \tag{B.37}$$

We can define the *within-class variance* as the weighted sum of the variances of each class:

$$\sigma_W^2(k) = \omega_0(k)\sigma_0{}^2(k) + \omega_1(k)\sigma_1{}^2(k) \tag{B.38}$$

The *Otsu method* finds the threshold k that minimizes the within-class variance, so as to make each cluster as tight as possible, which will in turn minimize their overlap. We could actually stop at this point; all we need to do is run through the full range of k values and pick the value that minimizes $\sigma_W^2(k)$. However, it is possible to develop a recursion relation that leads to a much faster calculation. The *total variance* of the combined distribution, σ_T^2, is given by

$$\sigma_T^2 = \sum_{i=0}^{L-1} [i - \mu_T]^2 \cdot P(i) \tag{B.39}$$

where

$$\mu_T = \sum_{i=0}^{L-1} i P(i) \tag{B.40}$$

Subtracting Equation (B.38) from Equation (B.39) gives the *between-class variance*, σ_B^2, the sum of the weighted squared distances between class means and grand mean, i.e.

$$\begin{aligned}\sigma_B^2 = \sigma_T^2 - \sigma_W^2 &= \omega(k) \cdot (\mu_0(k) - \mu_T)^2 - (1 - \omega(k)) \cdot (\mu_1(k) - \mu_T)^2 \\ &= \omega(k) \cdot (1 - \omega(k)) \cdot [\mu_0(k) - \mu_1(k)]^2\end{aligned} \tag{B.41}$$

Since the total variance, σ_T^2, is constant and independent of k, the effect of changing the threshold is merely to move the contributions between σ_W^2 and σ_B^2. Thus minimizing the within-class variance is equivalent to maximizing the between-class variance. The advantage of doing the latter is that we can compute the quantities in σ_B^2 recursively as we run through the k values. Initializing gives

$$\omega(1) = P(1); \quad \mu_0(0) = 0 \tag{B.42}$$

Then the recursive relation is

$$\omega(k+1) = \omega(k) + P(k+1) \tag{B.43a}$$

$$\mu_0(k+1) = (\omega(k) \cdot \mu_0(k) + (k+1) \cdot P(k+1))/(\omega(k+1)) \tag{B.43b}$$

$$\mu_1(k+1) = (\mu - \omega(k+1) \cdot \mu_0(k+1))/(1 - \omega(k+1)) \tag{B.43c}$$

This allows us to update σ_B^2, and look for the maximum, as we successively move through each threshold: σ_B^2 is always smooth and unimodal, which makes it easy to find the maximum.

Computer-based activities

Activity B.1 The positive predictive value

Open **discriminant.xls**, an Excel file. Look at formulation II and fill in the sensitivity, the specificity and the prior probability (denoted π_D) as the values in the worked example above. The contingency table updates immediately, showing the joint and marginal probabilities. Below that the conditional probabilities (Predicted | Actual), with the sensitivity and specificity highlighted in red, and (Actual | Predicted), with the positive and negative predictive probabilities highlighted in blue, are shown. Below that is a graph showing how the positive predictive value, variously referred to as PPV, P_+ or $P(A|B)$, changes with the prior probability.

Change the prior probability to 0.001 and observe the changes. Note especially that the PPV (or $P(A|B)$) changes from 4.7% to 33.3%, even though the test has not changed, i.e. the sensitivity and specificity have remained the same.

Activity B.2 ROC plots

Open **discriminant.xls** and look at formulation I: it assumes that both distributions are Gaussian, which is often the case in practice since many random factors are involved and the Central Limit Theorem is appropriate. Each can then be characterized by a mean and a standard deviation, and an area which corresponds to the prior probabilities, the fractions of the population which are either normal or diseased. Enter the healthy, non-diseased distribution as mean $\mu = 4$ and standard deviation $\sigma = 2$, and the diseased distribution as $\mu = 10$, $\sigma = 2$ (with the priors each equal to 0.5 and the loss factors both equal to 1). The program finds the optimal decision threshold by finding the intersection of the two suitably scaled Gaussians. The four mutually exclusive events can be found from the corresponding areas, from which the sensitivity and specificity and the posterior probabilities can be calculated. Note the optimal decision threshold of 7, which is intuitively reasonable, and the specificity, sensitivity and posterior probabilities (predictive values). The second page of the Excel file shows the distributions drawn to scale, and you can verify the intersection.

Change the standard deviation of the diseased distribution to 1. Note that the decision threshold increases to 7.8 (check the distributions drawn to scale), and observe how this affects the posterior probabilities. A range of thresholds above and below the optimal threshold can be taken and an ROC curve plotted. Scroll down to see the ROC curve, and note the value of AUC in cell E59.

Exercises

B.1 What is the truth table for the XOR operation?

B.2 What is the probability, when throwing two dice, of event C, that the white die should show a 1? What is the probability of event D, that the numbers on the dice add to 7?

B.3 Three coins are tossed simultaneously. What is the probability of them showing exactly two heads?

B.4 What is the probability of getting at least one double-6 in 24 throws of a pair of dice?

B.5 If three dice are thrown, what is the probability of event of getting at least one 6? (Hint: you can do this by looking at the complement. It is also instructive to imagine the sample space, as six slices, and pick out those outcomes with at least one 6 from each slice.)

B.6 Consider a family with two children. Given that one of the children is a boy, what is the probability that both children are boys?

B.7 Suppose that we have two envelopes in front of us, and that one contains twice the amount of money as the other. We are given one of the envelopes, and then asked if we would like to switch. Should we? (*Mathematics Magazine*, 1995.)

B.8 Suppose that 1% of the women of a certain age who participate in routine breast screening have breast cancer, 80% of those with breast cancer test positive (i.e. sensitivity $= 0.8$), and 9.6% of those without breast cancer test positive (note: $P(B|A) = 0.096$). If a woman receives a positive result from the test, what is the probability that she has breast cancer?

B.9 Use **discrimination.xls** with values for the distributions of 2 ± 3 and 6 ± 2. View the Gaussians, the contingency table and probabilities, and the ROC curve, and note the value of AUC. How good is this test?

Appendix C Shape and texture

Objects within an image have both shape and texture, the latter describing their contents. The properties can be described by *descriptors* or *features*, which can be used to aid segmentation and, after segmentation, to distinguish different objects and classify them.

C.1   Shape

Shape features include the following.

Area, A: the number of pixels in the object.
Perimeter, P: the number of pixels in the boundary of the object. This can be obtained easily from the *chain code* of an object (Fig. C.1), as

$$P = (\#\text{even codes}) + \sqrt{2}(\#\text{odd codes}) \qquad \text{(C.1)}$$

(The *curvature* and *binding energy* can also be extracted from the chain code).
Maximum Feret's diameter: the line between two points on the perimeter that are furthest apart, i.e. the longest dimension.
Eccentricity: the ratio of the maximum Feret's diameter to the maximum length perpendicular to it.
Circularity:

$$\text{circularity} = 4\pi A / P^2 \qquad \text{(C.2)}$$

and takes the maximum value of 1 for a circle.
Euler number: the number of connected components (i.e. objects) minus the number of holes in the image (Fig. C.2).
Fourier descriptors: the discrete Fourier transform (Chapter 7) of the (x, y) coordinates of the boundary. Often only a few low-order coefficients are sufficient to capture the gross shape.
Medial axis transform (Section 9.2.5) or points within it, such as branch points and end points.
Convex hull (Section 9.2.6)

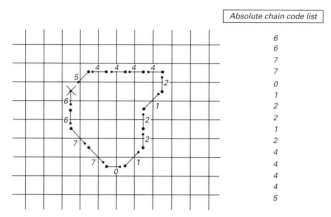

Absolute chain code list
6
6
7
7
0
1
2
2
1
2
4
4
4
4
5

Figure C.1   Eight-connectivity chain code of a boundary, starting at X. Each digit represents the direction to the next pixel on the boundary, with 0 indicating east, 1 indicating north-east, 2 indicating north, and so on, until 7, which indicates south-east. The path is generally traversed counter-clockwise.

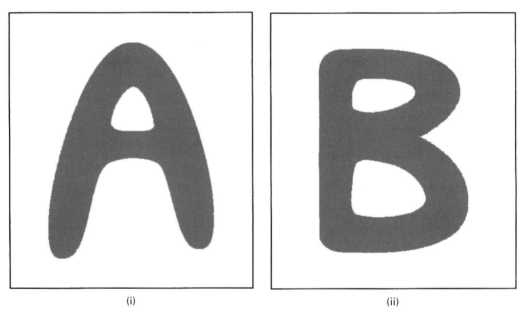

(i)   (ii)

Figure C.2   Objects with Euler numbers of (i) 0 (i.e. 1–1) and (ii) −1 (i.e. 1–2).

Another way to describe shape uses properties called *statistical moments*. The nth moment, m_n, of a 1-D discrete function, $f(x)$, such as a boundary, where $x = 1, 2, 3, \ldots , N$, is defined by

$$m_n = \sum_{x=1}^{N} x^n f(x) \qquad (C.3)$$

where the first moment, m_1, is the mean, μ.

The moments can be taken about the mean, in which case they are known as *central moments*, defined by

$$\mu_n = \sum_{x=1}^{N} (x - \mu)^n f(x) \tag{C.4}$$

The first central moment is zero, and the second central moment is the *variance*, the square root of which is the standard deviation, σ, which measures the spread of the function.

The central moments are commonly normalized by dividing by σ^n to give the normalized central moments, η_n. The (normalized) third central moment is the *skewness*, which measures asymmetry (a symmetric function has a skewness of 0), and the (normalized) fourth central moment is the *kurtosis*, which measures whether the function is peaked or flat relative to a normal distribution (which has a kurtosis of 3).

Moments can be extended to a 2-D discrete function, $f(x, y)$, such as a digital image with $M \times N$ pixels; the (m, n)th moment is defined as

$$m_{mn} = \sum_{x=1}^{M} \sum_{y=1}^{N} x^m y^n f(x, y) \tag{C.5}$$

where m_{00} is the sum of the pixels of an image: for a binary image it is equal to its area. The *centroid*, or *center of gravity*, of the image, (μ_x, μ_y), is given by $(m_{10}/m_{00}, m_{01}/m_{00})$. The central moments are given by

$$\mu_{mn} = \sum_{x=1}^{M} \sum_{y=1}^{N} (x - \mu_x)^m (y - \mu_y)^n f(x, y) \tag{C.6}$$

where μ_{20} and μ_{02} are the variances of x and y, respectively, and μ_{02} is the covariance between x and y. The *covariance matrix*, Σ or $\mathbf{cov}(x, y)$, is

$$\Sigma = \begin{bmatrix} \mu_{20} & \mu_{11} \\ \mu_{11} & \mu_{02} \end{bmatrix} \tag{C.7}$$

from which shape features can be computed. (The ratio of the eigenvalues of the covariance matrix gives the eccentricity, and the direction of the eigenvector gives the orientation.) The sequence of moments is analogous to the coefficients of a Fourier series: the first few give the general shape and the later terms fill in the details.

The central moments can be normalized to yield the normalized central moments:

$$\eta mn = \mu mn / \mu_{00}^{Y} \tag{C.8}$$

where

$$Y = (m + n)/2 + 1 \tag{C.9}$$

The matrix formed from the normalized central moment terms, analogous to the covariance matrix, is known as the *correlation matrix*.

Shape features which are invariant to translation, rotation and scale can be constructed from the normalized central moments and are the most useful for object recognition.

C.2   Fractals

Fractals are *self-similar* and *independent of scale*. They are complex shapes which are space-filling, and are characterized by a *fractal dimension* which is non-integral and larger than the topological dimension; the larger the fractal dimension, the more space-filling is the shape.

Iteration of a very simple rule can produce seemingly complex shapes with some highly unusual properties. One of the earliest mathematical fractals to be studied was the *Koch curve* (Fig. C.3). It is constructed using an iterative or recursive procedure: divide a simple line segment into thirds, and replace the middle segment by two equal segments forming part of an equilateral triangle. In the next stage, replace each of the four segments by four new segments with length one-third of their parent according to the original curve. Repeat this over and over again.

Unlike Euclidean shapes, this curve has detail on all length scales. Indeed, the closer you look the more detail you find. The curve possesses exact self-similarity, i.e. each small portion, when magnified, is the exact shape of a larger portion: the curve is said to be invariant under changes of scale. At each stage of its construction the length of the curve increases by 4/3. Thus, the limiting curve crams an infinite length into a finite area of the plane without intersecting itself. At successive iterations (i.e. successive magnification), one finds new detail and increasing length. And although it is easily computed, there is no algebraic formula that specifies the points of the curve.

A line segment of N identical parts can be scaled down by the ratio $r = 1/N$ from the whole. Similarly a square area can be divided into N self-similar parts each of which is scaled down by a factor $r = 1/\sqrt{N}$. A cube can be scaled down into N small cubes each of which is scaled down by a ratio $r = \sqrt[3]{N}$. In general, a D-dimensional self-similar object can be divided into N smaller copies of itself, each of which is scaled down by $\sqrt[D]{N}$, or

$$N = 1/r^D \tag{C.10}$$

Or, conversely, if we have a self-similar object of N parts scaled down by a ratio r from the whole, its *fractal dimension*, or Hausdorff dimension, is given by

$$D = \log N / \log(1/r) \tag{C.11}$$

So what is the fractal dimension of the Koch curve? Each segment comprises four sub-segments, each scaled down by 1/3 from its parent, so that

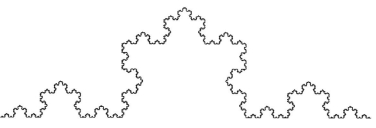

Figure C.3   The Koch curve.

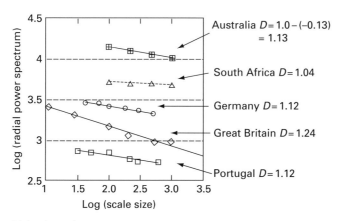

Figure C.4 Richardson plot.

$$D = \log(N)/\log(r)D = \log(4)/\log(3) = 1.26 \qquad (C.12)$$

Coastlines have a fractal property. Their measured lengths become larger as smaller scale rulers are used, since they are able to follow the irregularities better. Richardson (Mandelbrot, 1977) first noted the logarithmic relationship between the length of national boundaries, L, and scale size, s (Fig. C.4). The fractal dimension, D, of the boundary line can be obtained from the gradient, S, of the Richardson plot using

$$D = 1.0 - S \qquad (C.13)$$

The coastline of South Africa is very smooth with $D=1.04$: the "rougher" the line, the steeper the slope, and the larger is the fractal dimension. The fractal dimension of a line can vary between 1.0 (smooth) and 2.5 (random noise); and for a surface from 2.0 (smooth) to 4.0 (random noise).

Fractal models have long been considered appropriate for modeling texture in medical images, with fractal dimension commonly used as a compact descriptor. The fractal dimension describes how an object occupies space and is related to the complexity of its structure: it gives a numerical measure of the degree of boundary irregularity when applied to a line, or surface roughness when applied to a surface. Fractals have attractive properties, such as invariance to scale and projection, but real images of natural objects are not exactly self-similar like mathematical fractals, and fractalness is present only in a statistical sense and only over a limited range of scales.

C.3 Texture

The simplest features of an object or region based on its contents describe its general intensity properties, such as its mean gray value and the standard deviation of the mean. However these features depend on the gain of the imaging system, and change if the brightness or contrast of the image is changed. Texture is independent of gain. It describes roughness or smoothness, regularity (and hence, pattern) or irregularity. There are three principal approaches to describing the texture of a region in an image: (i) statistical, (ii) structural and (iii) spectral.

C.3.1   Statistical approaches

Since textures have some degree of order/disorder or regularity/irregularity, they can be described by their statistical properties. One of the simplest ways is to use *statistical moments* of the gray-level histogram (i.e. probability density function) of the region, i.e. use pixel values rather than pixel coordinates as used with shape. The *n*th *moment* is given by

$$m_n = \sum_{k=0}^{L-1} k^n P(k) \tag{C.14}$$

and the *n*th *central moment* is given by

$$\mu_n = \sum_{k=0}^{L-1} (k - \mu)^n P(k) \tag{C.15}$$

which are identical to Equations (C.3) and (C.4), except that we are using the normalized histogram, $P(k)$, and the gray value k, which takes values $0, 1, 2, \ldots, L-1$, and μ is the mean gray value rather than the mean position. Thus the first moment is the mean gray level or average brightness of the region, and the first central moment is zero. The second central moment is the *variance* of the gray values, and the normalized variance has been used as a simple measure of texture (Dougherty, 1996). Normalizing the variance ensures that it is independent of brightness.

Another statistical way to describe texture is by statistically sampling the occurrence of certain gray levels in relation to other gray levels. For a position operator p, we can define a matrix P_{ij} that counts the number of times a pixel with gray level i occurs at a position p from a pixel with gray level j. For example, if we have three distinct gray levels 0, 1 and 3, and the position operator is "lower right," then an image

$$\begin{matrix} 0\ 0\ 0\ 1\ 2 \\ 1\ 1\ 0\ 1\ 1 \\ 2\ 2\ 1\ 0\ 0 \\ 1\ 1\ 0\ 2\ 0 \\ 0\ 0\ 1\ 0\ 1 \end{matrix} \tag{C.16}$$

will give a counts matrix, P

$$P = \begin{bmatrix} P_{00} & P_{01} & P_{02} \\ P_{10} & P_{11} & P_{12} \\ P_{20} & P_{21} & P_{22} \end{bmatrix} = \begin{bmatrix} 4 & 2 & 1 \\ 2 & 3 & 2 \\ 0 & 2 & 0 \end{bmatrix} \tag{C.17}$$

If we normalize P by dividing each element by the total number of pixels, we get the *gray-level co-occurrence matrix*, C, where each term, C_{ij}, is between 0 and 1.

We can obtain various descriptors from the co-occurrence matrix including the maximum probability,

$$\max_{i,j}(C_{ij}) \tag{C.18}$$

the element difference moment of order k,

$$\sum_i \sum_j (i-j)^k C_{ij} \tag{C.19}$$

the inverse element difference moment of order k,

$$\sum_i \sum_j C_{ij}/(i-j)^k \tag{C.20}$$

entropy,

$$\sum_i \sum_j C_{ij} \log_2 C_{ij} \tag{C.21}$$

and uniformity,

$$\sum_i \sum_j C_{ij}^2 \tag{C.22}$$

Certain combinations of these moments are invariant to translation, rotation and scale (i.e. contrast) change, and can be used as texture descriptors.

Another approach applies the Sobel edge detection mask (Section 6.4.2) to the pixels in a region. Both the resulting "magnitude-of-the-edges" image and the "phase-of-the-edges" image are thresholded, and then a histogram of the "magnitude-of-the-edges" compiled for the various phase angles. Edgeness is akin to texture, and such plots have been used to visualize the directional texture in vertebral bone images (Caldwell *et al.*, 1995).

C.3.2 Structural approaches

The basic scheme is to build a grammar for the texture and then parse the texture to see if it matches the grammar. This involves defining *texture primitives*, simple patterns from which more complicated ones can be built.

C.3.3 Spectral approaches

Since texture has some degree of regularity, it can be described in terms of spatial frequencies. If the Fourier transform of an image $f(x, y)$ is expressed in polar coordinates, $S(r, \theta)$, one-dimensional functions can be obtained by summing over all directions to give $S(r)$, and all radii to give $S(\theta)$. The coordinate $S(r)$ gives the distribution of frequencies across all angles, and $S(\theta)$ gives the frequency content in specific directions. The mean and variance of these distributions are useful descriptors of texture.

A classical means of measuring the smoothness of a function $f(x)$ involves the Fourier transform. Thus the radial Fourier power spectrum, a plot of $|S(r)|^2$ against r, of rough (2-D) images will tend to fall as $1/r^2$, showing a gradient of -2 on a log–log plot; whilst smooth (2-D) images will fall as $1/r^4$ with a gradient of -4. At very low frequencies, corresponding to the bulk features of an object, the power spectrum may be fairly constant; at very high frequencies, approaching the Nyquist frequency, system noise will dominate and the power spectrum will become constant again. These general shapes have been reported in the power spectrum of MRI images of various organs (Fuderer, 1988). It should be noted that small images will give fewer data points and be subject to lack of resolution and quantization errors, and the power spectrum will be correspondingly jagged.

Natural textures can be considered as *statistical fractals* (Section C.2), whose *fractal dimension* can be used as a texture descriptor. There are many different models to describe fractals, and many ways to measure the fractal dimension of an image or a region within it. One of the most useful models for medical images is *fractional Brownian motion*, FBM, which is a generalization of the more familiar Brownian motion used to describe a random walk. (In Brownian motion, the mean square displacement, Δl^2, is proportional to the actual distance traveled, Δx, while in FBM Δl^2 is proportional to Δx^{2H}, where H is known as the Hurst parameter; FBM reduces to Brownian motion when $H = 1/2$.)

It has been shown (Stein and Hartt, 1988) that the scaling behavior of a statistically self-affine fractal results in a fractal dimension, D, given by

$$D = E + 1 - H \qquad (C.23)$$

where E is the topological (Euclidean) dimension of the fractal (i.e. $E = 2$ for a fractal surface or 2-D image, $E = 1$ for a boundary line).

Since there is a simple relationship between the Hurst parameter, H, and the magnitude of the slope of the Fourier power spectrum, β, i.e.

$$\beta = 2H + E \qquad (C.24)$$

then the fractal dimension of an image can be obtained from this slope using

$$D = 3E/2 + 1 - \beta/2 \qquad (C.25)$$

in general, or

$$D = 4 - \beta/2 \qquad (C.26)$$

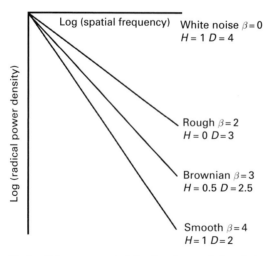

Figure C.5   Ideal radial power spectral density plots, and the relationship between the theoretical indices underpinning them.

in the case of a two-dimensional image ($E=2$), where D will be constrained to be between 2 (smooth) and 3 (rough). The relationships between the various indices are shown in Figure C.5, for the case of a 2-D image, $E=2$.

Thus the gradient of the radial power spectrum of the Fourier transform of an image or region within an image can be used to obtain its fractal dimension. Image blurring progressively filters out the higher spatial frequencies, resulting in a steeper power spectrum and a consequent underestimate of the fractal dimension; its effect would need to be reversed, using for example Wiener filtering (Section 8.4.1), prior to taking the Fourier transform of the image. If the radial power spectrum is not linear, then a *fractal signature* plotting fractal dimension against spatial frequency, rather than a global fractal dimension, will be obtained and can be used to distinguish regions (Dougherty and Henebry, 2001).

Although H was formally restricted to [0, 1], its range may be extended by taking the derivative of the FBM with $H=0$ to give white (Gaussian) noise with $H=-1$ (corresponding to a slope, β, of zero and a fractal dimension, D, of 4). Thus the range of values for the fractal dimension of a two-dimensional image normally extends from 2 (smooth) to 3 (rough), but can reach 4 (for white noise). And the fractal dimension of a one-dimensional boundary line normally ranges from 1 (smooth) to 2 (rough), but can reach 2.5 (for white noise).

Computer-based activities

Activity C.1 Fractal dimension and texture

Open **mri** in ImageJ and find its Fourier power spectrum (**Process/FFT**). Select the whole power spectrum image (**Edit/Selection/Select All**) and obtain the radial power plot (**Plugins/App.C Plugins/Radial Profile**). Save the coordinates as a text file, **radial_plot.txt**. Open the file as a tab delimited file in Microsoft Excel to see the (x, y) coordinates listed as columns. Take the logarithms of these columns and plot them: find the gradient of the best-fitting straight line (using Regression in the Data Analysis Toolpack, under **Tools/Data Analysis …**). Ignore the first few low-frequency points which are due to the dark frame around the head in the original image. Use the gradient to obtain the fractal dimension, which is a measure of the overall texture of the image. The image **mri** contains a variety of different textures: isolate several regions of different texture and find their fractal dimension. The regions chosen should be square and of size 2^n (e.g. 32×32) so that the FFT algorithm will work.

Exercises

C.1 Show that the central moments (Equation (C.6)) are translation invariant and the normalized central moments (Equations (C.8) and (C.9)) are both translation and scale invariant.

C.2 Open the standard texture images **grass** and **bubbles**, and find their fractal dimensions using the radial power spectrum.

Bibliography

Chapter 1

Cho, Z-H., Jones, J. P. and Singh, M. *Foundations of Medical Imaging*. Wiley, 1993.
Macovski, A. *Medical Imaging Systems*. Prentice-Hall, 1983.
Wolbarst, A. B. *Physics of Radiology*. Appleton and Lange, 1993.

Chapter 2

Barrett, H. H and Myers, K. J. *Foundations of Image Science*. Wiley Interscience, 2004.
Gonzalez, R. C. and Woods, R. E. *Digital Image Processing*, 2nd edn. Prentice-Hall, 2002.
Wolbarst, A. B. *Physics of Radiology*. Appleton and Lange, 1993.

Chapter 3

Cherry, S. R., Sorenson, J. A. and Phelps, M. E. *Physics in Nuclear Medicine*, 3rd edn. Elsevier
  Science, 2003.
Dendy, P. P. and Heaton, B. *Physics for Diagnostic Radiology*, 2nd edn, chapters 5, 7, 9 and 10.
  Institute of Physics Publishing Ltd, 1999.
International Commission on Radiological Protection (ICRP) Pergamon Press, NY. Publication 60:
  Recommendations of the ICRP, vol. **21**, 1991.
National Council on Radiation Protection and Measurements (NCRP), Bethesda, MD. Report
  No. 93: *Ionizing Radiation Exposure of the Population of the United States*, 1987.
Webb, A. *Introduction to Biomedical Imaging*. John Wiley & Sons, 2003.
Webster, J. G., editor. *Encyclopedia of Medical Devices and Instrumentation*, p. 834. Wiley,
  1988.
Wolbarst, A. B. *Physics of Radiology*. Appleton and Lange, 1993.

Chapter 4

Bushong, S. C. *Magnetic Resonance Imaging: Physical and Biological Principles*, 2nd edn.
  Mosby, 1996.
Curry T. S., Dowdy J. E. and Murray, R. C. *Christensen's Physics of Diagnostic Radiology*, 4th edn.
  Lippincott Williams & Wilkens, 1990.
Dendy, P. P. and Heaton, B. *Physics for Diagnostic Radiology*, 2nd edn, chapters 13 and 14.
  Institute of Physics Publishing Ltd, 1999.
Dhawan A. P. *Medical Image Analysis*, chapter 4. Wiley Interscience, 2003.
Prince J. L. and Links, J. L. *Medical Imaging Signals and Systems*, chapters 11 and 12. Pearson
  Prentice Hall, 2006.
Suetens, P. *Fundamentals of Medical Imaging*. Cambridge University Press, 2002.
Webb, A. *Introduction to Biomedical Imaging*. John Wiley & Sons, 2003.
Wolbarst, A. B. *Physics of Radiology*. Appleton and Lange, 1993.

Chapter 5

Baxes, G. A. *Digital Image Processing: Principles and Applications*. John Wiley & Sons, Inc., 1994.

Dougherty, G. and Henebry, G. M. "Fractal signature and lacunarity in the measurement of the texture of trabecular bone in clinical CT images," *Med. Eng. Phys.* **23**, 369–80, 2001.

Thiele, D. L., Kimme-Smith, C., Johnson, T. D., McCombs, M., and Basset, L. W. "Using tissue texture surrounding calcification clusters to predict benign vs. malignant outcomes," *Med. Phys.*, **23**(4), 549–55, 1996.

Pratt, W. K. *Digital Image Processing*, chapter 16. John Wiley & Sons, Inc., 2001.

Chapter 6

Gonzalez, R. C. and Woods, R. E. *Digital Image Processing*, 2nd edn, chapter 3. Prentice-Hall, 2002.

Jahne, B. *Digital Image Processing*, 5th edn. Springer-Verlag, 2002.

Marr, D. *Vision*. Freeman, 1982.

Seul, M., O'Gorman, L. and Sammon, M. J. *Practical Algorithms for Image Analysis: Description, Examples and Code*, chapter 3. Cambridge University Press, 2000.

Chapter 7

Ballani, N. and Dougherty, G. "The effect of finite spatial resolution on the measurement of cardiac phantom wall thickness in single photon emission computerized tomographic imaging," *Med. Principles and Practice*, **13**, 316–24, 2004.

Castleman, K. R. *Digital Image Processing*, chapter 14. Prentice-Hall, 1996.

Chui, C. K., Montefusco, L. and Puccio, L. *Wavelets: Theory, Algorithms, and Applications*. Academic Press, 1994.

Dougherty, G. and Newman, D. "Measurement of thickness and density of thin structures by computed tomography: a simulated study," *Med. Phys.*, **26**, 1341–8, 1999.

Gonzalez, R. C. and Woods, R. E. *Digital Image Processing*, 2nd edn, chapter 4, Prentice-Hall, 2002.

Newman, D. L., Dougherty, G., Al Obaid, A. and Al Hajrasy, H. "Limitations of clinical CT in assessing cortical thickness and density," *Phys. Med. Biol.*, **43**, 619–26, 1998.

Peters, T. M. and Williams, J., editors. *The Fourier Transform in Biomedical Engineering*. Birkhauser, 1998.

Prince J. L. and Links, J. L. *Medical Imaging Signals and Systems*, chapter 2. Pearson Prentice Hall, New Jersey, 2006.

Seul, M., O'Gorman, L. and Sammon, M. J. *Practical Algorithms for Image Analysis: Description, Examples and Code*, chapter 7. Cambridge University Press, 2000.

Suetens, P. *Fundamentals of Medical Imaging*, chapter 2. Cambridge University Press, 2005.

Yoo, T. S. *Insight into Images*, chapter 2. A. K. Peters, 2004.

Chapter 8

Brooks T. F. and Humphreys, W. F. The DAMAS algorithm, NASA-Langley Research Center. AIAA Paper 2004–2954.

Castleman, K. R. *Digital Image Processing*, chapter 11. Prentice-Hall, 1996.

Dougherty, G. and Kawaf, Z. "The point spread function revisited: image restoration using 2-D convolution," *Radiography*, **7**, 255–62, 2001.

Gonzalez, R. C. and Woods, R. E. *Digital Image Processing*, 2nd edn, chapter 5, Prentice-Hall, 2002.

Lehman, T. M., Gönner, C. and Spitzer, K. "Survey: Interpolation methods in medical imaging," *IEEE Trans. Medical Imaging*, **18**, 1049–76, 1999.

Pratt, W. K. *Digital Image Processing*, 3rd edn, chapters 10, 12 and 13. John Wiley and Sons Inc., 2001.

Starck, J. L., Murtagh, F. and Bijaoui, A. *Image Processing and Data Analysis*, chapter 3. Cambridge University Press, 1998.

Sorzano, C. O., Thévenaz, P. and Unser, M. "Elastic registration of biological images using vector-spline regularization," *IEEE Trans. Biomedical Engineering*, **52**, 652–63, 2005.

Young, I. T., Gerbrands, J.J and van Vliet, L. J. *Fundamentals of Image Processing*, 2nd edn, chapter 9. Delft University of Technology, The Netherlands, 1998.

Chapter 9

Baxes, G. A. *Digital Image Processing: Principles and Applications*, chapter 5. John Wiley & Sons, Inc., 1994.

Dougherty, G. and Johnson, M. K. "Clinical validation of three-dimensional tortuosity metrics based on the minimum curvature of approximating polynomial splines," *Med. Eng. Phys.* **30**, 190–8, 2008.

Fisher, R., Perkins, S., Walker, A. and Wolfart, E. Hypermedia Image Processing Reference (HIPR2), 2004: at http://homepages.inf.ed.ac.uk/rbf/HIPR2/hipr_top.htm

Gonzalez, R. C. and Woods, R. E. *Digital Image Processing*, 2nd edn, section 10.3, Prentice-Hall, 2002.

Johnson, M. K. and Dougherty, G. "Robust measures of three-dimensional vascular tortuosity based on the minimum curvature of approximating polynomial spline fits to the vessel mid-line," *Med. Eng. Phys.*, **29**, 677–90, 2007.

Lee, Y.-H., and Horng, S.-J. "The chessboard distance transform and the medial axis transform are interchangeable." *Proceedings of the 10th International Parallel Processing Symposium*, 424–8, 1996.

Pratt, W. K. *Digital Image Processing*, 3rd edn, chapters 14. John Wiley and Sons Inc., 2001.

Serra, J. *Image Analysis and Mathematical Morphometry*, Academic Press, 1982.

Seul, M., O'Gorman, L. and Sammon, M. J. *Practical Algorithms for Image Analysis: Description, Examples and Code*, chapter 3. Cambridge University Press, 2000.

Zhang, T. Y. and Suen, C. Y. "A fast parallel algorithm for thinning digital patterns." *Comm. ACM*, **27**, 236–9, 1984.

Chapter 10

Baxes, G. A. *Digital Image Processing: Principles and Applications*, chapter 5. John Wiley & Sons, Inc., 1994.

Castleman, K. R. *Digital Image Processing*, chapter 18. Prentice-Hall, 1996.

Gonzalez, R. C. and Woods, R. E. *Digital Image Processing*, 2nd edn, section 10.3, Prentice-Hall, 2002.

Kass, M., Witken, A. and Terzopoulos, D. "Snakes: active contour models," *Int. J. Comp. Vis.* **1**, 321–31, 1988.

Nixon, M. and Aguado, A. *Feature Extraction and Image Processing*. Newnes, 2002.

Otsu, N. "A threshold selection method from gray-level histograms," *IEEE Trans. Systems, Man and Cybernetics*, **SMC-9**, 62–6, 1979.

Pratt, W. K. *Digital Image Processing*, 3rd edn, chapters 17. John Wiley and Sons Inc., 2001.

Sahoo, P. K., Soltani, S., Wong, K. C. and Chen, Y. C. "A survey of thresholding techniques," *Computer Vision, Graphics, and Image Processing*, **41**, 233–60, 1988.

Sonka, M., Hlavac, V., and Boyle R. *Image Processing, Analysis, and Machine Vision*, 2nd edn, chapter 5. Brooks/Cole Publishing Company, 1999.

Chapter 11

Baumgartner, R., Ryder, L., Richter, W., Summers, R., Jarmasz, M. and Somorjai, R. "Comparison of two exploratory data analysis methods for fMRI: fuzzy clustering versus principal component analysis," *Mag. Resonance Imaging*, **18**, 89–94, 2000.

Duda, R. O., Hart, P. E. and Stork, D. G. *Pattern Classification*, 2nd edn. John Wiley and Sons, 2001.

Fisher, R. A. "The use of multiple measurements in taxonomic problems," *Ann. Eugenics*, **7**, 179–88, 1936.

Gonzalez, R. C. and Woods, R. E. *Digital Image Processing*, 2nd edn, chapter 12, Prentice-Hall, 2002.

Karssemeijer, N. "Adaptive noise equalization and recognition of microcalcification clusters in mammograms," *Int. J. Pattern Recognition Artificial Intell.* 1357–76, 1993.

Karssemeijer, N. and te Brake, G. "Detection of stellate distortions in mammograms," *IEEE Trans. Med. Imaging*, **15**, 611–19, 1996.

Kegelmeyer, W. P., Pruned, J. M. and Bourland, P. D. "Computer-aided mammographic screening for speculated lesions," *Radiology*, **191**, 331–7, 1994.

Li, H., Wang, Y., Lo, S. and Freedman, M. "Computerized radiographic mass detection – part 2," *IEEE Trans. Med. Imaging*, **20**, 302–13, 2001.

Ogiela, M. R. and Tadeusiewicz, R. "Syntactic reasoning and pattern recognition for analysis of coronary artery images," *Artificial Intelligence Med.*, **670**, 1–15, 2002.

Qian, W., Sun, X. Song, D. and Clark, R. A. "Digital mammography – wavelet transform and Kalman-filtering neural network in mass segmentation and detection," *Acad. Radiol. 8*, **11**, 1074–82, 2001.

Russ, J. C. *The Image Processing Handbook*, 4th edn, chapter 10. CRC Press, 2002.

Sahiner, B., Chan, H. P., Petrick, N., Wei, D., Helvie, M. A., Adler, D. and Goodsitt, M. M. "Classification of mass and normal breast tissue: a convolution neural network classifier with spatial domain and texture images," *IEEE Trans. Med. Imaging*, **15**, 598–610, 1996.

Sonka, M., Hlavac, V., and Boyle R. *Image Processing, Analysis, and Machine Vision*, 2nd edn, chapter 7. Brooks/Cole Publishing Company, 1999.

Therrien, C. W. *Decision Estimation and Classification*, chapters 2 and 3. John Wiley and Sons, 1989.

Zhu, Y. and Yan, H. "Computerized tumor boundary detection using a Hopfield neural network," *Proc. IEEE Joint Int. Conf. Neural Networks, Houston*, **3**, 2467–72, 1997.

Chapter 12

Dhawan, A. P. *Medical Image Analysis*, chapter 10. Wiley-Interscience, 2003.

Lorensen, W. E. and Cline, H. E. "Marching cubes: a high resolution 3D surface construction algorithm," *Computer Graphics (Proceedings of SIGGRAPH)*, **21**, 163–9, 1987.

Robb, R. A. *Biomedical Imaging, Visualization, and Analysis*, chapter 4. Wiley-Liss, 2000.

Udupa, J. K. "Three-dimensional visualization: principles and approaches," in *Handbook of Medical Imaging, Vol. 3: Display and PACS* (Kim, Y. and Horii, S. C., eds.). SPIE, 2000.

Chapter 13

Bankman, L. N., Christens-Barry, W. A., Kim, D. W., Weinberg, I. N., Gatewood, O. B. and Brody, W. R. "Automated recognition of microcalcification clusters in mammograms," *Proc. SPIE*, **1905**, 1993.

Bick, U., Giger, M. L., Schmidt, R. A., Nishikawa, R. M. and Doi, K. "Density correction of peripheral breast tissue on digital mammograms," *Radiographics*, **16**, 1403–11, 1996.

Breen, J. F., Sheedy, P. F., Schwartz, R. S., Stanson, A., Kaufman, R., Moll, P. and Run, J. "Coronary artery calcification detected with ultrafast CT as an indication of coronary artery disease," *Radiology*, **185**, 435–9, 1992.

Caldwell, C. B., Willett, K., Cuncins, A. V. and Hearn, T. C. "Characterization of vertebral strength using digital radiographic analysis of bone structure," *Med. Phys.* **22**, 611–15, 1995.

Capowski, J. J., Kylstra, J. A. and Freedman, S. F. "A numeric index based on spatial frequency for the tortuosity of retinal vessels and its application to plus disease in retinopathy," *Retina*, **15**, 490–500, 1995.

Chang, Y. H., Zheng, B., Wood, W. F. and Gur, D. "Identification of clustered microcalcifications on digitized mammograms using morphology and topography-based computer-aided detection schemes: a preliminary experiment," *Invest. Radiol.* **33**, 746–51, 1998.

Chen, S. Y. J. and Carroll, J. D. "3D coronary angiography: improving visualization strategy for coronary interventions," in *What's New in Cardiovascular Imaging?* (J. H. C. Reiber and E. E. van der Wall, eds.), vol. 24 of *Developments in Cardiovascular Medicine*, pp. 61–78. Kluwer, 1998.

Diab, K. M., Sevastik, J. A., Hedlund, R., and Suliman, I. A. "Accuracy and applicability of measurement of the scoliotic angle at the frontal plane by Cobb's method, by Ferguson's method and by a new method," *Eur. Spine J.*, **4**, 291–5, 1995.

Dougherty, G. "Quantitative indices for ranking the severity of hepatocellular carcinoma," *Comp. Med. Imaging and Graphics*, **19**, 329–38, 1995.

Dougherty, G. "Quantitative CT in the measurement of bone quantity and bone quality for assessing osteoporosis," *Med. Eng. Phys.* **18**, 557–68, 1996.

Dougherty, G. "Quantitative assessment of abdominal aortic atherosclerosis observed in CT scans," *Comp. Med. Imaging and Graphics*, **21**, 185–93, 1997.

Dougherty, G. "Computerized evaluation of mammographic image quality using phantom images," *Comput. Med. Imaging and Graphics*, **22**, 365–73, 1998.

Dougherty, G. "A comparison of the texture of computed tomography and projection radiography images of vertebral trabecular bone using fractal signature and lacunarity," *Med. Eng. Phys.* **23**, 313–21, 2001.

Dougherty, G. and Henebry, G. M. "Fractal signature and lacunarity in the measurement of the texture of trabecular bone in clinical CT images," *Med. Eng. Phys.* **23**, 369–80, 2001.

Dougherty, G. and Henebry, G. M. "Lacunarity analysis of spatial pattern in CT images of vertebral trabecular bone for assessing osteoporosis," *Med. Eng. Phys.* **24**, 129–38, 2002.

Dougherty, G. and Johnson, M. J., "Clinical validation of three-dimensional tortuosity metrics based on the minimum curvature of approximating polynomial splines," *Med. Eng. Phys.*, **30**, 190–8, 2008a.

Dougherty, G. and Johnson, M. J., "The measurement of retinal vascular tortuosity and its application to retinal pathologies," *Med. Eng. Phys.*, 2008b, in press.

Dougherty, G. and Johnson, M. J., "Assessment of scoliosis by direct measurement of the curvature of the spine," *Med. Eng. Phys.*, 2008c, in press.

Dougherty, G. and Kawaf, Z. "A simplified method for densitometric determination of vessel stenosis from angiographic images," *Radiography*, **7**, 187–91, 2001.

Dougherty G. and Varro J. "A quantitative index for the measurement of the tortuosity of blood vessels," *Med. Eng. Phys.* **22**, 567–74, 2000.

Fazzalari, N. L. and Parkinson, J. H. "Fractal dimension and architecture of trabecular bone," *J. Path.*, **178**, 100–5, 1996.

Giger, M. L., Yin, F,-F., Doi, K., Metz, C. E., Schmidt, R. A. and Vyborny, C. J. "Investigation of methods for the computerized detection and analysis of mammographic masses," *Proc. SPIE*, **1233**, 183–4, 1990.

Giger, M. L., Vyborny, C. J. and Schmidt, R. A. "Computerized characterization of mammographic masses: analysis of spiculations," *Cancer Letters*, **77**, 201–11, 1994.

Goldstein, S. A., Goulet, R. and McCubbrey, D. "Measurement and significance of three-dimensional architecture to the mechanical integrity of bone," *Calcif. Tissue Int.*, **53**, 5127–33, 1993.

Goto, M., Morikawa, A., Fujita, H., Hara, T. and Endo, T. "Detection of spicules on mammograms based on multi-stage pendulum filter," in *Digital Mammography* (N. Karresmeijer *et al.*, eds.). Kluwer Academic Publishers, 1998.

Grisan, E., Forrachia, M., and Ruggeri, A. "A novel method for the automatic evaluation of retinal vessel tortuosity," *Proc. Ann. Int. Conf., IEEE Eng. Med. Biol. Soc.*, Cancun, Mexico, 2003.

Hart, W. E., Goldbaum, M., Côté, B., Kube, P. and Nelson, M. R. "Measurements and classification of retinal vascular tortuosity," *Intl J. Med. Informatics*, **53**, 239–52, 1999.

Hoffman, K. R., Chen, Y., Esthappen, J., Chen, S. Y. J. and Carroll. J. D., "Pincushion correction techniques and their effects on calculated 3D positions and imaging geometries," in *Medical Imaging 1996: Image Processing* (M. H. Loew and K. M. Hanson, eds.), pp. 462–7. SPIE, 1996.

Hoover, A., Kouznetsova, V. and Goldbaum, M. "Locating blood vessels in retinal images by piece-wise threshold probing of a matched filter response," *IEEE Trans. Med. Imaging*, **19**, 203–10, 2000.

Huo, Z., Giger, M. L., Vyborny, C. J., Bick, U., Lu, P., Wolverton, D. E. and Schmidt, R. A. "Analysis of spiculation in the computerized classification of mammographic masses," *Med. Phys.* **22**, 1569–79, 1995.

Huo, Z., Giger, M. L., Vyborny, C. J., Wolverton, D. E., Schmidt, R. A. and Doi, K. "Automated computerized classification of malignant and benign mass lesions on digitized mammograms," *Acad. Radiol.*, **5**, 155–68, 1998.

Jiang, Y., Nishikawa, R. M., Schmidt, R. A., Metz, C. E., Giger, M. L. and Doi, K. "Improving breast cancer diagnosis with computer-aided diagnosis," *Acad. Radiol.*, **6**, 22–33, 1999.

Karssemeijer, N. "Recognition of stellate lesions in digital mammograms," in *Digital Mammography* (A. C. Gale, S. M. Astley, D. R. Dance and A. Y. Cairns, eds.). Elsevier, 1994.

Kobatake, H. and Murakami, M. "Adaptive filter to detect rounded convex regions: Iris filter," *Proc. Int. Conf. on Pattern Recognition*, **2**, 340–4, 1996.

Kopans, D. "The positive predictive value of mammography," *Am. J. Roentgen*, **158**, 521–6, 1992.

Martin, J. E., Moskowitz, M. and Milbrath, J. R. "Breast cancers missed by mammography", *Am. J. Roentgen*, **132**, 737, 1979.

Miles, K. A. "Tumour angiogenesis and its relation to contrast enhancement on computed tomography: a review," *Eur. J. Radiol.*, **30**, 198–205, 1999.

Millard, J., Augat, P., Link, T. *et al.*, "Power spectral analysis of trabecular bone structure from radiographs: correlation with bone mineral density and biomechanics," *Calcif. Tissue Int.*, **63**, 482–9, 1998.

Morton. B. C., Gill, J. B., Roberts, R. S., Larocque, B. G., Jozwiak, L. A. and Cairns, J. A. "Does it matter how coronary projections are combined to assess restenosis following PCTA?," *Int. J. Cardiac Imaging*, **11**, 145–9, 1995.

Nash C. L. Jr., Gregg E. C., Brown R. H. and Pillai K. "Risks of exposure to x-rays in patients undergoing long-term treatment for scoliosis," *J. Bone Joint Surg. (Am.)* **61**, 371–4, 1979.

Nishikawa, R. M., Giger, M. L., Doi, K., Vyborny, and Schmidt, R. A. "Use of morphological filters in the computerized detcection of microcalcifications in digital mammograms," *Med. Phys.*, **17**, 524, 1990.

Nishikawa, R. M., Giger, M. L., Doi, K., Schmidt, R. A., Vyborny, C. J., Ema, T., Zhang, W. and Nagel, R. H. "A noise reduction filter for use in a computerized scheme for the detection of clustered microcalcifications," *Radiology*, **189**P, 218, 1993a.

Nishikawa, R. M., Giger, M. L., Doi, K., Vyborny, and Schmidt, R. A. "Computer-aided detection of clustered microcalcifications: an improved method for grouping detected signals," *Med. Phys.* **20**, 1661–6, 1993b.

Parr, T., Zwiggelaar, R., Astley, S., Boggis, C. and Taylor, C. "Comparison of methods for combining evidence for speculated lesions," in *Digital Mammography* (N. Karresmeijer *et al.*, eds.). Kluwer Academic Publishers, 1998.

Robb, R. A. *Biomedical Imaging, Visualization, and Analysis*, chapter 7. Wiley-Liss, 2000.

Sallam, M. and Bowyer, K. "Detecting abnormal densities in mammograms by comparison to previous screening," in *Digital Mammography*, **96**, 417–20, Elsevier, 1996.

Schaefer, P., Lev, M. H., Buchbinder, B. and Gonzalez, R. G. "Clinical applications of functional MRI," in *Radiology: Diagnosis/Imaging/Interventional* (J. M. Taveras and T. M. Ferucci, eds.), p. 3. Lippincott-Raven, 1997.

Smedby, Ö., Högman, N., Nilsson, S., Erikson, U., Olsson A. G., and Walldius, G., "Two-dimensional tortuosity of the superficial femoral artery in early atherosclerosis," *J. Vasc. Res.* **30**, 181–91, 1993.

Sonka, M., Winniford, M. D. and Collins, S. M. "Robust simultaneous detection of coronary borders in complex images," *IEEE Trans. Med. Imaging*, **14**, 151–61, 1995.

Swets, J. A., Getty, D. J., Pickett, R. M., D'Orsi, C. J., Seltzer, S. E. and McNeil, B. J. "Enhancing and evaluating diagnostic accuracy," *Med. Decision Making*, **11**, 9–18, 1991.

Van der Zwet, P. and Reiber, J. "The influence of image enhancement and reconstruction on quantitative coronary arteriography," *Int. J. Cardiac Imaging*, **11**, 211–21, 1995.

Wolf, Y. G., Tillich, M., Lee, W. A., Rubin, G. D., Fogarty, T. J. and Zarius, C. K. "Impact of aortoiliac tortuosity on endovascular repair of abdominal aortic aneurysm: evaluation of 3D computer-based assessment," *J. Vasc. Surg.*, **34**, 394–9, 2001.

Yin, F. F., Giger, M. L., Doi, K., Vyborny, C. J. and Schmidt, R. A. "Computerized detection of masses in digital mammograms: automated alignment of breast images and its effect on bilateral-subtraction technique," *Med. Phys.*, **21**, 445–52, 1994.

Zheng, B., Chang, Y. H., Wang, X. H., Good, W. F. and Gur, D. "Feature selection for computerized mass detection in digitized mammograms by using a genetic algorithm," *Acad. Radiol.*, **6**, 327–32, 1999.

Chapter 14

Cameron, B. M. and Robb, R. A. "Virtual-reality-assisted interventional procedures," *Clin. Orthop. Relat. Res.*, **442**, 63–73, 2006.

Carts-Powell, Y. "Small wonders," *Engin. & Technol.*, **1**, 32–5, 2006.

Ciccarelli, O., Werring D. J., Barker G. J., *et al.*, "A study of the mechanisms of normal-appearing white matter damage in multiple sclerosis using diffusion tensor imaging – evidence of Wallerian degeneration," *J. Neurol.*, **250**, 287–92, 2003.

Dhawan, A. P. *Medical Image Analysis*, chapter 11. Wiley Interscience, 2003.

Huber, D. and Hebert, M. "Fully automatic registration of multiple 3D data sets," *Image and Vision Computing*, **21**, 637–50, 2003.

Liu, Z., Ding, L. and He, B. "Integration of EEG/MEG with MRI and fMRI," *IEEE Eng. Med. Biol. Mag.*, **25**, 46–54, 2006.

Meder, R., de Visser S. K., Bowden J. C., Bostrom T. and Pope J. M. "Diffusion tensor imaging of articular cartilage as a measure of tissue microstructure," *Osteoarthritis and Cartilage*, **14**, 875–81, 2006.

Robb, R. A. *Biomedical Imaging, Visualization, and Analysis*, chapter 7. Wiley-Liss, 2000.

Russ, J. C. *The Image Processing Handbook*, 4th edn, chapter 12. CRC Press, 2002.

Suetens, P. *Fundamentals of Medical Imaging*, chapter 10. Cambridge University Press, 2002.

Van Leemput, K., Maes, F., Vandermeulen, D. and Suetens, P. "Automated model-based tissue classification of MR images of the brain," *IEEE Trans. Med. Imaging*, **18**, 897–908, 1999.

Way, T. W., Hadjiiski, L. M., Sahiner, B., Chan, H. P., Cascade, P. N., Kazerooni, E. A., Bogot, N. and Zhou, C. "Computer-aided diagnosis of pulmonary nodules on CT scans: segmentation and classification using 3D active contours," *Med. Phys.*, **33**, 2323–37, 2006.

Appendix A

Randall, R. B. *Frequency Analysis*. Bruel and Kjaer, 1987.

Appendix B

Gonzalez, R. C. and Woods, R. E. Digital Image Processing, 3rd edn, chapter 11. Prentice-Hall, 2008.

Mathematics Magazine, **68**, 29, 1995.

Appendix C

Caldwell, C. B., Willett, K., Cuncins, A. V. and Hearn, T. C. "Characterization of vertebral strength using digital radiographic analysis of bone structure," *Med. Phys.* **22**, 611–15, 1995.

Dougherty, G. "Quantitative CT in the measurement of bone quantity and bone quality for assessing osteoporosis," *Med. Eng. Phys.*, **18**, 557–68, 1996.

Dougherty, G. and Henebry, G. M. "Fractal signature and lacunarity in the measurement of the texture of trabecular bone in clinical CT images," *Med. Eng. Phys.*, **23**, 369–80, 2001.

Fuderer, M. "The information content of MR images," *IEEE Trans. Med. Imag.*, **7**, 368–80, 1988.

Gonzalez, R. C. and Woods, R. E. *Digital Image Processing*, 3rd edn, chapter 11. Prentice-Hall, 2008.

Mandelbrot, B. B. *The Fractal Geometry of Nature*. W. H. Freeman, 1977.

Pratt, W. K. *Digital Image Processing*, 3rd edn, chapter 16. John Wiley and Sons Inc., 2001.

Sonka, M., Hlavac, V. and Boyle R. *Image Processing, Analysis, and Machine Vision*, 2nd edn, chapter 6. Brooks/Cole Publishing Company, 1999.

Stein, M. C. and Hartt, K. D. "Non-parametric estimation of fractal dimension," *Proc. SPIE Vis. Commun. Image Process.*, **1001**, 132–7, 1988.

Index